Skill Checklists to Accompany

Taylor's Clinical Nursing Skills:

A NURSING PROCESS APPROACH

Skill Checklists to Accompany

Taylor's Clinical Nursing Skills:

A NURSING PROCESS APPROACH

2ND EDITION

Pamela Lynn, RN, MSN
Faculty
School of Nursing
Gwynedd-Mercy College
Gwynedd Valley, Pennsylvania

Marilee LeBon, BA
Developmental Editor
Mountaintop, Pennsylvania

Wolters Kluwer | Lippincott Williams & Wilkins
Health
Philadelphia · Baltimore · New York · London
Buenos Aires · Hong Kong · Sydney · Tokyo

Ancillary Editor: Audrey Lickwar
Senior Production Editor: Sandra Cherrey Scheinin
Director of Nursing Production: Helen Ewan
Senior Managing Editor/Production: Erika Kors
Senior Manufacturing Manager: William Alberti
Compositor: Techbooks
Printer: Victor Graphics

9 8 7 6 5 4 3 2

ISBN 13: 978-0-7817-6405-6
ISBN 10: 0-7817-6405-X

Care has been taken to confirm the accuracy of the information presented and to describe generally accepted practices. However, the authors, editors, and publisher are not responsible for errors or omissions or for any consequences from application of the information in this book and make no warranty, express or implied, with respect to the content of the publication.

The authors, editors, and publisher have exerted every effort to ensure that drug selection and dosage set forth in this text are in accordance with the current recommendations and practice at the time of publication. However, in view of ongoing research, changes in government regulations, and the constant flow of information relating to drug therapy and drug reactions, the reader is urged to check the package insert for each drug for any change in indications and dosage and for added warnings and precautions. This is particularly important when the recommended agent is a new or infrequently employed drug.

Some drugs and medical devices presented in this publication have Food and Drug Administration (FDA) clearance for limited use in restricted research settings. It is the responsibility of the health care provider to ascertain the FDA status of each drug or device planned for use in his or her clinical practice.

LWW.com

Introduction

Developing clinical competency is a major challenge for each fundamentals student. To facilitate the mastery of nursing skills, we are happy to provide Skill Checklists for each skill in *Taylor Clinical Nursing Skills: A Nursing Process Approach,* 2nd edition. The skill checklists follow each step of the skill to provide a complete evaluative tool. Students can use the checklists to facilitate self-evaluation, and faculty will find them useful in measuring and recording student performance. Three-hole punched and perforated, these checklists can be easily reproduced and brought to the simulation laboratory or clinical area. The checklists are designed to record an evaluation of each step of the skill.

- Checkmark in the "Excellent" column denotes mastering the skill.
- Checkmark in the "Satisfactory" column indicates use of the recommended technique.
- Checkmark in the "Needs Practice" column indicates use of *some but not all* of each recommended technique.

The Comments section allows you to highlight suggestions that will improve skills. Space is available at the top of each checklist to record a final pass/fail evaluation, date, and the signature of the student and evaluating faculty member.

List of Skills by Chapter

List of Skills in Alphabetical Order

Skill Checklists to Accompany Taylor's Clinical Nursing Skills:
A Nursing Process Approach, 2nd edition

Name _____   Date _____

Unit _____   Position _____

Instructor/Evaluator: _____   Position _____

Excellent	Satisfactory	Needs Practice	SKILL 1-1 **Assessing Body Temperature** **Goal:** The patient's temperature is assessed accurately without injury and the patient experiences minimal discomfort.	Comments
___	___	___	1. Check physician's order or nursing care plan for frequency and route. More frequent temperature measurement may be appropriate based on nursing judgment.	
___	___	___	2. Identify the patient. Discuss procedure with patient and assess patient's ability to assist with the procedure.	
___	___	___	3. Ensure the electronic or digital thermometer is in working condition.	
___	___	___	4. Close curtains around bed and close door to room if possible.	
___	___	___	5. **Perform hand hygiene and put on gloves if appropriate or indicated.**	
___	___	___	6. Select the appropriate site based on previous assessment data.	
___	___	___	7. Follow the steps as outlined below for the appropriate type of thermometer.	
___	___	___	8. When measurement is completed, remove gloves, if worn. Perform hand hygiene.	
			Measuring a Tympanic Membrane Temperature	
___	___	___	1. If necessary, push the "on" button and wait for the "ready" signal on the unit.	
___	___	___	2. Attach tympanic probe covering.	
___	___	___	3. **Insert the probe snugly into the external ear using gentle but firm pressure, angling the thermometer toward the patient's jaw line. Pull pinna up and back to straighten the ear canal in an adult.**	
___	___	___	4. Activate the unit by pushing the trigger button. The reading is immediate (usually within 2 seconds). Note the reading.	
___	___	___	5. Discard the probe cover in an appropriate receptacle by pushing the probe-release button or use rim of cover to remove from probe. Replace the thermometer in its charger, if necessary.	

Assessing Body Temperature *(Continued)*

Excellent	Satisfactory	Needs Practice		Comments

Assessing Oral Temperature

1. Remove the electronic unit from the charging unit, and remove the probe from within the recording unit.

2. Cover thermometer probe with disposable probe cover and slide it on until it snaps into place.

3. **Place the probe beneath the patient's tongue in the posterior sublingual pocket. Ask the patient to close his or her lips around the probe.**

4. **Continue to hold the probe until you hear a beep.** Note the temperature reading.

5. Remove the probe from the patient's mouth. Dispose of the probe cover by holding the probe over an appropriate receptacle and pressing the probe release button.

6. Return the thermometer probe to the storage place within the unit. Return the electronic unit to the charging unit, if appropriate.

Assessing Rectal Temperature

1. Place the bed at an appropriate working height. Put on nonsterile gloves.

2. Assist the patient to a side-lying position. Pull back the covers enough to expose only the buttocks.

3. Remove the rectal probe from within the recording unit of the electronic thermometer. Cover the probe with a disposable probe cover and slide it into place until it snaps in place.

4. **Lubricate about 1″ of the probe with a water-soluble lubricant.**

5. Reassure the patient. Separate the buttocks until the anal sphincter is clearly visible.

6. **Insert the thermometer probe into the anus about 1.5″ in an adult or 1″ in a child.**

7. Hold the probe in place until you hear a beep, then carefully remove the probe. Note the temperature reading on the display.

8. Dispose of the probe cover by holding the probe over an appropriate waste receptacle and pressing the release button.

9. Using toilet tissue, wipe the anus of any feces or excess lubricant. Dispose of the toilet tissue.

Excellent	Satisfactory	Needs Practice		Comments

SKILL 1-1

Assessing Body Temperature *(Continued)*

—— —— —— 10. Cover the patient and help him or her to a position of comfort.

—— —— —— 11. Remove gloves and discard them. Perform hand hygiene.

—— —— —— 12. Place the bed in the lowest position; elevate rails as needed.

—— —— —— 13. Return the thermometer to the charging unit.

Assessing Axillary Temperature

—— —— —— 1. Place the bed at an appropriate working height.

—— —— —— 2. Move the patient's clothing to expose only the axilla.

—— —— —— 3. Remove the probe from the recording unit of the electronic thermometer. Place a disposable probe cover on by sliding it on and snapping it securely.

—— —— —— 4. **Place the end of the probe in the center of the axilla. Have the patient bring the arm down and close to the body.**

—— —— —— 5. Hold the probe in place until you hear a beep, and then carefully remove the probe. Note the temperature reading.

—— —— —— 6. Cover the patient and help him or her to a position of comfort.

—— —— —— 7. Dispose of the probe cover by holding the probe over an appropriate waste receptacle and pushing the release button.

—— —— —— 8. Place the bed in the lowest position and elevate rails as needed. Leave the patient clean and comfortable.

—— —— —— 9. Return the electronic thermometer to the charging unit.

Skill Checklists to Accompany Taylor's Clinical Nursing Skills:
A Nursing Process Approach, 2nd edition

Name _____   Date _____

Unit _____   Position _____

Instructor/Evaluator: _____   Position _____

Excellent	Satisfactory	Needs Practice	SKILL 1-2 **Assessing a Peripheral Pulse by Palpation**	Comments
			Goal: The patient's pulse is assessed accurately without injury and the patient experiences minimal discomfort.	
___	___	___	1. Check physician's order or nursing care plan for frequency of pulse assessment. More frequent pulse measurement may be appropriate based on nursing judgment.	
___	___	___	2. Identify the patient.	
___	___	___	3. Explain the procedure to the patient.	
___	___	___	4. Close curtains around bed and close door to room if possible.	
___	___	___	5. Perform hand hygiene and put on gloves as appropriate.	
___	___	___	6. Select the appropriate peripheral site based on assessment data.	
___	___	___	7. Move the patient's clothing to expose only the site chosen.	
___	___	___	8. Place your first, second, and third fingers over the artery. **Lightly compress the artery so pulsations can be felt and counted.**	
___	___	___	9. **Using a watch with a second hand, count the number of pulsations felt for 30 seconds. Multiply this number by 2 to calculate the rate for 1 minute. If the rate, rhythm, or amplitude of the pulse is abnormal in any way, palpate and count the pulse for 1 minute or longer.**	
___	___	___	10. **Note the rhythm and amplitude of the pulse.**	
___	___	___	11. Cover the patient and help him or her to a position of comfort.	
___	___	___	12. Remove gloves, if necessary. Perform hand hygiene.	

Skill Checklists to Accompany Taylor's Clinical Nursing Skills:
A Nursing Process Approach, 2nd edition

Name _____ Date _____

Unit _____ Position _____

Instructor/Evaluator: _____ Position _____

SKILL 1-3
Assessing the Apical Pulse by Auscultation

Goal: The patient's pulse is assessed accurately without injury and the patient experiences minimal discomfort.

Excellent	Satisfactory	Needs Practice		Comments
___	___	___	1. Check physician's order or nursing care plan for frequency of pulse assessment. More frequent pulse measurement may be appropriate based on nursing judgment. Identify the need to obtain an apical pulse measurement.	
___	___	___	2. Identify the patient.	
___	___	___	3. Explain the procedure to the patient.	
___	___	___	4. Close curtains around bed and close door to room if possible.	
___	___	___	5. Perform hand hygiene and put on gloves as appropriate.	
___	___	___	6. Use alcohol swab to clean the diaphragm of the stethoscope. Use another swab to clean the earpieces if necessary.	
___	___	___	7. Assist patient to a sitting or reclining position and expose chest area.	
___	___	___	8. Move the patient's clothing to expose only the apical site.	
___	___	___	9. Hold the stethoscope diaphragm against the palm of your hand for a few seconds.	
___	___	___	10. **Palpate the space between the fifth and sixth ribs (fifth intercostal space), and move to the left midclavicular line.** Place the diaphragm over the apex of the heart.	
___	___	___	11. Listen for heart sounds ("lub-dub"). Each "lub-dub" counts as one beat.	
___	___	___	12. **Using a watch with a second hand, count the heartbeat for 1 minute.**	
___	___	___	13. Cover the patient and help him or her to a position of comfort.	
___	___	___	14. Clean diaphragm of the stethoscope with an alcohol swab.	
___	___	___	15. Remove gloves, if necessary. Perform hand hygiene.	

Skill Checklists to Accompany Taylor's Clinical Nursing Skills:
A Nursing Process Approach, 2nd edition

Name _____ Date _____

Unit _____ Position _____

Instructor/Evaluator: _____ Position _____

Excellent	Satisfactory	Needs Practice	SKILL 1-4 **Assessing Respiration**	Comments
			Goal: The patient's respirations are assessed accurately without injury and the patient experiences minimal discomfort.	
——	——	——	1. **While your fingers are still in place for the pulse measurement, after counting the pulse rate, observe the patient's respirations.**	
——	——	——	2. Note the rise and fall of the patient's chest.	
——	——	——	3. Using a watch with a second hand, count the number of respirations for 30 seconds. Multiply this number by 2 to calculate the respiratory rate per minute.	
——	——	——	4. If respirations are abnormal in any way, count the respirations for at least 1 full minute.	
——	——	——	5. Note the depth and rhythm of the respirations.	
——	——	——	6. Perform hand hygiene.	

Skill Checklists to Accompany Taylor's Clinical Nursing Skills:
A Nursing Process Approach, 2nd edition

Name _____   Date _____

Unit _____   Position _____

Instructor/Evaluator: _____   Position _____

Excellent	Satisfactory	Needs Practice	SKILL 1-5 **Assessing a Brachial Artery Blood Pressure**	Comments
			Goal: The patient's blood pressure is measured accurately without injury.	
___	___	___	1. Check physician's order or nursing care plan for frequency of blood pressure measurement. More frequent measurement may be appropriate based on nursing judgment.	
___	___	___	2. Identify the patient.	
___	___	___	3. Explain the procedure to the patient.	
___	___	___	4. Perform hand hygiene and put on gloves if appropriate or indicated.	
___	___	___	5. Close curtains around bed and close door to room if possible.	
___	___	___	6. **Select the appropriate arm for application of cuff.**	
___	___	___	7. Have the patient assume a comfortable lying or sitting position with the forearm supported at the level of the heart and the palm of the hand upward.	
___	___	___	8. Expose the brachial artery by removing garments, or move a sleeve, if it is not too tight, above the area where the cuff will be placed.	
___	___	___	9. Palpate the location of the brachial artery. **Center the bladder of the cuff over the brachial artery, about midway on the arm, so that the lower edge of the cuff is about 2.5 to 5 cm (1″–2″) above the inner aspect of the elbow. Line the artery marking on the cuff up with the patient's brachial artery. The tubing should extend from the edge of the cuff nearer the patient's elbow.**	
___	___	___	10. Wrap the cuff around the arm smoothly and snugly, and fasten it. Do not allow any clothing to interfere with the proper placement of the cuff.	
___	___	___	11. Check that the needle on the aneroid gauge is within the zero mark. If using a mercury manometer, check to see that the manometer is in the vertical position and that the mercury is within the zero level with the gauge at eye level.	
			Estimating Systolic Pressure	
___	___	___	12. **Palpate the pulse at the brachial or radial artery by pressing gently with the fingertips.**	

Excellent	Satisfactory	Needs Practice	SKILL 1-5 **Assessing a Brachial Artery Blood Pressure** *(Continued)*
			Comments

Excellent	Satisfactory	Needs Practice		Comments
——	——	——	13. Tighten the screw valve on the air pump.	
——	——	——	14. **Inflate the cuff while continuing to palpate the artery. Note the point on the gauge where the pulse disappears.**	
——	——	——	15. Deflate the cuff and wait 15 seconds.	
			Obtaining Blood Pressure Measurement	
——	——	——	16. **Assume a position that is no more than 3 feet away from the gauge.**	
——	——	——	17. Place the stethoscope earpieces in your ears. Direct the earpieces forward into the canal and not against the ear itself.	
——	——	——	18. **Place the bell or diaphragm of the stethoscope firmly but with as little pressure as possible over the brachial artery. Do not allow the stethoscope to touch clothing or the cuff.**	
——	——	——	19. Pump the pressure 30 mm Hg above the point at which the systolic pressure was palpated and estimated. Open the valve on the manometer and allow air to escape slowly (allowing the gauge to drop 2–3 mm per heartbeat).	
——	——	——	20. **Note the point on the gauge at which the first faint, but clear, sound appears that slowly increases in intensity. Note this number as the systolic pressure.**	
——	——	——	21. Read the pressure to the closest even number.	
——	——	——	22. Do not reinflate the cuff once the air is being released to recheck the systolic pressure reading.	
——	——	——	23. **Note the pressure at which the sound first becomes muffled. Also observe the point at which the sound completely disappears. These may occur separately or at the same point.**	
——	——	——	24. Allow the remaining air to escape quickly. Repeat any suspicious reading, but wait 30 to 60 seconds between readings to allow normal circulation to return in the limb. Deflate the cuff completely between attempts to check the blood pressure.	
——	——	——	25. Remove the cuff, and clean and store the equipment.	
——	——	——	26. Remove gloves, if worn. Perform hand hygiene.	

Skill Checklists to Accompany Taylor's Clinical Nursing Skills:
A Nursing Process Approach, 2nd edition

Name _____   Date _____

Unit _____   Position _____

Instructor/Evaluator: _____   Position _____

Excellent	Satisfactory	Needs Practice	SKILL 1-6 **Using a Bed Scale**	Comments
			Goal: The patient's weight is assessed accurately, without injury, and the patient experiences minimal discomfort.	
____	____	____	1. Check physician's order or nursing care plan for frequency of weight measurement. More frequent pulse measurement may be appropriate based on nursing judgment. Obtain the assistance of a second caregiver, based on patient's mobility and ability to cooperate with procedure.	
____	____	____	2. Identify the patient.	
____	____	____	3. Explain the procedure to the patient.	
____	____	____	4. Close curtains around bed and close door to room if possible.	
____	____	____	5. Perform hand hygiene.	
____	____	____	6. Place a cover over the sling of the bed scale.	
____	____	____	7. Attach the sling to the bed scale. Lay the sheet or bath blanket in the sling. Turn the scale on. **Adjust the dial so that weight reads 0.0.**	
____	____	____	8. Raise bed to a comfortable working level. Position one caregiver on each side of the bed, if two caregivers are present. Raise side rail on the opposite side of the bed from where the scale is located, if not already in place. Cover the patient with the sheet or bath blanket. Remove other covers and any pillows.	
____	____	____	9. Turn patient onto side facing side rail, keeping his or her body covered with the sheet or blanket. Remove the sling from the scale. Roll sling long ways. Place rolled sling under patient, making sure the patient is centered in the sling.	
____	____	____	10. Roll patient back over sling and onto other side. Pull sling through, as if placing sheet under patient, unrolling sling as it is pulled through.	
____	____	____	11. Roll scale over the bed so that arms of scale are directly over patient. **Spread the base of the scale.** Lower arms of the scale and place arm hooks into holes on the sling.	
____	____	____	12. Once scale arms are hooked onto the sling, begin to crank scale so that patient is lifted up off of the bed. **Assess all tubes and drains, making sure that none have tension**	

Excellent	Satisfactory	Needs Practice		Comments
			SKILL 1-6 **Using a Bed Scale** *(Continued)*	

Excellent	Satisfactory	Needs Practice		Comments
			placed on them as the scale is lifted. Once the sling is no longer touching the bed, ensure that nothing else is hanging onto the sling (eg, ventilator tubing, IV tubing). If any tubing is connected to the patient, raise it up so that it is not adding any weight to the patient.	
——	——	——	13. Note weight reading on the scale. Slowly and gently, lower patient back onto the bed. Disconnect scale arms from sling. Close base of scale and pull it away from the bed.	
——	——	——	14. Raise side rail. Turn patient to side rail. Roll the sling up against the patient's backside.	
——	——	——	15. Raise the other side rail. Roll patient back over the sling and up facing the other side rail. Remove sling from bed.	
——	——	——	16. Cover the patient and help him or her to a position of comfort. **Place the bed in the lowest position.**	
——	——	——	17. Remove disposable cover from sling and discard in appropriate receptacle. Replace scale and sling in appropriate spot. Plug scale into electrical outlet.	
——	——	——	18. Document weight and scale used.	

Skill Checklists to Accompany Taylor's Clinical Nursing Skills:
A Nursing Process Approach, 2nd edition

Name _____   Date _____

Unit _____   Position _____

Instructor/Evaluator: _____   Position _____

Excellent	Satisfactory	Needs Practice	SKILL 1-7 **Monitoring Temperature Using an** **Overhead Radiant Warmer**	Comments
			Goal: The infant's temperature is maintained within normal limits without injury.	
____	____	____	1. Check physician's order or nursing care plan for the use of a radiant warmer.	
____	____	____	2. Identify the patient.	
____	____	____	3. Explain the procedure to the family.	
____	____	____	4. Gather equipment.	
____	____	____	5. Perform hand hygiene.	
____	____	____	6. Plug the warmer in. Turn the warmer to the manual setting. Allow the blankets to warm before placing the infant under the warmer.	
____	____	____	7. **Switch the warmer setting to automatic.** Place the infant under the warmer. Attach probe to the infant's skin but not on a bony area. Cover with a foil patch.	
____	____	____	8. **Adjust the temperature as ordered.**	
____	____	____	9. **Continue to monitor the axillary temperature as ordered.** The temperature may need to be monitored more frequently in the beginning.	
____	____	____	10. Adjust the warmer's temperature as needed according to the axillary temperatures.	

Skill Checklists to Accompany Taylor's Clinical Nursing Skills:
A Nursing Process Approach, 2nd edition

Name _____ Date _____

Unit _____ Position _____

Instructor/Evaluator: _____ Position _____

Excellent	Satisfactory	Needs Practice	SKILL 2-1 **Performing Integumentary Assessment**	Comments
			Goal: The assessment is completed without the patient experiencing anxiety or discomfort, the findings are documented, and the appropriate referral is made to the physician as needed for further evaluation.	
____	____	____	1. Identify the patient.	
____	____	____	2. Explain the purpose of the integumentary examination and answer any questions.	
____	____	____	3. Ask the patient to remove all clothing and put on an examination gown (if appropriate). The patient remains in the sitting position for most of the examination but will need to stand or lie on the side when the posterior part of the body is examined exposing only the body part being examined.	
____	____	____	4. Perform hand hygiene.	
____	____	____	5. Inspect the overall skin coloration.	
____	____	____	6. Inspect skin for vascularity, bleeding, or bruising.	
____	____	____	7. Inspect the skin for lesions. Note bruises, scratches, cuts, inspect bites, and wounds. If present, note size, shape, color, exudates, and distribution/pattern.	
____	____	____	8. Palpate skin using the backs of your hands to assess temperature. Wear gloves when palpating any potentially open area of the skin.	
____	____	____	9. Palpate for texture and moisture.	
____	____	____	10. Assess for skin turgor by gently pinching the skin under the clavicle.	
____	____	____	11. Palpate for edema (which is characterized by swelling, with taut and shiny skin over the edematous area).	
____	____	____	12. If lesions are present, put on gloves and palpate the lesion.	
____	____	____	13. Inspect the nail angle noting if any clubbing is present, as well as the shape and color of the nails.	
____	____	____	14. Palpate nails for texture and capillary refill.	
____	____	____	15. Inspect the hair and scalp. Wear gloves for palpation if lesions or infestation is suspected or if hygiene is poor.	
____	____	____	16. If wearing gloves, discard gloves. Perform hand hygiene.	

Skill Checklists to Accompany Taylor's Clinical Nursing Skills:
A Nursing Process Approach, 2nd edition

Name _____   Date _____

Unit _____   Position _____

Instructor/Evaluator: _____   Position _____

Excellent	Satisfactory	Needs Practice	SKILL 2-2 **Assessing the Head and Neck** **Goal:** The assessment is completed, the findings are documented, and the appropriate referral is made to the physician as needed, for further evaluation.	Comments
___	___	___	1. Identify the patient.	
___	___	___	2. Explain the purpose of the head and neck examination and answer any questions.	
___	___	___	3. Perform hand hygiene.	
___	___	___	4. Inspect the head and then the face for color, symmetry, lesions, and distribution of facial hair. Note facial expression. Palpate the skull.	
___	___	___	5. Inspect the external eye structures (eyelids, eyelashes, eyeball, eyebrows), cornea, conjunctiva, and sclera. Note color, edema, symmetry, and alignment.	
___	___	___	6. **Examine the pupils for equality of size, shape, reaction to light by darkening the room and using a penlight to shine the light on each pupil.**	
___	___	___	7. To test for pupillary accommodation and convergence, ask the patient to focus on an object as you bring it closer to the nose.	
___	___	___	8. Using an ophthalmoscope, check the red reflex.	
___	___	___	9. Test the patient's visual acuity with a Snellen chart. Ask the patient to read the smallest possible line of letters, first with both eyes and then with one eye at a time.	
___	___	___	10. With the patient about 2 feet away, ask the patient to focus on your finger and move the patient's eyes through the six cardinal positions of gaze.	
___	___	___	11. Inspect the external ear bilaterally for shape, size, and lesions. Palpate the ear and mastoid process.	
___	___	___	12. Perform an otoscopic examination. For an adult, pull the auricle up and back; for a child, pull the auricle down and back. Note cerumen (wax), edema, discharge, or foreign bodies and condition of the tympanic membrane.	
___	___	___	13. Use a whispered voice to test hearing. Stand about 1 to 2 feet away from the patient, out of her line of vision. Ask the patient to cover the ear not being tested. Perform test on each ear.	

Excellent	Satisfactory	Needs Practice		Comments
			SKILL 2-2 **Assessing the Head and Neck** *(Continued)*	
——	——	——	14. Use a tuning fork to perform Weber's test and Rinne's test if the patient reports diminished hearing in either ear.	
——	——	——	15. Inspect and palpate the external nose.	
——	——	——	16. Palpate and lightly percuss over the frontal and maxillary sinuses. Transilluminate the sinuses if the patient reports tenderness.	
——	——	——	17. Occlude one nostril externally with a finger while patient breathes through the other; repeat for the other side.	
——	——	——	18. Inspect the internal nostrils using an otoscope with a nasal speculum attachment.	
——	——	——	19. Palpate the temporomandibular joint by placing your index finger over the front of each ear as you ask the patient to open and close the mouth.	
——	——	——	20. Perform hand hygiene and don gloves. Inspect the lips, oral mucosa, hard and soft palates, gingivae, teeth, and salivary gland openings by asking the patient to open the mouth wide using a tongue blade and penlight.	
——	——	——	21. Inspect the tongue. Ask the patient to stick out the tongue. Place a tongue blade at the side of the tongue while patient pushes it to the left and right with the tongue. Inspect the uvula by asking the patient to say "ahh" while sticking out the tongue. Palpate the tongue for muscle tone and tenderness. Remove gloves.	
——	——	——	22. Palpate from the forehead to the posterior triangle of the neck for the posterior cervical lymph nodes using the fingerpads in a slow, circular motion.	
——	——	——	23. Inspect and palpate in front of and behind the ears, under the chin, and in the anterior triangle for the anterior cervical lymph nodes.	
——	——	——	24. Inspect and palpate the left and then the right carotid arteries. **Only palpate one carotid artery at a time.** Use the bell of the stethoscope to auscultate the arteries.	
——	——	——	25. Inspect and palpate the trachea.	
——	——	——	26. Palpate the thyroid gland. Then, if enlarged, auscultate the thyroid gland using the bell of the stethoscope.	
——	——	——	27. Inspect and palpate the supraclavicular area.	
——	——	——	28. Inspect the ability of the patient to move his neck. Ask the patient to touch his chin to chest and to each shoulder, each ear to the corresponding shoulder, and then tip head back as far as possible.	
——	——	——	29. Perform hand hygiene.	

Skill Checklists to Accompany Taylor's Clinical Nursing Skills:
A Nursing Process Approach, 2nd edition

Name _____   Date _____

Unit _____   Position _____

Instructor/Evaluator: _____   Position _____

SKILL 2-3

Assessing the Thorax and Lungs

Excellent	Satisfactory	Needs Practice	**Goal:** The assessment is completed without causing the patient to experience anxiety or discomfort, the findings are documented, and the appropriate referral is made to the physician as needed, for further evaluation.	**Comments**
____	____	____	1. Identify the patient.	
____	____	____	2. Explain the purpose of the respiratory system examination and answer any questions.	
____	____	____	3. Perform hand hygiene.	
____	____	____	4. Help the patient undress if needed and provide a patient gown. Assist the patient to a sitting position and expose the posterior thorax.	
____	____	____	5. Inspect the posterior thorax. Examine the skin, bones, and muscles of the spine, shoulder blades, and back as well as symmetry of expansion and accessory muscle use during respirations.	
____	____	____	6. Assess the anteroposterior and lateral diameters of the thorax.	
____	____	____	7. Palpate over the spine and posterior thorax.	
____	____	____	a. Use the palmar surface of the hand to palpate for temperature, tenderness, muscle development, and masses.	
____	____	____	b. Instruct patient to take a deep breath. Assess for tactile fremitus by using the ball of the hands to palpate over the posterior thorax and while the patient says "ninety-nine."	
____	____	____	8. Assess thoracic expansion by standing behind the patient, placing both thumbs on either side of the patient's spine at the level of T9 or T10. Ask the patient to take a deep breath and note movement of examiner's hands.	
____	____	____	9. Percuss over the posterior and lateral lung fields for tone using a zigzag pattern, starting above the scapulae to the bases of the lungs. Note intensity, pitch, duration, and quality of sounds produced. Percuss for diaphragmatic excursion on each side of the posterior thorax.	
____	____	____	10. **Auscultate the lungs across and down the posterior thorax to the bases of lungs as the patient breathes slowly and deeply through the mouth.**	

Excellent	Satisfactory	Needs Practice	SKILL 2-3 **Assessing the Thorax and Lungs** *(Continued)*	
				Comments
——	——	——	11. Examine the anterior thorax. With the patient sitting, rearrange the gown so the anterior chest is exposed. Inspect the skin, bones, and muscles, as well as symmetry of lung expansion and accessory muscle use.	
——	——	——	12. Palpate the anterior thorax. Palpate for tactile fremitus (as the patient repeats the word "ninety-nine").	
——	——	——	13. Percuss over the anterior thorax.	
——	——	——	14. **Auscultate the lungs through the anterior thorax as the patient breathes slowly and deeply through the mouth.**	
——	——	——	15. Inspect the breasts and axillae with the patient's hands resting on both sides of the body, placed on the hips, and then raised above the head.	
——	——	——	16. Palpate the axillae with the patient's arms resting against the side of the body. Assist the patient into a supine position. Place a small pillow or towel under the patient's back. Palpate the breasts and nipples. Wear gloves if there is any discharge from the nipples or if a lesion is present.	
——	——	——	17. Assist the patient in replacing the gown. Perform hand hygiene.	

Skill Checklists to Accompany Taylor's Clinical Nursing Skills:
A Nursing Process Approach, 2nd edition

Name _____ Date _____

Unit _____ Position _____

Instructor/Evaluator: _____ Position _____

Excellent	Satisfactory	Needs Practice	SKILL 2-4 **Assessing the Cardiovascular System** **Goal:** The assessment is completed without causing the patient to experience anxiety or discomfort, the findings are documented, and the appropriate referral for further evaluation is made to the physician as needed.	Comments
——	——	——	1. Identify the patient.	
——	——	——	2. Explain the purpose of the cardiovascular examination and answer any questions.	
——	——	——	3. Perform hand hygiene.	
——	——	——	4. Assist the patient to a supine position with the head elevated about 30 to 45 degrees and expose anterior chest.	
——	——	——	5. Inspect and palpate the left and then the right carotid arteries. **Only palpate one carotid artery at a time.** Use the bell of the stethoscope to auscultate the arteries.	
——	——	——	6. **Inspect the neck for jugular vein distention, observing for pulsations.**	
——	——	——	7. Inspect the precordium for contour, pulsations, and heaves. Observe for the apical impulse at the 4th to 5th intercostal spaces (ICS).	
——	——	——	8. Using the palmar surface with the four fingers held together, palpate the precordium gently for pulsations. Remember that hands should be warm. Palpation proceeds in a systematic manner, with assessment of specific cardiac landmarks—the aortic, pulmonic, tricuspid, and mitral areas and Erb's point. **Palpate the apical impulse in the mitral area.** Note size, duration, force, and location in relationship to the midclavicular line.	
——	——	——	9. **Use systematic auscultation, beginning at the aortic area, moving to the pulmonic area, then to Erb's point, then to the tricuspid area, and finally to the mitral area.** Ask the patient to breathe normally. The stethoscope diaphragm is first used to listen to high-pitched sounds, followed by use of the bell to listen to low-pitched sounds. Focus on the overall rate and rhythm of the heart and the normal heart sounds.	
——	——	——	10. Replace the patient's gown and assist the patient to a comfortable position.	
——	——	——	11. Perform hand hygiene.	

Skill Checklists to Accompany Taylor's Clinical Nursing Skills:
A Nursing Process Approach, 2nd edition

Name _____   Date _____

Unit _____   Position _____

Instructor/Evaluator: _____   Position _____

SKILL 2-5
Assessing the Abdomen

Goal: The assessment is completed without causing the patient to experience anxiety or discomfort, the findings are documented, and the appropriate referral is made to the physician as needed, for further evaluation.

Excellent	Satisfactory	Needs Practice		Comments
――	――	――	1. Identify the patient.	
――	――	――	2. Explain the purpose of the abdominal examination and answer any questions.	
――	――	――	3. Perform hand hygiene.	
――	――	――	4. Help the patient undress if needed and provide a patient gown. Assist the patient to a supine position and expose the abdomen.	
――	――	――	5. Inspect the abdomen for skin color, contour, pulsations, the umbilicus, and other surface characteristics (rashes, lesions, masses, scars).	
――	――	――	6. **Auscultate all four quadrants of the abdomen for bowel sounds by using the diaphragm of the stethoscope.** Use a systematic method.	
――	――	――	7. **Auscultate the abdomen for vascular sounds by using the bell of the stethoscope.**	
――	――	――	8. Percuss the abdomen for tones.	
――	――	――	9. Palpate the abdomen lightly in all four quadrants and then palpate using deep palpation technique. If the patient complains of pain or discomfort in a particular area of the abdomen, palpate that area last.	
――	――	――	10. Palpate for the kidneys on each side of the abdomen. Palpate the liver at the right costal border. Palpate for the spleen at the left costal border.	
――	――	――	11. **Assess for rebound tenderness last if the patient reports pain by pressing deeply and gently into the abdomen with the hand and fingers downward and then withdrawing the hand rapidly.**	
――	――	――	12. **Palpate and then auscultate the femoral pulses in the groin.**	
――	――	――	13. Replace the patient's gown and assist the patient to a comfortable position.	
――	――	――	14. Perform hand hygiene.	

Skill Checklists to Accompany Taylor's Clinical Nursing Skills:
A Nursing Process Approach, 2nd edition

Name _____   Date _____

Unit _____   Position _____

Instructor/Evaluator: _____   Position _____

Excellent	Satisfactory	Needs Practice	SKILL 2-6 **Assessing the Neurologic, Musculoskeletal, and Peripheral Vascular Systems**	Comments
			Goal: The assessment is completed, the findings are documented, and the appropriate referral for further evaluation is made to the physician, as needed.	
——	——	——	1. Identify the patient.	
——	——	——	2. Explain the purpose of the neurologic, musculoskeletal, and peripheral vascular examination and answer any questions.	
——	——	——	3. Instruct the patient to void if possible. Collect a urine specimen if ordered.	
——	——	——	4. Perform hand hygiene.	
——	——	——	5. Help the patient undress if needed and provide a patient gown. Assist the patient to a sitting position.	
——	——	——	6. Begin with a survey of the patient's overall hygiene and physical appearance.	
——	——	——	7. Assess the patient's mental status.	
——	——	——	a. Evaluate the patient's orientation to person, place, and time.	
——	——	——	b. Evaluate level of consciousness.	
——	——	——	c. Assess memory (immediate recall and past memory).	
——	——	——	d. Assess abstract reasoning by asking the patient to explain a proverb, such as "The early bird catches the worm."	
——	——	——	e. Evaluate the patient's ability to understand spoken and written word.	
——	——	——	8. Test cranial nerve (CN) function.	
——	——	——	a. Ask the patient to close the eyes, occlude one nostril, and then identify the smell of different substances, such as coffee, chocolate, or alcohol. Repeat with other nostril.	
——	——	——	b. Test visual acuity and pupillary constriction.	
——	——	——	c. Move the patient's eyes through the six cardinal positions of gaze.	
——	——	——	d. Ask the patient to smile, frown, wrinkle forehead, and puff out cheeks.	
——	——	——	e. Test hearing.	

SKILL 2-6

Assessing the Neurologic, Musculoskeletal, and Peripheral Vascular Systems *(Continued)*

Excellent	Satisfactory	Needs Practice		Comments
——	——	——	f. Test the gag reflex by touching the posterior pharynx with the tongue depressor. Explain to patient that this may be uncomfortable.	
——	——	——	g. Place your hands on the patient's shoulders while he or she shrugs against resistance. Then place your hand on the patient's left cheek, then the right cheek, and have the patient push against it.	
——	——	——	9. Inspect the ability of the patient to move his neck. Ask the patient to touch his or her chin to chest and to each shoulder, each ear to the corresponding shoulder, and then tip head back as far as possible.	
——	——	——	10. Inspect the upper extremities. Observe for skin color, presence of lesions, rashes, and muscle mass. Palpate for skin temperature, texture, and presence of masses.	
——	——	——	11. Ask patient to extend arms forward and then rapidly turn palms up and down.	
——	——	——	12. Ask patient to flex upper arm and to resist examiner's opposing force.	
——	——	——	13. Inspect and palpate the hands, fingers, wrists, and elbow joints; palpate the hands.	
——	——	——	14. Palpate the radial and brachial pulses.	
——	——	——	15. Have the patient squeeze two of your fingers.	
——	——	——	16. Ask the patient to close his/her eyes. Using your finger or applicator, trace a one-digit number on the patient's palm and ask him or her to identify the number. Repeat on the other hand with a different number.	
——	——	——	17. Ask the patient to close his/her eyes. Place a familiar object such as a key in the patient's hand and ask him or her to identify the object. Repeat using another object for the other hand.	
——	——	——	18. Assist the patient to a supine position. Examine the lower extremities. Inspect the legs and feet for color, lesions, varicosities, hair growth, nail growth, edema, and muscle mass.	
——	——	——	19. Test for pitting edema in the pretibial area by pressing fingers into the skin of the pretibial area. If an indentation remains in the skin after the fingers have been lifted, pitting edema is present.	
——	——	——	20. Palpate for pulses and skin temperature at the posterior tibial, dorsalis pedis, and popliteal areas.	

Excellent	Satisfactory	Needs Practice	SKILL 2-6 **Assessing the Neurologic, Musculoskeletal, and Peripheral Vascular Systems** *(Continued)*	Comments
——	——	——	21. Have the patient perform the straight leg test with one leg at a time.	
——	——	——	22. Ask the patient to move one leg laterally with the knee straight to test abduction and medially to test adduction of the hips.	
——	——	——	23. Ask the patient to raise the thigh against the resistance of your hand; next have the patient push outward against the resistance of your hand; then have the patient pull backward against the resistance of your hand. Repeat on the opposite side.	
——	——	——	24. Assess the patient's deep tendon reflexes (DTRs).	
——	——	——	a. Place your fingers above the patient's wrist and tap with a reflex hammer; repeat on the other arm.	
——	——	——	b. Place your fingers over the antecubital area and tap with a reflex hammer; repeat on the other side.	
——	——	——	c. Place your fingers over the triceps tendon area and tap with a reflex hammer; repeat on the other side.	
——	——	——	d. Tap just below the patella with a reflex hammer; repeat on the other side.	
——	——	——	e. Tap over the Achilles tendon area with reflex hammer; repeat on the other side.	
——	——	——	25. Stroke the sole of the patient's foot with the end of a reflex hammer handle or other hard object such as a key; repeat on the other side.	
——	——	——	26. Ask patient to dorsiflex and then plantarflex both feet against opposing resistance.	
——	——	——	27. As needed, assist the patient to a standing position. Observe the patient as he or she walks with a regular gait, on the toes, on the heels, and then heel to toe.	
——	——	——	28. Perform the Romberg's test; ask the patient to stand straight with feet together, both eyes closed with arms at side. Wait 20 seconds and observe for patient swaying and ability to maintain balance. Nurse must be alert to prevent patient fall or injury related to losing balance during this assessment.	
——	——	——	29. Assist the patient to a comfortable position.	
——	——	——	30. Perform hand hygiene.	

Skill Checklists to Accompany Taylor's Clinical Nursing Skills:
A Nursing Process Approach, 2nd edition

Name _____   Date _____

Unit _____   Position _____

Instructor/Evaluator: _____   Position _____

Excellent	Satisfactory	Needs Practice	SKILL 3-1 **Fall Prevention**	Comments
			Goal: The patient does not experience a fall and remains free of injury.	
___	___	___	1. Identify the patient. Explain the rationale for fall prevention interventions to the patient and family/significant others.	
___	___	___	2. Provide adequate lighting.	
___	___	___	3. Remove excess equipment, supplies, furniture, and other objects from rooms and walkways. Pay particular attention to high traffic areas and the route to the bathroom.	
___	___	___	4. Orient patient and significant others to new surroundings, including use of the telephone, call signal, patient bed, and room illumination. Indicate the location of the patient bathroom.	
___	___	___	5. Provide nonskid foot wear.	
___	___	___	6. Provide a bedside commode, if appropriate. Ensure that it is near the bed at all times.	
___	___	___	7. Ensure that the call signal, bedside table, telephone, and other personal items are within the patient's reach at all times.	
___	___	___	8. Confer with physician or primary care provider regarding appropriate exercise and physical therapy.	
___	___	___	9. Encourage the patient to rise or change position slowly and sit for several minutes before standing.	
___	___	___	10. Evaluate the appropriateness of elastic stockings for lower extremities.	
___	___	___	11. Review medications for potential hazards.	
___	___	___	12. Keep the bed in the lowest position during use. If elevated to provide care (to reduce caregiver strain), ensure that it is lowered when care is completed.	
___	___	___	13. Make sure locks on the bed or wheelchair are secured at all times.	
___	___	___	14. Use bed rails according to facility policy, when appropriate.	
___	___	___	15. Anticipate patient needs and provide assistance with activities instead of waiting for the patient to ask.	
___	___	___	16. Consider the use of an electronic bed or chair alarm.	
___	___	___	17. Include the patient's family and/or significant others in the plan of care.	

Skill Checklists to Accompany Taylor's Clinical Nursing Skills:
A Nursing Process Approach, 2nd edition

Name _____ Date _____

Unit _____ Position _____

Instructor/Evaluator: _____ Position _____

SKILL 3-2

Applying an Extremity Restraint

Goal: The patient is constrained by the restraint, remains free from injury, and the restraint does not interfere with therapeutic devices.

Excellent	Satisfactory	Needs Practice		Comments
——	——	——	1. Determine need for restraints. Assess patient's physical condition, behavior, and mental status. Refer to the review boxes at the beginning of the chapter.	
——	——	——	2. Confirm agency policy for application of restraints. **Secure a physician's order, or validate that the order has been obtained within the past 24 hours.**	
——	——	——	3. Identify the patient.	
——	——	——	4. Explain reason for use to patient and family. Clarify how care will be given and how needs will be met. Explain that restraint is a temporary measure.	
——	——	——	5. Perform hand hygiene.	
——	——	——	6. Apply restraint according to manufacturer's directions:	
——	——	——	a. Choose the least restrictive type of device that allows the greatest possible degree of mobility.	
——	——	——	b. Pad bony prominences.	
——	——	——	c. Wrap the restraint around the extremity with the soft part in contact with the skin. If hand mitt is being used, pull over hand with cushion to the palmar aspect of hand. Secure in place with the Velcro® straps or reverse clove hitch.	
——	——	——	7. **Ensure that two fingers can be inserted between the restraint and patient's wrist or ankle.**	
——	——	——	8. Maintain restrained extremity in normal anatomic position. **Use a quick-release knot to tie the restraint to the bed frame, not side rail. The restraint may also be attached to chair frame. The site should not be readily accessible to patient.**	
——	——	——	9. Assess the patient at least every hour or according to facility policy. Assessment should include: the placement of the restraint, neurovascular assessment of the affected extremity, and skin integrity. In addition, assess for signs of sensory deprivation, such as increased sleeping, daydreaming, anxiety, panic, and hallucinations.	

Excellent	Satisfactory	Needs Practice		Comments

SKILL 3-2
Applying an Extremity Restraint *(Continued)*

___	___	___	10. **Remove restraint at least every 2 hours, or according to agency policy and patient need.** Perform range-of-motion exercises.	
___	___	___	11. Evaluate patient for continued need of restraint. Reapply restraint only if continued need is evident and order is still valid.	
___	___	___	12. Reassure patient at regular intervals. Provide continued explanation of rationale for interventions, reorientation if necessary, and plan of care. **Keep call bell within easy reach.**	
___	___	___	13. Perform hand hygiene.	

Skill Checklists to Accompany Taylor's Clinical Nursing Skills:
A Nursing Process Approach, 2nd edition

Name _____ Date _____

Unit _____ Position _____

Instructor/Evaluator: _____ Position _____

Excellent	Satisfactory	Needs Practice	SKILL 3-3 **Applying a Jacket or Vest Restraint**	Comments
			Goal: The patient is constrained by the restraint, remains free from injury, and the restraint does not interfere with therapeutic devices.	
___	___	___	1. Determine need for restraints. Assess patient's physical condition, behavior, and mental status.	
___	___	___	2. Confirm agency policy for application of restraints. **Secure a physician's order, or validate that the order has been obtained within the past 24 hours.**	
___	___	___	3. Identify the patient.	
___	___	___	4. Explain reason for use to patient and family. Clarify how care will be given and how needs will be met. Explain that restraint is a temporary measure.	
___	___	___	5. Perform hand hygiene.	
___	___	___	6. Apply restraint according to manufacturer's directions:	
___	___	___	a. Choose the correct size of the least restrictive type of device that allows the greatest possible degree of mobility.	
___	___	___	b. Pad bony prominences that may be affected by the vest.	
___	___	___	c. Assist patient to a sitting position, if not contraindicated.	
___	___	___	d. **Place vest on patient over gown, with flaps crisscrossing over the abdomen if appropriate. The V opening should be on the patient's front.**	
___	___	___	e. Pull the tabs secure. **Ensure that there are no wrinkles in the vest behind the patient.**	
___	___	___	f. **Insert fist between restraint and patient to ensure that breathing is not constricted. Assess respirations after restraint is applied.**	
___	___	___	7. **Use a quick-release knot to tie the restraint to the bed frame, not side rail.** If patient is in a wheelchair, lock the wheels and place the restraints under the arm rests and tie behind the chair. Site should not be readily accessible to the patient.	

Excellent	Satisfactory	Needs Practice	SKILL 3-3 **Applying a Jacket or Vest Restraint** *(Continued)*	Comments
____	____	____	8. Assess the patient at least every hour or according to facility policy as required. An assessment should include: the placement of the restraint, respiratory assessment, and skin integrity. Assess for signs of sensory deprivation, such as increased sleeping, daydreaming, anxiety, panic, and hallucinations.	
____	____	____	9. **Remove restraint at least every 2 hours or according to agency policy and patient need.** Perform range-of-motion exercises.	
____	____	____	10. Evaluate patient for continued need of restraint. Reapply restraint only if continued need is evident and order is still valid.	
____	____	____	11. Reassure patient at regular intervals. Provide continued explanation of rationale for interventions, reorientation if necessary, and plan of care. **Keep call bell within easy reach.**	
____	____	____	12. Perform hand hygiene.	

Skill Checklists to Accompany Taylor's Clinical Nursing Skills:
A Nursing Process Approach, 2nd edition

Name _____ Date _____

Unit _____ Position _____

Instructor/Evaluator: _____ Position _____

Excellent	Satisfactory	Needs Practice	SKILL 3-4 **Applying an Elbow Restraint**	Comments
			Goal: The patient is constrained by the restraint, remains free from injury, and the restraint does not interfere with therapeutic devices.	
___	___	___	1. Determine need for restraints. Assess patient's physical condition, behavior, and mental status.	
___	___	___	2. Confirm agency policy for application of restraints. **Secure a physician's order, or validate that the order has been obtained within the past 24 hours.**	
___	___	___	3. Identify the patient.	
___	___	___	4. Explain reason for use to patient and family. Clarify how care will be given and how needs will be met. Explain that restraint is a temporary measure.	
___	___	___	5. Perform hand hygiene.	
___	___	___	6. Apply restraint according to manufacturer's directions:	
___	___	___	a. Choose the correct size of the least restrictive type of device that allows the greatest possible degree of mobility.	
___	___	___	b. Pad bony prominences that may be affected by the restraint.	
___	___	___	c. Spread elbow restraint out flat. Place middle of elbow restraint behind patient's elbow. **The restraint should not extend below the wrist or place pressure on the axilla.**	
___	___	___	d. **Wrap restraint snugly around patient's arm, but make sure that two fingers can easily fit under restraint.**	
___	___	___	e. Wrap Velcro straps around restraint.	
___	___	___	f. Apply restraint to opposite arm if patient can move arm.	
___	___	___	g. Thread Velcro strap from one elbow restraint across the back and into the loop on the opposite elbow restraint.	
___	___	___	7. **Assess circulation to fingers and hand.**	
___	___	___	8. Assess the patient at least every hour or according to facility policy is required. An assessment should include: the placement of the restraint, neurovascular assessment, and skin integrity. Assess for signs of sensory deprivation, such as increased sleeping, daydreaming, anxiety, inconsolable crying, and panic.	

Excellent	Satisfactory	Needs Practice		Comments

SKILL 3-4
Applying an Elbow Restraint *(Continued)*

Excellent	Satisfactory	Needs Practice		
——	——	——	9. Remove restraint at least every 2 hours for children ages 9–17 years and at least every 1 hour for children under age 9, or according to agency policy and patient need. Perform range-of-motion exercises.	
——	——	——	10. Evaluate patient for continued need of restraint. Reapply restraint only if continued need is evident.	
——	——	——	11. Reassure patient at regular intervals. **Keep call bell within easy reach.**	
——	——	——	12. Perform hand hygiene.	

Skill Checklists to Accompany Taylor's Clinical Nursing Skills:
A Nursing Process Approach, 2nd edition

Name _____ Date _____

Unit _____ Position _____

Instructor/Evaluator: _____ Position _____

Excellent	Satisfactory	Needs Practice	SKILL 3-5 **Applying a Mummy Restraint** **Goal:** The patient is constrained by the restraint remains free from injury, and the restraint does not interfere with therapeutic devices.	Comments
——	——	——	1. Determine need for restraints. Assess patient's physical condition, behavior, and mental status.	
——	——	——	2. Confirm agency policy for application of restraints.	
——	——	——	3. Identify the patient.	
——	——	——	4. Explain reason for use to patient and family. Clarify how care will be given and how needs will be met. Explain that restraint is a temporary measure.	
——	——	——	5. Perform hand hygiene.	
——	——	——	6. Open the blanket or sheet. Fold one corner to the center. Place the child on the blanket, shoulders at the fold, and feet toward the opposite corner.	
——	——	——	7. Position the child's right arm alongside his body. Left arm should not be constrained at this time. Pull the right side of the blanket tightly over the child's right shoulder and chest. Secure under the left side of his body.	
——	——	——	8. Position the left arm along side the child's body. Pull the left side of the blanket tightly over the child's left shoulder and chest. Secure under the right side of his body.	
——	——	——	9. Fold the lower corner up and pull over the child's body. Secure under the child's body on each side or with safety pins.	
——	——	——	10. Stay with child while mummy wrap is in place. Reassure child and parents at regular intervals. Once examination or treatment is completed, unwrap child.	
——	——	——	11. Perform hand hygiene.	

Skill Checklists to Accompany Taylor's Clinical Nursing Skills:
A Nursing Process Approach, 2nd edition

Name _____   Date _____

Unit _____   Position _____

Instructor/Evaluator: _____   Position _____

Excellent	Satisfactory	Needs Practice	SKILL 3-6 **Applying Leather Restraints**	
			Goal: The patient is constrained by the restraint, remains free from injury, and the restraint does not interfere with therapeutic devices.	**Comments**
――	――	――	1. Determine need for restraints. Assess patient's physical condition, behavior, and mental status.	
――	――	――	2. Confirm agency policy for application of restraints. **Secure a physician's order, or validate that the order has been obtained within the past 24 hours.**	
――	――	――	3. Identify the patient.	
――	――	――	4. Explain reason for use to patient and family. Clarify how care will be given and how needs will be met. Explain that restraint is a temporary measure.	
――	――	――	5. Perform hand hygiene.	
――	――	――	6. Apply restraints according to manufacturer's directions:	
――	――	――	a. Pad bony prominences.	
――	――	――	b. Wrap the restraint around the extremity with the soft part in contact with the skin. Secure in place with the buckles.	
――	――	――	c. **Ensure that two fingers can be inserted between the restraint and patient's wrist or ankle.** Maintain restrained extremity in normal anatomic position.	
――	――	――	d. **If using locking leather restraints, ensure that key is available at all times.**	
――	――	――	7. **Fasten restraint to bed frame, not side rail.** Leather restraints have leather straps with buckles to secure to the bed frame. Site should not be readily accessible to the patient.	
――	――	――	8. Assessment of the patient at least every hour or according to facility policy is required. An assessment should include: the placement of the restraint, neurovascular assessment of the affected extremity, and skin integrity. Assess for signs of sensory deprivation, such as increased sleeping, daydreaming, anxiety, panic, and hallucinations.	

Excellent	Satisfactory	Needs Practice		Comments
			SKILL 3-6 **Applying Leather Restraints** *(Continued)*	
___	___	___	9. **Remove restraint at least every 2 hours, or according to agency policy and patient need.** Perform range-of-motion exercises.	
___	___	___	10. Evaluate patient for continued need of restraint. Reapply restraint only if continued need is evident and order is valid.	
___	___	___	11. Reassure patient at regular intervals. **Keep call bell within easy reach.**	
___	___	___	12. Perform hand hygiene.	

Skill Checklists to Accompany Taylor's Clinical Nursing Skills:
A Nursing Process Approach, 2nd edition

Name _____ Date _____

Unit _____ Position _____

Instructor/Evaluator: _____ Position _____

Excellent	Satisfactory	Needs Practice	SKILL 4-1 **Performing Hand Hygiene Using Soap and Water (Handwashing)** **Goal:** The hands will be free of visible soiling and transient microorganisms will be eliminated.	Comments
——	——	——	1. Gather the necessary supplies. Stand in front of the sink. Do not allow your clothing to touch the sink during the washing procedure.	
——	——	——	2. Remove jewelry, if possible, and secure in a safe place. A plain wedding band may remain in place.	
——	——	——	3. Turn on water and adjust force. Regulate the temperature until the water is warm.	
——	——	——	4. Wet the hands and wrist area. Keep hands lower than elbows to allow water to flow toward fingertips.	
——	——	——	5. Use about 1 teaspoon liquid soap from dispenser or rinse bar of soap and lather thoroughly. Cover all areas of hands with the soap product. Rinse soap bar again and return to soap dish.	
——	——	——	6. With firm rubbing and circular motions, wash the palms and backs of the hands, each finger, the areas between the fingers, and the knuckles, wrists, and forearms. **Wash at least 1″ above area of contamination.** If hands are not visibly soiled, wash to 1″ above the wrists.	
——	——	——	7. Continue this friction motion for at least 15 seconds.	
——	——	——	8. Use fingernails of the opposite hand or a clean orangewood stick to clean under fingernails.	
——	——	——	9. Rinse thoroughly with water flowing toward fingertips.	
——	——	——	10. Pat hands dry with a paper towel, beginning with the fingers and moving upward toward forearms, and discard it immediately. Use another clean towel to turn off the faucet. Discard towel immediately without touching other clean hand.	
——	——	——	11. Use oil-free lotion on hands if desired.	

Skill Checklists to Accompany Taylor's Clinical Nursing Skills:
A Nursing Process Approach, 2nd edition

Name _____ Date _____

Unit _____ Position _____

Instructor/Evaluator: _____ Position _____

Excellent	Satisfactory	Needs Practice	SKILL 4-2 **Performing Hand Hygiene Using an Alcohol-Based Hand Rub**	
			Goal: Transient microorganisms will be eliminated from the hands.	**Comments**
——	——	——	1. Remove jewelry, if possible, and secure in a safe place. A plain wedding band may remain in place.	
——	——	——	2. Check the product labeling for correct amount of product needed.	
——	——	——	3. Apply the correct amount of product to the palm of one hand. Rub hands together, covering all surfaces of hands and fingers.	
——	——	——	4. Rub hands together until they are dry.	
——	——	——	5. Use oil-free lotion on hands if desired.	

Skill Checklists to Accompany Taylor's Clinical Nursing Skills:
A Nursing Process Approach, 2nd edition

Name _____   Date _____

Unit _____   Position _____

Instructor/Evaluator: _____   Position _____

Excellent	Satisfactory	Needs Practice	SKILL 4-3 **Preparing a Sterile Field Using a Packaged Sterile Drape** **Goal:** The sterile field is created without evidence of contamination and the patient remains free of exposure to potential infection-causing microorganisms.	Comments
——	——	——	1. Identify the patient. Explain the procedure to the patient.	
——	——	——	2. Perform hand hygiene.	
——	——	——	3. Check that packaged sterile drape is dry and unopened. Also note expiration date, making sure that the date is still valid.	
——	——	——	4. Select a work area that is waist level or higher.	
——	——	——	5. Open the outer covering of the drape. Remove sterile drape, lifting it carefully by its corners. Hold away from body and above the waist and work surface.	
——	——	——	6. Continue to hold only by the corners. Allow the drape to unfold, away from your body and any other surface.	
——	——	——	7. Position the drape on the work surface with the moisture-proof side down. This would be the shiny or blue side. Avoid touching any other surface or object with the drape.	
——	——	——	8. Place additional sterile items on field as needed. Refer to Skill 4-5. Continue with the procedure as indicated.	

Skill Checklists to Accompany Taylor's Clinical Nursing Skills:
A Nursing Process Approach, 2nd edition

Name _____   Date _____

Unit _____   Position _____

Instructor/Evaluator: _____   Position _____

SKILL 4-4

Preparing a Sterile Field Using a Commercially Prepared Sterile Kit or Tray

Excellent	Satisfactory	Needs Practice	**Goal:** A sterile field is created without evidence of contamination, the contents of the package remain sterile, and the patient remains free of exposure to potential infection-causing microorganisms.	Comments
___	___	___	1. Identify the patient. Explain the procedure to the patient.	
___	___	___	2. Perform hand hygiene.	
___	___	___	3. Check that packaged kit or tray is dry and unopened. Also note expiration date, making sure that the date is still valid.	
___	___	___	4. Select a work area that is waist level or higher.	
___	___	___	5. Open the outside cover of the package and remove the kit or tray. Place in the center of the work surface.	
___	___	___	6. Reach around the package and grasp the outer surface of the end of the topmost flap, holding no more than one inch from the border of the flap. Pull open away from the body, keeping the arm outstretched and away from the inside of the wrapper. Allow the wrapper to lie flat on the work surface.	
___	___	___	7. Reach around the package and grasp the outer surface of the first side flap, holding no more than one inch from the border of the flap. Pull open to the side of the package, keeping the arm outstretched and away from the inside of the wrapper. Allow the wrapper to lie flat on the work surface.	
___	___	___	8. Reach around the package and grasp the outer surface of the remaining side flap, holding no more than one inch from the border of the flap. Pull open to the side of the package, keeping the arm outstretched and away from the inside of the wrapper. Allow the wrapper to lie flat on the work surface.	

Excellent	Satisfactory	Needs Practice	SKILL 4-4 **Preparing a Sterile Field Using a Commercially Prepared Sterile Kit or Tray** *(Continued)*	Comments
——	——	——	9. Stand away from the package and work surface. Grasp the outer surface of the remaining flap closest to the body, holding not more than one inch from the border of the flap. Pull the flap back toward the body, keeping arm outstretched and away from the inside of the wrapper. Allow the wrapper to lie flat on the work surface.	
——	——	——	10. The outer wrapper of the package has become a sterile field with the package's supplies in the center. Do not touch or reach over the sterile field. Place additional sterile items on field as needed. Refer to Skill 4-5. Continue with the procedure as indicated.	

Skill Checklists to Accompany Taylor's Clinical Nursing Skills:
A Nursing Process Approach, 2nd edition

Name _____   Date _____

Unit _____   Position _____

Instructor/Evaluator: _____   Position _____

SKILL 4-5
Adding Sterile Items to a Sterile Field

Excellent	Satisfactory	Needs Practice	**Goal:** The sterile field is created without evidence of contamination, the sterile supplies are not contaminated, and the patient remains free of exposure to potential infection-causing microorganisms.	**Comments**
____	____	____	1. Identify the patient. Explain the procedure to the patient.	
____	____	____	2. Perform hand hygiene.	
____	____	____	3. Check that the sterile, packaged drape and supplies are dry and unopened. Also note expiration date, making sure that the date is still valid.	
____	____	____	4. Select a work area that is waist level or higher.	
____	____	____	5. Prepare sterile field as described in Skill 4-3 or Skill 4-4.	
____	____	____	6. Add sterile item:	
			To Add an Agency-Wrapped and Sterilized Item	
____	____	____	a. Hold agency-wrapped item in the dominant hand, with top flap opening away from the body. With other hand, reach around the package and unfold top flap and both sides.	
____	____	____	b. Keep a secure hold on item through the wrapper with the dominant hand. Grasp the remaining flap of the wrapper closest to the body, taking care not to touch the inner surface of the wrapper or the item. Pull the flap back toward the wrist, so the wrapper covers the hand and wrist.	
____	____	____	c. Grasp all the corners of the wrapper together with the nondominant hand and pull back toward wrist, covering hand and wrist. Hold in place.	
____	____	____	d. Hold the item 6″ above the surface of the sterile field and drop onto the field. Be careful to avoid touching the surface or other items or dropping onto the 1″ border.	
			To Add a Commercially Wrapped and Sterilized Item:	
____	____	____	a. Hold package in one hand. Pull back top cover with other hand. Alternately, carefully peel the edges apart using both hands.	

Excellent	Satisfactory	Needs Practice	

Comments

Excellent	Satisfactory	Needs Practice	
⸺	⸺	⸺	b. After top cover or edges are partially separated, hold the item 6″ above the surface of the sterile field. Continue opening the package and drop the item onto the field. Be careful to avoid touching the surface or other items or dropping onto the 1″ border.
⸺	⸺	⸺	c. Discard wrapper.
			To Add a Sterile Solution:
⸺	⸺	⸺	a. Obtain appropriate solution and check expiration date.
⸺	⸺	⸺	b. Open solution container according to directions and **place cap on table with edges up.**
⸺	⸺	⸺	c. If bottle has previously been opened, "lip" it by pouring a small amount of solution into waste container.
⸺	⸺	⸺	d. Hold bottle outside the edge of the sterile field with the label side facing the palm of your hand and prepare to pour from a height of 4″ to 6″ (10 to 15 cm). The tip of the bottle should never touch a sterile container or dressing.
⸺	⸺	⸺	e. Pour required amount of solution steadily into sterile container positioned at side of sterile field or onto dressings. **Avoid splashing any liquid.**
⸺	⸺	⸺	f. Touch only the outside of the lid when recapping. Label solution with date and time of opening.
⸺	⸺	⸺	7. Continue with procedure as indicated.

Skill Checklists to Accompany Taylor's Clinical Nursing Skills:
A Nursing Process Approach, 2nd edition

Name _____ Date _____

Unit _____ Position _____

Instructor/Evaluator: _____ Position _____

SKILL 4-6

Putting on Sterile Gloves and Removing Soiled Gloves

Excellent	Satisfactory	Needs Practice	**Goal:** The gloves are applied and removed without contamination.	Comments
___	___	___	1. Identify the patient. Explain the procedure to the patient.	
___	___	___	2. Perform hand hygiene.	
___	___	___	3. Check that the sterile glove package is dry and unopened. Also note expiration date, making sure that the date is still valid.	
___	___	___	4. Place sterile glove package on clean, dry surface at or above your waist.	
___	___	___	5. Open the outside wrapper by carefully peeling the top layer back. Remove inner package, handling only the outside of it.	
___	___	___	6. Place the inner package on the work surface with the side labeled "cuff end" closest to the body.	
___	___	___	7. Carefully open the inner package. Fold open the top flap, then the bottom and sides. Take care not to touch the inner surface of the package or the gloves.	
___	___	___	8. With the thumb and forefinger of the nondominant hand, grasp the folded cuff of the glove for dominant hand, touching only the exposed inside of the glove.	
___	___	___	9. Keeping the hands above the waistline, lift and hold the glove up and off the inner package with fingers down. **Be careful it does not touch any unsterile object.**	
___	___	___	10. Carefully insert dominant hand palm up into glove and pull glove on. Leave the cuff folded until the opposite hand is gloved.	
___	___	___	11. Hold the thumb of the gloved hand outward. Place the fingers of the gloved hand inside the cuff of the remaining glove. Lift it from the wrapper, taking care not to touch anything with the gloves or hands.	
___	___	___	12. Carefully insert nondominant hand into glove. Pull the glove on, taking care that the skin does not touch any of the outer surfaces of the gloves.	

Excellent	Satisfactory	Needs Practice		Comments

SKILL 4-6

Putting on Sterile Gloves and Removing Soiled Gloves *(Continued)*

Excellent	Satisfactory	Needs Practice		Comments
——	——	——	13. Slide the fingers of one hand under the cuff of the other and fully extend the cuff down the arm, touching only the sterile outside of the glove. Repeat for the remaining hand.	
——	——	——	14. Adjust gloves on both hands if necessary, touching only sterile areas with other sterile areas.	
——	——	——	15. Continue with procedure as indicated.	
			Removing Soiled Gloves	
——	——	——	16. Use dominant hand to grasp the opposite glove near cuff end on the outside exposed area. Remove it by pulling it off, inverting it as it is pulled, keeping the contaminated area on the inside. Hold the removed glove in the remaining gloved hand.	
——	——	——	17. Slide fingers of ungloved hand between the remaining glove and the wrist. Take care to avoid touching the outside surface of the glove. Remove it by pulling it off, inverting it as it is pulled, keeping the contaminated area on the inside, and securing the first glove inside the second.	
——	——	——	18. Discard gloves in appropriate container and perform hand hygiene.	

Skill Checklists to Accompany Taylor's Clinical Nursing Skills:
A Nursing Process Approach, 2nd edition

Name _____ Date _____

Unit _____ Position _____

Instructor/Evaluator: _____ Position _____

Excellent	Satisfactory	Needs Practice	SKILL 4-7 **Using Personal Protective Equipment**	Comments
			Goal: The transmission of microorganisms is prevented.	
____	____	____	1. Check physician's order for type of precautions and review precautions in infection-control manual.	
____	____	____	2. Plan nursing activities before entering patient's room.	
____	____	____	3. Provide instruction about precautions to patient, family members, and visitors.	
____	____	____	4. Perform hand hygiene.	
____	____	____	5. Put on gown, gloves, mask, and protective eyewear, based on the type of exposure anticipated and category of isolation precautions.	
____	____	____	a. Put on the gown, with the opening in the back. Tie gown securely at neck and waist.	
____	____	____	b. Put on the mask or respirator over your nose, mouth, and chin. Secure ties or elastic bands at the middle of the head and neck. If respirator is used, perform a fit check. Inhale; the respirator should collapse. Exhale; air should not leak out.	
____	____	____	c. Put on goggles. Place over eyes and adjust to fit. Alternately, a face shield could be used to take the place of the mask and goggles.	
____	____	____	d. Put on clean disposable gloves. Extend gloves to cover wrists of gown.	
____	____	____	6. Remove PPE: Except for respirator, remove PPE at the doorway or in anteroom. Remove respirator after leaving the patient room and closing door.	
____	____	____	a. If impervious gown has been tied in front of the body at the waistline, untie waist strings before removing gloves.	
____	____	____	b. Grasp the outside of one glove with the opposite gloved hand and peel off, turning the glove inside out as you pull it off. Hold the removed glove in the remaining gloved hand.	
____	____	____	c. Slide fingers of ungloved hand under the remaining glove at the wrist, taking care not to touch the outer surface of the glove.	

Excellent	Satisfactory	Needs Practice	SKILL 4-7 **Using Personal Protective Equipment** *(Continued)*	
				Comments

Excellent	Satisfactory	Needs Practice		Comments
___	___	___	d. Peel off the glove over the first glove, containing the one glove inside the other. Discard in appropriate container.	
___	___	___	e. To remove the goggles: Handle by the headband or earpieces. Lift away from the face. Place in designated receptacle for reprocessing or in an appropriate waste container.	
___	___	___	f. To remove gown: Unfasten ties, if at the neck and back. Allow the gown to fall away from shoulders. Touching only the inside of the gown, pull away from the torso. Keeping hands on the inner surface of the gown, pull from arms. Turn gown inside out. Fold or roll into a bundle and discard.	
___	___	___	g. To remove mask or respirator: Grasp the neck ties or elastic, then top ties or elastic and remove. Take care to avoid touching front of mask or respirator. Discard in waste container. If using a respirator, save for future use in the designated area.	
___	___	___	7. Perform hand hygiene immediately after removing all PPE.	

Skill Checklists to Accompany Taylor's Clinical Nursing Skills:
A Nursing Process Approach, 2nd edition

Name _____ Date _____

Unit _____ Position _____

Instructor/Evaluator: _____ Position _____

Excellent	Satisfactory	Needs Practice	SKILL 5-1 **Administering Oral Medications**	Comments
			Goal: The patient will swallow the medication.	
___	___	___	1. Gather equipment. Check each medication order against the original physician's order according to agency policy. Clarify any inconsistencies. Check the patient's chart for allergies.	
___	___	___	2. Know the actions, special nursing considerations, safe dose ranges, purpose of administration, and adverse effects of the medications to be administered. Consider the appropriateness of the medication for this patient.	
___	___	___	3. Perform hand hygiene.	
___	___	___	4. Move the medication cart to the outside of the patient's room or prepare for administration in the medication area.	
___	___	___	5. Unlock the medication cart or drawer. Enter pass code and scan employee identification, if required.	
___	___	___	6. **Prepare medications for one patient at a time.**	
___	___	___	7. Read the MAR and select the proper medication from the patient's medication drawer or unit stock.	
___	___	___	8. Compare the label with the MAR. Check expiration dates and perform calculations, if necessary. Scan the bar code on the package, if required.	
___	___	___	9. Prepare the required medications:	
___	___	___	a. *Unit dose packages:* Place unit dose-packaged medications in a disposable cup. **Do not open wrapper until at the bedside.** Keep narcotics and medications that require special nursing assessments in a separate container.	
___	___	___	b. *Multidose containers:* When removing tablets or capsules from a multidose bottle, pour the necessary number into the bottle cap and then place the tablets in a medication cup. Break only scored tablets, if necessary, to obtain the proper dosage. Do not touch tablets with hands.	

Excellent	Satisfactory	Needs Practice		Comments
			SKILL 5-1 **Administering Oral Medications** *(Continued)*	

Excellent	Satisfactory	Needs Practice		Comments
___	___	___	c. *Liquid medication in multidose bottle:* When pouring liquid medications in a multidose bottle, hold the bottle so the label is against the palm. Use the appropriate measuring device when pouring liquids, and read the amount of medication at the bottom of the meniscus at eye level. Wipe the lip of the bottle with a paper towel.	
___	___	___	10. **When all medications for one patient have been prepared, recheck the label with the MAR before taking them to the patient. Replace any multidose containers in the patient's drawer or unit stock. Lock the medication cart before leaving it.**	
___	___	___	11. Transport medications to the patient's bedside carefully, and keep the medications in sight at all times.	
___	___	___	12. **Ensure that the patient receives the medications at the correct time.**	
___	___	___	13. **Identify the patient.** Usually, the patient should be identified using two methods. Compare information with the MAR or CMAR.	
___	___	___	a. Check the name and identification number on the patient's identification band.	
___	___	___	b. Ask the patient to state his or her name.	
___	___	___	c. If the patient cannot identify him or herself, verify the patient's identification with a staff member who knows the patient for the second source.	
___	___	___	14. **Complete necessary assessments before administering medications. Check allergy bracelet or ask patient about allergies. Explain the purpose and action of each medication to the patient.**	
___	___	___	15. Scan the patient's bar code on the identification band, if required.	
___	___	___	16. Assist the patient to an upright or lateral position.	
___	___	___	17. Administer medications:	
___	___	___	a. Offer water or other permitted fluids with pills, capsules, tablets, and some liquid medications.	
___	___	___	b. Ask whether the patient prefers to take the medications by hand or in a cup.	
___	___	___	18. **Remain with the patient until each medication is swallowed. Never leave medication at the patient's bedside.**	

Excellent	Satisfactory	Needs Practice	SKILL 5-1 **Administering Oral Medications** *(Continued)*	Comments
___	___	___	19. Perform hand hygiene. Leave the patient in a comfortable position.	
___	___	___	20. Check on the patient within 30 minutes, or time appropriate for drug(s), to verify response to medication.	

Skill Checklists to Accompany Taylor's Clinical Nursing Skills:
A Nursing Process Approach, 2nd edition

Name _____ Date _____

Unit _____ Position _____

Instructor/Evaluator: _____ Position _____

Excellent	Satisfactory	Needs Practice	SKILL 5-2 **Removing Medication From an Ampule**	Comments
			Goal: The medication will be removed in a sterile manner, be free from glass shards, and be prepared in the proper dose.	
——	——	——	1. Gather equipment. Check the medication order against the original physician's order according to agency policy. Clarify any inconsistencies. Check the patient's chart for allergies.	
——	——	——	2. Know the actions, special nursing considerations, safe dose ranges, purpose of administration, and adverse effects of the medications to be administered. Consider the appropriateness of the medication for this patient.	
——	——	——	3. Perform hand hygiene.	
——	——	——	4. Move the medication cart to the outside of the patient's room or prepare for administration in the medication area.	
——	——	——	5. Unlock the medication cart or drawer. Enter pass code and scan employee identification, if required.	
——	——	——	6. **Prepare medications for one patient at a time.**	
——	——	——	7. Read the MAR and select the proper medication from the patient's medication drawer or unit stock.	
——	——	——	8. Compare the label with the MAR. Check expiration dates and perform calculations, if necessary. Scan the bar code on the package, if required.	
——	——	——	9. Tap the stem of the ampule or twist your wrist quickly while holding the ampule vertically.	
——	——	——	10. **Wrap a small gauze pad around the neck of the ampule.**	
——	——	——	11. Use a snapping motion to break off the top of the ampule along the scored line at its neck. Always break away from your body.	
——	——	——	12. Attach filter needle to syringe. **Remove the cap from the filter needle by pulling it straight off. Insert the filter needle into the ampule, being careful not to touch the rim.**	
——	——	——	13. Withdraw medication in the amount ordered plus a small amount more (approximately 30%). **Do not inject air into the solution.** Use either of the following methods:	

			SKILL 5-2

SKILL 5-2
Removing Medication From an Ampule *(Continued)*

Excellent	Satisfactory	Needs Practice		Comments
——	——	——	a. Insert the tip of the needle into the ampule, which is upright on a flat surface, and withdraw fluid into the syringe. **Touch plunger at knob only.**	
——	——	——	b. Insert the tip of the needle into the ampule and invert the ampule. Keep the needle centered and not touching the sides of the ampule. Withdraw fluid into syringe. **Touch plunger at knob only.**	
——	——	——	14. **Wait until the needle has been withdrawn to tap the syringe and expel the air carefully by pushing on the plunger. Check the amount of medication in the syringe with the medication dose and discard any surplus according to facility policy.**	
——	——	——	15. **Recheck the label with the MAR.**	
——	——	——	16. Engage safety guard on filter needle and remove. Discard the filter needle in a suitable container. Attach appropriate administration device to syringe.	
——	——	——	17. Discard the ampule in a suitable container.	
——	——	——	18. Lock the medication cart before leaving it.	
——	——	——	19. Perform hand hygiene.	
——	——	——	20. Proceed with administration, based on prescribed route.	

Skill Checklists to Accompany Taylor's Clinical Nursing Skills:
A Nursing Process Approach, 2nd edition

Name _____ Date _____

Unit _____ Position _____

Instructor/Evaluator: _____ Position _____

SKILL 5-3
Removing Medication From a Vial

Excellent	Satisfactory	Needs Practice		Comments

Goal: Withdrawal of the medication into a syringe in a sterile manner with the proper dose prepared.

Excellent	Satisfactory	Needs Practice		Comments
——	——	——	1. Gather equipment. Check the medication order against the original physician's order according to agency policy.	
——	——	——	2. Know the actions, special nursing considerations, safe dose ranges, purpose of administration, and adverse effects of the medications to be administered. Consider the appropriateness of the medication for this patient.	
——	——	——	3. Perform hand hygiene.	
——	——	——	4. Move the medication cart to the outside of the patient's room or prepare for administration in the medication area.	
——	——	——	5. Unlock the medication cart or drawer. Enter pass code and scan employee identification, if required.	
——	——	——	6. **Prepare medications for one patient at a time.**	
——	——	——	7. Read the MAR and select the proper medication from the patient's medication drawer or unit stock.	
——	——	——	8. Compare the label with the MAR. Check expiration dates and perform calculations, if necessary. Scan the bar code on the package, if required.	
——	——	——	9. Remove the metal or plastic cap on the vial that protects the rubber stopper.	
——	——	——	10. **Swab the rubber top with the antimicrobial swab and allow to dry.**	
——	——	——	11. Remove the cap from the needle or blunt cannula by pulling it straight off. Touch the plunger at the knob only. Draw back an amount of air into the syringe that is equal to the specific dose of medication to be withdrawn. Some agencies recommend use of a filter needle when withdrawing premixed medication from multidose vials.	
——	——	——	12. Hold the vial on a flat surface. Pierce the rubber stopper in the center with the needle tip and inject the measured air into the space above the solution. Do not inject air into the solution.	
——	——	——	13. **Invert the vial. Keep the tip of the needle or blunt cannula below the fluid level.**	

Excellent	Satisfactory	Needs Practice	SKILL 5-3 **Removing Medication From a Vial** *(Continued)*	Comments
——	——	——	14. Hold the vial in one hand and use the other to withdraw the medication. Touch the plunger at the knob only. **Draw up the prescribed amount of medication while holding the syringe vertically and at eye level.**	
——	——	——	15. If any air bubbles accumulate in the syringe, tap the barrel of the syringe sharply and move the needle past the fluid into the air space to reinject the air bubble into the vial. Return the needle tip to the solution and continue withdrawal of the medication.	
——	——	——	16. After the correct dose is withdrawn, remove the needle from the vial and carefully replace the cap over the needle. If a filter needle has been used to draw up the medication, remove it and attach the appropriate administration device. Some agencies recommend changing the needle, if one was used to withdraw the medication, before administering the medication.	
——	——	——	17. **Check the amount of medication in the syringe with the medication dose and discard any surplus.**	
——	——	——	18. **Recheck the label with the MAR.**	
——	——	——	19. **If a multidose vial is being used, label the vial with the date and time opened, and store the vial containing the remaining medication according to agency policy.**	
——	——	——	20. Lock the medication cart before leaving it.	
——	——	——	21. Perform hand hygiene.	
——	——	——	22. Proceed with administration, based on prescribed route.	

Skill Checklists to Accompany Taylor's Clinical Nursing Skills:
A Nursing Process Approach, 2nd edition

Name _____   Date _____

Unit _____   Position _____

Instructor/Evaluator: _____   Position _____

Excellent	Satisfactory	Needs Practice	SKILL 5-4 **Mixing Medications From Two Vials in One Syringe**	Comments
			Goal: The accurate withdrawal of the medication into a syringe in a sterile manner with the proper dose prepared.	
____	____	____	1. Gather equipment. Check medication order against the original physician's order according to agency policy.	
____	____	____	2. Know the actions, special nursing considerations, safe dose ranges, purpose of administration, and adverse effects of the medications to be administered. Consider the appropriateness of the medication for this patient.	
____	____	____	3. Perform hand hygiene.	
____	____	____	4. Move the medication cart to the outside of the patient's room or prepare for administration in the medication area.	
____	____	____	5. Unlock the medication cart or drawer. Enter pass code and scan employee identification, if required.	
____	____	____	6. **Prepare medications for one patient at a time.**	
____	____	____	7. Read the MAR and select the proper medications from the patient's medication drawer or unit stock.	
____	____	____	8. Compare the labels with the MAR. Check expiration dates and perform calculations, if necessary. Scan the bar code on the package, if required.	
____	____	____	9. If necessary, remove the cap that protects the rubber stopper on each vial.	
____	____	____	10. **If insulin is a suspension (eg, NPH, Lente), roll and agitate the vial to mix it well.**	
____	____	____	11. Cleanse the rubber tops with antimicrobial swabs.	
____	____	____	12. Remove cap from needle by pulling it straight off. Touch the plunger at the knob only. Draw back an amount of air into the syringe that is equal to the dose of modified insulin to be withdrawn.	
____	____	____	13. Hold the modified vial on a flat surface. Pierce the rubber stopper in the center with the needle tip and inject the measured air into the space above the solution. Do not inject air into the solution. Withdraw the needle.	
____	____	____	14. Draw back an amount of air into the syringe that is equal to the dose of unmodified insulin to be withdrawn.	

Mixing Medications From Two Vials in One Syringe *(Continued)*

Excellent	Satisfactory	Needs Practice		Comments
——	——	——	15. Hold the unmodified vial on a flat surface. Pierce the rubber stopper in the center with the needle tip and inject the measured air into the space above the solution. Do not inject air into the solution. Keep the needle in the vial.	
——	——	——	16. Invert vial of unmodified insulin. Hold the vial in one hand and use the other to withdraw the medication. Touch the plunger at the knob only. **Draw up the prescribed amount of medication while holding the syringe at eye level and vertically.** Turn the vial over and then remove needle from vial.	
——	——	——	17. Check that there are no air bubbles in the syringe.	
——	——	——	18. **Check the amount of medication in the syringe with the medication dose and discard any surplus.**	
——	——	——	19. **Recheck the vial label with the MAR.**	
——	——	——	20. Calculate the endpoint on the syringe for the combined insulin amount by adding the number of units for each dose together.	
——	——	——	21. Insert the needle into the modified vial and invert it, taking care not to push the plunger and inject medication from the syringe into the vial. Invert vial of modified insulin. Hold the vial in one hand and use the other to withdraw the medication. Touch the plunger at the knob only. **Draw up the prescribed amount of medication while holding the syringe at eye level and vertically. Take care to only withdraw the prescribed amount.** Turn the vial over and then remove needle from vial. Carefully recap the needle. Carefully replace the cap over the needle.	
——	——	——	22. **Check the amount of medication in the syringe with the medication dose.**	
——	——	——	23. **Recheck the vial label with the MAR.**	
——	——	——	24. **Label the vials with the date and time opened, and store the vials containing the remaining medication according to agency policy.**	
——	——	——	25. Lock medication cart before leaving it.	
——	——	——	26. Perform hand hygiene.	
——	——	——	27. Proceed with administration, based on prescribed route.	

Name _____   Date _____

Unit _____   Position _____

Instructor/Evaluator: _____   Position _____

Excellent	Satisfactory	Needs Practice	SKILL 5-5 **Administering an Intradermal Injection**	Comments
			Goal: Appearance of a wheal at the site of injection.	
——	——	——	1. Gather equipment. Check each medication order against the original physician's order according to agency policy. Clarify any inconsistencies. Check the patient's chart for allergies.	
——	——	——	2. Know the actions, special nursing considerations, safe dose ranges, purpose of administration, and adverse effects of the medications to be administered. Consider the appropriateness of the medication for this patient.	
——	——	——	3. Perform hand hygiene.	
——	——	——	4. Move the medication cart to the outside of the patient's room or prepare for administration in the medication area.	
——	——	——	5. Unlock the medication cart or drawer. Enter pass code and scan employee identification, if required.	
——	——	——	6. **Prepare medications for one patient at a time.**	
——	——	——	7. Read the MAR and select the proper medication from the patient's medication drawer or unit stock.	
——	——	——	8. Compare the label with the MAR. Check expiration dates and perform calculations, if necessary. Scan the bar code on the package, if required.	
——	——	——	9. If necessary, withdraw medication from an ampule or vial as described in Skills 5-2 and 5-3.	
——	——	——	10. **When all medications for one patient have been prepared, recheck the label with the MAR before taking them to the patient.**	
——	——	——	11. Lock the medication cart before leaving it.	
——	——	——	12. Transport medications to the patient's bedside carefully, and keep the medications in sight at all times.	
——	——	——	13. **Ensure that the patient receives the medications at the correct time.**	
——	——	——	14. **Identify the patient.** Usually, the patient should be identified using two methods. Compare information with the MAR or CMAR.	
——	——	——	a. Check the name and identification number on the patient's identification band.	

Excellent	Satisfactory	Needs Practice	SKILL 5-5 **Administering an Intradermal Injection** *(Continued)*	
				Comments
—— —— ——			b. Ask the patient to state his or her name.	
—— —— ——			c. If the patient cannot identify him or herself, verify the patient's identification with a staff member who knows the patient for the second source.	
—— —— ——			15. Close the door to the room or pull the bedside curtain.	
—— —— ——			16. Complete necessary assessments before administering medications. Check allergy bracelet or ask patient about allergies. Explain the purpose and action of the medication to the patient.	
—— —— ——			17. Scan the patient's bar code on the identification band, if required.	
—— —— ——			18. Perform hand hygiene and put on clean gloves.	
—— —— ——			19. Select an appropriate administration site. Assist the patient to the appropriate position for the site chosen. Drape as needed to expose only area of site to be used.	
—— —— ——			20. Cleanse the site with an antimicrobial swab while wiping with a firm, circular motion and moving outward from the injection site. Allow the skin to dry.	
—— —— ——			21. Remove the needle cap with the nondominant hand by pulling it straight off.	
—— —— ——			22. Use the nondominant hand to spread the skin taut over the injection site.	
—— —— ——			23. Hold the syringe in the dominant hand, between the thumb and forefinger with the bevel of the needle up.	
—— —— ——			24. Hold the syringe at a 10-to-15 degree angle from the site. **Place the needle almost flat against the patient's skin, bevel side up, and insert the needle into the skin so that the point of the needle can be seen through the skin. Insert the needle only about 1/8″ with entire bevel under the skin.**	
—— —— ——			25. Once the needle is in place, steady the lower end of the syringe. Slide your dominant hand to the end of the plunger.	
—— —— ——			26. Slowly inject the agent while watching for a small wheal or blister to appear.	
—— —— ——			27. Withdraw the needle quickly at the same angle that it was inserted.	
—— —— ——			28. **Do not massage area after removing needle. Tell patient not to rub or scratch site. If necessary, gently blot the site with a dry gauze square. Do not apply pressure or rub the site.**	

SKILL 5-5

Administering an Intradermal Injection *(Continued)*

Excellent	Satisfactory	Needs Practice		Comments
——	——	——	29. Do not recap the used needle. Engage the safety shield or needle guard, if present. Discard the needle and syringe in the appropriate receptacle.	
——	——	——	30. Assist the patient to a position of comfort.	
——	——	——	31. Remove gloves and dispose of them properly. Perform hand hygiene.	
——	——	——	32. Observe the area for signs of a reaction at determined intervals after administration. Inform the patient of the need for inspection.	

Skill Checklists to Accompany Taylor's Clinical Nursing Skills:
A Nursing Process Approach, 2nd edition

Name _____ Date _____

Unit _____ Position _____

Instructor/Evaluator: _____ Position _____

Excellent	Satisfactory	Needs Practice	SKILL 5-6 **Administering a Subcutaneous Injection**	Comments
			Goal: The patient receives medication via the subcutaneous route.	
——	——	——	1. Gather equipment. Check each medication order against the original physician's order according to agency policy. Clarify any inconsistencies. Check the patient's chart for allergies.	
——	——	——	2. Know the actions, special nursing considerations, safe dose ranges, purpose of administration, and adverse effects of the medications to be administered. Consider the appropriateness of the medication for this patient.	
——	——	——	3. Perform hand hygiene.	
——	——	——	4. Move the medication cart to the outside of the patient's room or prepare for administration in the medication area.	
——	——	——	5. Unlock the medication cart or drawer. Enter pass code and scan employee identification, if required.	
——	——	——	6. **Prepare medications for one patient at a time.**	
——	——	——	7. Read the MAR and select the proper medication from the patient's medication drawer or unit stock.	
——	——	——	8. Compare the label with the MAR. Check expiration dates and perform calculations, if necessary. Scan the bar code on the package, if required.	
——	——	——	9. If necessary, withdraw medication from an ampule or vial as described in Skills 5-2 and 5-3.	
——	——	——	10. **When all medications for one patient have been prepared, recheck the label with the MAR before taking them to the patient.**	
——	——	——	11. Lock the medication cart before leaving it.	
——	——	——	12. Transport medications to the patient's bedside carefully, and keep the medications in sight at all times.	
——	——	——	13. **Ensure that the patient receives the medications at the correct time.**	
——	——	——	14. **Identify the patient.** Usually, the patient should be identified using two methods. Compare information with the MAR or CMAR.	

Excellent	Satisfactory	Needs Practice	SKILL 5-6 **Administering a Subcutaneous Injection** *(Continued)*	Comments
——	——	——	a. Check the name and identification number on the patient's identification band.	
——	——	——	b. Ask the patient to state his or her name.	
——	——	——	c. If the patient cannot identify him or herself, verify the patient's identification with a staff member who knows the patient for the second source.	
——	——	——	15. Close the door to the room or pull the bedside curtain.	
——	——	——	16. Complete necessary assessments before administering medications. Check allergy bracelet or ask patient about allergies. Explain the purpose and action of the medication to the patient.	
——	——	——	17. Scan the patient's bar code on the identification band, if required.	
——	——	——	18. Perform hand hygiene and put on clean gloves.	
——	——	——	19. Select an appropriate administration site.	
——	——	——	20. Assist the patient to the appropriate position for the site chosen. Drape as needed to expose only area of site to be used.	
——	——	——	21. Identify the appropriate landmarks for the site chosen.	
——	——	——	22. Clean the area around the injection site with an antimicrobial swab. Use a firm, circular motion while moving outward from the injection site. Allow area to dry.	
——	——	——	23. Remove the needle cap with the nondominant hand, pulling it straight off.	
——	——	——	24. Grasp and bunch the area surrounding the injection site or spread the skin taut at the site.	
——	——	——	25. **Hold the syringe in the dominant hand between the thumb and forefinger. Inject the needle quickly at a 45–90 degree angle.**	
——	——	——	26. After the needle is in place, release the tissue. If you have a large skin fold pinched up, ensure that the needle stays in place as the skin is released. Immediately move your nondominant hand to steady the lower end of the syringe. Slide your dominant hand to the end of the plunger. Avoid moving the syringe.	
——	——	——	27. Inject the medication slowly (at a rate of 10 seconds per milliliter).	
——	——	——	28. Withdraw the needle quickly at the same angle at which it was inserted, while supporting the surrounding tissue with your nondominant hand.	

Administering a Subcutaneous Injection *(Continued)*

Excellent	Satisfactory	Needs Practice		Comments
——	——	——	29. Using a gauze square, apply gentle pressure to the site after the needle is withdrawn. Do not massage the site.	
——	——	——	30. Do not recap the used needle. Engage the safety shield or needle guard, if present. Discard the needle and syringe in the appropriate receptacle.	
——	——	——	31. Assist the patient to a position of comfort.	
——	——	——	32. Remove gloves and dispose of them properly. Perform hand hygiene.	
——	——	——	33. Evaluate the response of the patient to the medication within an appropriate time frame for the particular medication.	

Skill Checklists to Accompany Taylor's Clinical Nursing Skills:
A Nursing Process Approach, 2nd edition

Name _____   Date _____

Unit _____   Position _____

Instructor/Evaluator: _____   Position _____

SKILL 5-7

Administering an Intramuscular Injection

Goal: The patient receives the medication via the intramuscular route.

Excellent	Satisfactory	Needs Practice		Comments
⎯⎯	⎯⎯	⎯⎯	1. Gather equipment. Check each medication order against the original physician's order according to agency policy. Clarify any inconsistencies. Check the patient's chart for allergies.	
⎯⎯	⎯⎯	⎯⎯	2. Know the actions, special nursing considerations, safe dose ranges, purpose of administration, and adverse effects of the medications to be administered. Consider the appropriateness of the medication for this patient.	
⎯⎯	⎯⎯	⎯⎯	3. Perform hand hygiene.	
⎯⎯	⎯⎯	⎯⎯	4. Move the medication cart to the outside of the patient's room or prepare for administration in the medication area.	
⎯⎯	⎯⎯	⎯⎯	5. Unlock the medication cart or drawer. Enter pass code and scan employee identification, if required.	
⎯⎯	⎯⎯	⎯⎯	6. **Prepare medications for one patient at a time.**	
⎯⎯	⎯⎯	⎯⎯	7. Read the MAR and select the proper medication from the patient's medication drawer or unit stock.	
⎯⎯	⎯⎯	⎯⎯	8. Compare the label with the MAR. Check expiration dates and perform calculations, if necessary. Scan the bar code on the package, if required.	
⎯⎯	⎯⎯	⎯⎯	9. If necessary, withdraw medication from an ampule or vial as described in Skills 5-2 and 5-3.	
⎯⎯	⎯⎯	⎯⎯	10. **When all medications for one patient have been prepared, recheck the label with the MAR before taking them to the patient.**	
⎯⎯	⎯⎯	⎯⎯	11. Lock the medication cart before leaving it.	
⎯⎯	⎯⎯	⎯⎯	12. Transport medications to the patient's bedside carefully, and keep the medications in sight at all times.	
⎯⎯	⎯⎯	⎯⎯	13. **Ensure that the patient receives the medications at the correct time.**	
⎯⎯	⎯⎯	⎯⎯	14. **Identify the patient.** Usually, the patient should be identified using two methods. Compare information with the MAR or CMAR.	

Excellent	Satisfactory	Needs Practice		Comments
——	——	——	a. Check the name and identification number on the patient's identification band.	
——	——	——	b. Ask the patient to state his or her name.	
——	——	——	c. If the patient cannot identify him or herself, verify the patient's identification with a staff member who knows the patient for the second source.	
——	——	——	15. Close the door to the room or pull the bedside curtain.	
——	——	——	16. Complete necessary assessments before administering medications. Check allergy bracelet or ask patient about allergies. Explain the purpose and action of the medication to the patient.	
——	——	——	17. Scan the patient's bar code on the identification band, if required.	
——	——	——	18. Perform hand hygiene and put on clean gloves.	
——	——	——	19. Select an appropriate administration site.	
——	——	——	20. Assist the patient to the appropriate position for the site chosen. Drape as needed to expose only area of site to be used.	
——	——	——	21. **Identify the appropriate landmarks for the site chosen.**	
——	——	——	22. Clean the area around the injection site with an antimicrobial swab. Use a firm, circular motion while moving outward from the injection site. Allow area to dry.	
——	——	——	23. Remove the needle cap by pulling it straight off. Hold the syringe in your dominant hand between the thumb and forefinger.	
——	——	——	24. Displace the skin in a Z-track manner by pulling the skin down or to one side about 1″ (2.5 cm) with your nondominant hand and hold the skin and tissue in this position.	
——	——	——	25. Quickly dart the needle into the tissue so that the needle is perpendicular to the patient's body. This should ensure that it is given using an angle of injection between 72 to 90 degrees.	
——	——	——	26. As soon as the needle is in place, use your thumb and forefinger of your nondominant hand to hold the lower end of the syringe. Slide your dominant hand to the end of the plunger.	
——	——	——	27. **Aspirate by slowly (for at least 5 seconds) pulling back on the plunger to determine whether the needle is in a blood vessel. Watch for a flash of pink or red in the syringe.**	

Excellent	Satisfactory	Needs Practice	SKILL 5-7 **Administering a Subcutaneous Injection** *(Continued)*	
				Comments
⎯	⎯	⎯	28. If no blood is aspirated, inject the solution slowly (10 seconds per milliliter of medication).	
⎯	⎯	⎯	29. Once the medication has been instilled, wait 10 seconds before withdrawing the needle.	
⎯	⎯	⎯	30. Withdraw the needle smoothly and steadily at the same angle at which it was inserted, supporting tissue around the injection site with your nondominant hand.	
⎯	⎯	⎯	31. **Apply gentle pressure at the site with a dry gauze.**	
⎯	⎯	⎯	32. Do not recap the used needle. Engage the safety shield or needle guard, if present. Discard the needle and syringe in the appropriate receptacle.	
⎯	⎯	⎯	33. Assist the patient to a position of comfort.	
⎯	⎯	⎯	34. Remove gloves and dispose of them properly. Perform hand hygiene.	
⎯	⎯	⎯	35. Evaluate patient's response to medication within an appropriate time frame. Assess site, if possible, within 2 to 4 hours after administration.	

Skill Checklists to Accompany Taylor's Clinical Nursing Skills:
A Nursing Process Approach, 2nd edition

Name _____   Date _____

Unit _____   Position _____

Instructor/Evaluator: _____   Position _____

Excellent	Satisfactory	Needs Practice	SKILL 5-8 **Administering Continuous Subcutaneous Infusion: Applying an Insulin Pump**	Comments
			Goal: The device is applied successfully and medication is administered.	
___	___	___	1. Gather equipment. Check each medication order against the original physician's order according to agency policy. Clarify any inconsistencies. Check the patient's chart for allergies.	
___	___	___	2. Know the actions, special nursing considerations, safe dose ranges, purpose of administration, and adverse effects of the medications to be administered. Consider the appropriateness of the medication for this patient.	
___	___	___	3. Perform hand hygiene.	
___	___	___	4. Move the medication cart to the outside of the patient's room or prepare for administration in the medication area.	
___	___	___	5. Unlock the medication cart or drawer. Enter pass code and scan employee identification, if required.	
___	___	___	6. **Prepare medications for one patient at a time.**	
___	___	___	7. Read the MAR and select the proper medication from the patient's medication drawer or unit stock.	
___	___	___	8. Compare the label with the MAR. Check expiration dates and perform calculations, if necessary. Scan the bar code on the package, if required.	
___	___	___	9. Attach blunt-ended needle or small-gauge needle to syringe. Follow Skill 5-3 to remove insulin from vial. Remove enough insulin to last patient 2 to 3 days, plus 30 units for priming tubing.	
___	___	___	10. **When all medications for one patient have been prepared, recheck the label with the MAR before taking them to the patient.**	
___	___	___	11. Lock the medication cart before leaving it.	
___	___	___	12. Transport medications to the patient's bedside carefully, and keep the medications in sight at all times.	
___	___	___	13. **Ensure that the patient receives the medications at the correct time.**	
___	___	___	14. **Identify the patient.** Usually, the patient should be identified using two methods. Compare information with the MAR or CMAR.	

62

Excellent	Satisfactory	Needs Practice		Comments

Administering Continuous Subcutaneous Infusion: Applying an Insulin Pump *(Continued)*

Excellent	Satisfactory	Needs Practice		Comments
——	——	——	a. Check the name and identification number on the patient's identification band.	
——	——	——	b. Ask the patient to state his or her name.	
——	——	——	c. If the patient cannot identify him or herself, verify the patient's identification with a staff member who knows the patient.	
——	——	——	15. Close the door to the room or pull the bedside curtain.	
——	——	——	16. Complete necessary assessments before administering medications. Check allergy bracelet or ask patient about allergies. Explain the purpose and action of the medication to the patient.	
——	——	——	17. Scan the patient's bar code on the identification band, if required.	
——	——	——	18. Perform hand hygiene.	
——	——	——	19. Attach sterile tubing to syringe. Prime the tubing by pushing the plunger of syringe until insulin is coming from introducer needle. **Check for any bubbles in tubing.**	
——	——	——	20. Program pump according to manufacturer's recommendations following physician's orders. Open pump and place syringe in compartment according to manufacturer's directions. Close pump.	
——	——	——	21. Activate delivery device. Place needle between prongs of insertion device with sharp edge facing out. Push insertion set down until click is heard.	
——	——	——	22. Put on clean gloves.	
——	——	——	23. Select an appropriate administration site.	
——	——	——	24. Assist the patient to the appropriate position for the site chosen. Drape as needed to expose only area of site to be used.	
——	——	——	25. Identify the appropriate landmarks for the site chosen.	
——	——	——	26. Clean area around injection site with antimicrobial swab. Use a firm, circular motion while moving outward from insertion site. Allow antiseptic to dry.	
——	——	——	27. Remove paper from adhesive backing. Remove needle guard. Pinch skin at insertion site, press insertion device on site, and press release button to insert needle. Remove triggering device.	
——	——	——	28. **While holding needle hub, turn it a quarter-turn and remove needle.** Do not recap the used needle. Engage the safety shield or needle guard, if present.	

Copyright © 2008 by Lippincott Williams & Wilkins. *Skill Checklists to Accompany Taylor's Clinical Nursing Skills: A Nursing Process Approach*, 2nd edition, by Pamela Lynn and Marilee LeBon.

SKILL 5-8

Administering Continuous Subcutaneous Infusion: Applying an Insulin Pump *(Continued)*

Excellent	Satisfactory	Needs Practice		Comments
——	——	——	29. Apply sterile occlusive dressing over insertion site. Attach the pump to patient's clothing.	
——	——	——	30. Discard the needle and syringe in the appropriate receptacle.	
——	——	——	31. Assist the patient to a position of comfort.	
——	——	——	32. Remove gloves and dispose of them properly. Perform hand hygiene.	
——	——	——	33. Evaluate patient's response to medication within appropriate time frame. Monitor the patient's blood glucose levels as appropriate or as ordered.	

64

Skill Checklists to Accompany Taylor's Clinical Nursing Skills: A Nursing Process Approach, 2nd edition

Name _____   Date _____

Unit _____   Position _____

Instructor/Evaluator: _____   Position _____

Excellent	Satisfactory	Needs Practice	SKILL 5-9 **Adding Medications to an Intravenous (IV) Solution Container**	Comments
			Goal: The medication is added to an adequate amount of compatible solution and mixed appropriately.	
——	——	——	1. Gather equipment. Check medication order against the original physician's order according to agency policy. Clarify any inconsistencies. Check the patient's chart for allergies. Verify the compatibility of the medication and IV fluid. Calculate the infusion rate.	
——	——	——	2. Know the actions, special nursing considerations, safe dose ranges, purpose of administration, and adverse effects of the medications to be administered. Consider the appropriateness of the medication for this patient.	
——	——	——	3. Perform hand hygiene.	
——	——	——	4. Move the medication cart to the outside of the patient's room or prepare for administration in the medication area.	
——	——	——	5. Unlock the medication cart or drawer. Enter pass code and scan employee identification, if required.	
——	——	——	6. **Prepare medication for one patient at a time.**	
——	——	——	7. Read the MAR and select the proper medication from the patient's medication drawer or unit stock.	
——	——	——	8. Compare the label with the MAR. Check expiration dates and perform calculations, if necessary. Scan the bar code on the package, if required.	
——	——	——	9. If necessary, withdraw medication from an ampule or vial as described in Skills 5-2 and 5-3.	
——	——	——	10. **Recheck the label with the MAR before taking it to the patient.**	
——	——	——	11. Lock the medication cart before leaving it.	
——	——	——	12. Transport medications and equipment to the patient's bedside carefully, and keep the medications in sight at all times.	
——	——	——	13. Perform hand hygiene.	
——	——	——	14. **Identify the patient.** Usually, the patient should be identified using two methods. Compare information with the MAR or CMAR.	

Adding Medications to an Intravenous (IV) Solution Container *(Continued)*

Excellent	Satisfactory	Needs Practice		Comments
___	___	___	a. Check the name and identification number on the patient's identification band.	
___	___	___	b. Ask the patient to state his or her name.	
___	___	___	c. If the patient cannot identify him or herself, verify the patient's identification with a staff member who knows the patient for the second source.	
___	___	___	15. Close the door to the room or pull the bedside curtain.	
___	___	___	16. Complete necessary assessments before administering medications. Check allergy bracelet or ask patient about allergies. Explain the purpose and action of the medication to the patient.	
___	___	___	17. Scan the patient's bar code on the identification band, if required.	
___	___	___	18. **Check that the volume in the current IV infusion is adequate.**	
___	___	___	19. Close the clamp between the solution container and roller clamp on the infusion tubing and pause the IV pump, if appropriate.	
___	___	___	20. Clean the medication port with an antimicrobial swab.	
___	___	___	21. Steady the container and uncap the needle or needleless device. Insert it into the port. Inject the medication. Withdraw the needle or needleless device. Do not recap the used needle. Engage the safety shield or needle guard, if present.	
___	___	___	22. Remove the container from the IV pole and gently rotate the container to mix the medication and solution.	
___	___	___	23. Rehang the container on the pole. **Attach the label to the container so that the dose of medication that has been added is apparent.**	
___	___	___	24. Open the clamp, and readjust the flow rate or check the pump settings for correct infusion rate and restart pump.	
___	___	___	25. Discard the needle and syringe in the appropriate receptacle.	
___	___	___	26. Perform hand hygiene.	
___	___	___	27. Evaluate the patient's response to medication within the appropriate time frame.	

Skill Checklists to Accompany Taylor's Clinical Nursing Skills:
A Nursing Process Approach, 2nd edition

Name _____   Date _____

Unit _____   Position _____

Instructor/Evaluator: _____   Position _____

Excellent	Satisfactory	Needs Practice	SKILL 5-10 **Administering Medications by Intravenous Bolus or Push Through an Intravenous Infusion**	
			Goal: The medication is given safely.	**Comments**
——	——	——	1. Gather equipment. Check medication order against the original physician's order according to agency policy. Clarify any inconsistencies. Check the patient's chart for allergies. Verify the compatibility of the medication and IV fluid. Check a drug resource to clarify whether medication needs to be diluted before administration. Check the infusion rate.	
——	——	——	2. Know the actions, special nursing considerations, safe dose ranges, purpose of administration, and adverse effects of the medications to be administered. Consider the appropriateness of the medication for this patient.	
——	——	——	3. Perform hand hygiene.	
——	——	——	4. Move the medication cart to the outside of the patient's room or prepare for administration in the medication area.	
——	——	——	5. Unlock the medication cart or drawer. Enter pass code and scan employee identification, if required.	
——	——	——	6. **Prepare medication for one patient at a time.**	
——	——	——	7. Read the MAR and select the proper medication from the patient's medication drawer or unit stock.	
——	——	——	8. Compare the label with the MAR. Check expiration dates and perform calculations, if necessary. Scan the bar code on the package, if required.	
——	——	——	9. If necessary, withdraw medication from an ampule or vial as described in Skills 5-2 and 5-3.	
——	——	——	10. **Recheck the label with the MAR before taking it to the patient.**	
——	——	——	11. Lock the medication cart before leaving it.	
——	——	——	12. Transport medications and equipment to the patient's bedside carefully, and keep the medications in sight at all times.	
——	——	——	13. Perform hand hygiene.	
——	——	——	14. **Identify the patient.** Usually, the patient should be identified using two methods. Compare information with the MAR or CMAR.	

Excellent

Satisfactory

Needs Practice

SKILL 5-10

Administering Medications by Intravenous Bolus or Push Through an Intravenous Infusion (Continued)

Comments

Excellent	Satisfactory	Needs Practice		
___	___	___	a. Check the name and identification number on the patient's identification band.	
___	___	___	b. Ask the patient to state his or her name.	
___	___	___	c. If the patient cannot identify him or herself, verify the patient's identification with a staff member who knows the patient for the second source.	
___	___	___	15. Close the door to the room or pull the bedside curtain.	
___	___	___	16. Complete necessary assessments before administering medications. Check allergy bracelet or ask patient about allergies. Explain the purpose and action of the medication to the patient.	
___	___	___	17. Scan the patient's bar code on the identification band, if required.	
___	___	___	18. **Assess IV site for presence of inflammation or infiltration.**	
___	___	___	19. If IV infusion is being administered via an infusion pump, pause the pump.	
___	___	___	20. Put on clean gloves.	
___	___	___	21. Select injection port on tubing that is closest to venipuncture site. Clean port with antimicrobial swab.	
___	___	___	22. Uncap syringe. Steady port with your nondominant hand while inserting syringe, needleless device, or needle into center of port.	
___	___	___	23. Move your nondominant hand to section of IV tubing just above the injection port. Fold tubing between your fingers.	
___	___	___	24. Pull back slightly on plunger just until blood appears in tubing.	
___	___	___	25. **Inject medication at recommended rate.**	
___	___	___	26. Release the tubing. Remove the syringe. Do not recap the used needle. Engage the safety shield or needle guard, if present. Release the tubing and allow the IV fluid to flow. Discard the needle and syringe in the appropriate receptacle.	
___	___	___	27. Check IV fluid infusion rate. Restart infusion pump, if appropriate.	
___	___	___	28. Remove gloves and perform hand hygiene.	
___	___	___	29. Evaluate patient's response to medication within appropriate time frame.	

Skill Checklists to Accompany Taylor's Clinical Nursing Skills:
A Nursing Process Approach, 2nd edition

Name _____   Date _____

Unit _____   Position _____

Instructor/Evaluator: _____   Position _____

Excellent	Satisfactory	Needs Practice	SKILL 5-11 **Administering a Piggyback Intermittent Intravenous Infusion of Medication**	Comments
			Goal: The medication is delivered via the parenteral route using sterile technique.	
——	——	——	1. Gather equipment. Check each medication order against the original physician's order according to agency policy. Clarify any inconsistencies. Check the patient's chart for allergies.	
——	——	——	2. Know the actions, special nursing considerations, safe dose ranges, purpose of administration, and adverse effects of the medications to be administered. Consider the appropriateness of the medication for this patient.	
——	——	——	3. Perform hand hygiene.	
——	——	——	4. Move the medication cart to the outside of the patient's room or prepare for administration in the medication area.	
——	——	——	5. Unlock the medication cart or drawer. Enter pass code and scan employee identification, if required.	
——	——	——	6. **Prepare medications for one patient at a time.**	
——	——	——	7. Read the MAR and select the proper medication from the patient's medication drawer or unit stock.	
——	——	——	8. Compare the label with the MAR. Check expiration dates. Confirm the prescribed or appropriate infusion rate. Calculate the drip rate if using gravity system. Scan the bar code on the package, if required.	
——	——	——	9. **When all medications for one patient have been prepared, recheck the label with the MAR before taking them to the patient.**	
——	——	——	10. Lock the medication cart before leaving it.	
——	——	——	11. Transport medications to the patient's bedside carefully, and keep the medications in sight at all times.	
——	——	——	12. **Ensure that the patient receives the medications at the correct time.**	
——	——	——	13. **Identify the patient.** Usually, the patient should be identified using two methods. Compare information with the MAR or CMAR.	

SKILL 5-11

Administering a Piggyback Intermittent Intravenous Infusion of Medication *(Continued)*

Excellent	Satisfactory	Needs Practice		Comments
___	___	___	a. Check the name and identification number on the patient's identification band.	
___	___	___	b. Ask the patient to state his or her name.	
___	___	___	c. If the patient cannot identify him or herself, verify the patient's identification with a staff member who knows the patient for the second source.	
___	___	___	14. Close the door to the room or pull the bedside curtain.	
___	___	___	15. Perform hand hygiene.	
___	___	___	16. Complete necessary assessments before administering medications. Check allergy bracelet or ask patient about allergies. Explain the purpose and action of the medication to the patient.	
___	___	___	17. Scan the patient's bar code on the identification band, if required.	
___	___	___	18. Assess the IV site for the presence of inflammation or infiltration.	
___	___	___	19. Close the clamp on the short secondary infusion tubing. Using aseptic technique, remove the cap on the tubing spike and the cap on the port of the medication container, taking care to not contaminate either end.	
___	___	___	20. Attach infusion tubing to the medication container by inserting the tubing spike into the port with a firm push and twisting motion, taking care to not contaminate either end.	
___	___	___	21. **Hang piggyback container on IV pole, positioning it higher than primary IV according to manufacturer's recommendations.** Use metal or plastic hook to lower primary IV fluid container.	
___	___	___	22. Place label on tubing with appropriate date.	
___	___	___	23. Squeeze drip chamber and release. Fill to the line or about half full. Open clamp and prime tubing. Close clamp. Place needleless connector or needle on the end of the tubing, using sterile technique, if required.	
___	___	___	24. Use an antimicrobial swab to clean the access port or stopcock above the roller clamp on the primary IV infusion tubing.	
___	___	___	25. Connect piggyback setup to the access port or stopcock. If using, turn the stopcock to the open position.	
___	___	___	26. Use strip of tape to secure secondary tubing to primary infusion tubing, if a needle is used to connect.	

Administering a Piggyback Intermittent Intravenous Infusion of Medication *(Continued)*

Excellent	Satisfactory	Needs Practice		Comments
——	——	——	27. Open clamp on the secondary tubing. Use the roller clamp on the primary infusion tubing to regulate flow at prescribed delivery rate or set rate for secondary infusion on infusion pump. Monitor medication infusion at periodic intervals.	
——	——	——	28. Clamp tubing on piggyback set when solution is infused. Follow agency policy regarding disposal of equipment.	
——	——	——	29. Replace primary IV fluid container to original height. **Readjust flow rate of primary IV or check primary infusion rate on infusion pump.**	
——	——	——	30. Perform hand hygiene.	
——	——	——	31. Evaluate patient's response to medication within appropriate time frame. Monitor IV site at periodic intervals.	

Skill Checklists to Accompany Taylor's Clinical Nursing Skills:
A Nursing Process Approach, 2nd edition

Name _____   Date _____

Unit _____   Position _____

Instructor/Evaluator: _____   Position _____

Excellent	Satisfactory	Needs Practice	SKILL 5-12 **Administering an Intermittent Intravenous Infusion of Medication via a Mini-Infusion Pump** Goal: The medication is delivered via the parenteral route using sterile technique.	Comments
___	___	___	1. Gather equipment. Check each medication order against the original physician's order according to agency policy. Clarify any inconsistencies. Check the patient's chart for allergies.	
___	___	___	2. Know the actions, special nursing considerations, safe dose ranges, purpose of administration, and adverse effects of the medications to be administered. Consider the appropriateness of the medication for this patient.	
___	___	___	3. Perform hand hygiene.	
___	___	___	4. Move the medication cart to the outside of the patient's room or prepare for administration in the medication area.	
___	___	___	5. Unlock the medication cart or drawer. Enter pass code and scan employee identification, if required.	
___	___	___	6. **Prepare medications for one patient at a time.**	
___	___	___	7. Read the MAR and select the proper medication from the patient's medication drawer or unit stock.	
___	___	___	8. Compare the label with the MAR. Check expiration dates. Confirm the prescribed or appropriate infusion rate. Calculate the drip rate if using gravity system. Scan the bar code on the package, if required.	
___	___	___	9. **When all medications for one patient have been prepared, recheck the label with the MAR before taking them to the patient.**	
___	___	___	10. Lock the medication cart before leaving it.	
___	___	___	11. Transport medications to the patient's bedside carefully, and keep the medications in sight at all times.	
___	___	___	12. **Ensure that the patient receives the medications at the correct time.**	
___	___	___	13. **Identify the patient.** Usually, the patient should be identified using two methods. Compare information with the MAR or CMAR.	
___	___	___	a. Check the name and identification number on the patient's identification band.	

Excellent	Satisfactory	Needs Practice	SKILL 5-12 **Administering an Intermittent Intravenous Infusion of Medication via a Mini-Infusion Pump** *(Continued)*	Comments
——	——	——	b. Ask the patient to state his or her name.	
——	——	——	c. If the patient cannot identify him or herself, verify the patient's identification with a staff member who knows the patient for the second source.	
——	——	——	14. Close the door to the room or pull the bedside curtain.	
——	——	——	15. Perform hand hygiene.	
——	——	——	16. Complete necessary assessments before administering medications. Check allergy bracelet or ask patient about allergies. Explain the purpose and action of the medication to the patient.	
——	——	——	17. Scan the patient's bar code on the identification band, if required.	
——	——	——	18. Assess the IV site for the presence of inflammation or infiltration.	
——	——	——	19. Using aseptic technique, remove the cap on the tubing and the cap on the syringe, taking care to not contaminate either end.	
——	——	——	20. Attach infusion tubing to the syringe, taking care to not contaminate either end.	
——	——	——	21. Place label on tubing with appropriate date and attach needle or needleless device to end of tubing according to manufacturer's directions.	
——	——	——	22. Fill tubing with medication by applying gentle pressure to syringe plunger. Place needleless connector or needle on the end of the tubing, using sterile technique, if required.	
——	——	——	23. Insert syringe into mini-infusion pump according to manufacturer's directions.	
——	——	——	24. Use antimicrobial swab to clean the access port or stopcock below the roller clamp on the primary IV infusion tubing, usually the port closest to the IV insertion site.	
——	——	——	25. Connect the secondary infusion to the primary infusion at the cleansed port.	
——	——	——	26. Program pump to the appropriate rate and begin infusion. Set alarm if recommended by manufacturer.	
——	——	——	27. Clamp tubing on secondary set when solution is infused. Remove secondary tubing from access port and replace connector or needle with a new, capped one, if reusing. Follow agency policy regarding disposal of equipment.	
——	——	——	28. Check rate of primary infusion.	

Administering an Intermittent Intravenous Infusion of Medication via a Mini-Infusion Pump *(Continued)*

Excellent	Satisfactory	Needs Practice		Comments
⎯	⎯	⎯	29. Perform hand hygiene.	
⎯	⎯	⎯	30. Evaluate patient's response to medication within appropriate time frame. Monitor IV site at periodic intervals.	

Skill Checklists to Accompany Taylor's Clinical Nursing Skills:
A Nursing Process Approach, 2nd edition

Name _____ Date _____

Unit _____ Position _____

Instructor/Evaluator: _____ Position _____

SKILL 5-13

Administering an Intermittent Intravenous Infusion of Medication via a Volume-Control Administration Set

Goal: The medication is delivered via the parenteral route using sterile technique.

Excellent	Satisfactory	Needs Practice		Comments
——	——	——	1. Gather equipment. Check medication order against the original physician's order according to agency policy. Clarify any inconsistencies. Check the patient's chart for allergies. Verify the compatibility of the medication and IV fluid.	
——	——	——	2. Know the actions, special nursing considerations, safe dose ranges, purpose of administration, and adverse effects of the medications to be administered. Consider the appropriateness of the medication for this patient.	
——	——	——	3. Perform hand hygiene.	
——	——	——	4. Move the medication cart to the outside of the patient's room or prepare for administration in the medication area.	
——	——	——	5. Unlock the medication cart or drawer. Enter pass code and scan employee identification, if required.	
——	——	——	6. **Prepare medication for one patient at a time.**	
——	——	——	7. Read the MAR and select the proper medication from the patient's medication drawer or unit stock.	
——	——	——	8. Compare the label with the MAR. Check expiration dates and perform calculations, if necessary. Scan the bar code on the package, if required. Check the infusion rate.	
——	——	——	9. If necessary, withdraw medication from an ampule or vial as described in Skills 5-2 and 5-3. Attach needleless connector or needle to end of syringe, if necessary.	
——	——	——	10. **Recheck the label with the MAR before taking it to the patient.**	
——	——	——	11. Prepare medication label including name of medication, dose, total volume, including diluent, and time of administration.	
——	——	——	12. Lock the medication cart before leaving it.	
——	——	——	13. Transport medications and equipment to the patient's bedside carefully, and keep the medications in sight at all times.	

SKILL 5-13
Administering an Intermittent Intravenous Infusion of Medication via a Volume-Control Administration Set (Continued)

Excellent	Satisfactory	Needs Practice		Comments
——	——	——	14. Perform hand hygiene.	
——	——	——	15. **Identify the patient.** Usually, the patient should be identified using two methods. Compare information with the MAR or CMAR.	
——	——	——	a. Check the name and identification number on the patient's identification band.	
——	——	——	b. Ask the patient to state his or her name.	
——	——	——	c. If the patient cannot identify him or herself, verify the patient's identification with a staff member who knows the patient for the second source.	
——	——	——	16. Close the door to the room or pull the bedside curtain.	
——	——	——	17. Complete necessary assessments before administering medications. Check allergy bracelet or ask patient about allergies. Explain the purpose and action of the medication to the patient.	
——	——	——	18. Scan the patient's bar code on the identification band, if required.	
——	——	——	19. **Assess IV site for presence of inflammation or infiltration.**	
——	——	——	20. Fill the volume-control administration set with the prescribed amount of IV fluid by opening the clamp between IV solution and the volume-control administration set. Follow manufacturer's instructions and fill with prescribed amount of IV solution. Close clamp.	
——	——	——	21. Check to make sure the air vent on the volume-control administration set chamber is open.	
——	——	——	22. Use antimicrobial swab to clean access port on volume-control administration set chamber.	
——	——	——	23. Insert the needle or blunt needleless device into port while holding syringe steady. Inject medication into the chamber. Gently rotate the chamber.	
——	——	——	24. Attach the medication label to the volume-control device.	
——	——	——	25. Use antimicrobial swab to clean the access port or stopcock below the roller clamp on the primary IV infusion tubing, usually the port closest to the IV insertion site.	
——	——	——	26. Connect the secondary infusion to the primary infusion at the cleansed port.	
——	——	——	27. Use the roller clamp on the volume-control administration set tubing to adjust the infusion to the prescribed rate.	

SKILL 5-13
Administering an Intermittent Intravenous Infusion of Medication via a Volume-Control Administration Set *(Continued)*

Excellent	Satisfactory	Needs Practice		Comments
____	____	____	28. Do not recap the used needle. Engage the safety shield or needle guard, if present. Discard the needle and syringe in the appropriate receptacle.	
____	____	____	29. Clamp tubing on secondary set when solution is infused. Remove secondary tubing from access port and replace connector or needle with a new, capped one, if reusing. Follow agency policy regarding disposal of equipment.	
____	____	____	30. Check rate of primary infusion.	
____	____	____	31. Perform hand hygiene.	
____	____	____	32. Evaluate patient's response to medication within appropriate time frame. Monitor IV site at periodic intervals.	

*Skill Checklists to Accompany Taylor's Clinical Nursing Skills:
A Nursing Process Approach, 2nd edition*

Name _____ Date _____

Unit _____ Position _____

Instructor/Evaluator: _____ Position _____

SKILL 5-14

Introducing Drugs Through a Medication or Drug Infusion Lock Using the Saline Flush (Intermittent Peripheral Venous Access Device)

Goal: The medication is delivered via the parenteral route using sterile technique.

Excellent	Satisfactory	Needs Practice		Comments
___	___	___	1. Gather equipment. Check medication order against the original physician's order according to agency policy. Clarify any inconsistencies. Check the patient's chart for allergies. Verify the compatibility of the medication and IV fluid. Check a drug resource to clarify whether medication needs to be diluted before administration. Check the infusion rate.	
___	___	___	2. Know the actions, special nursing considerations, safe dose ranges, purpose of administration, and adverse effects of the medications to be administered. Consider the appropriateness of the medication for this patient.	
___	___	___	3. Perform hand hygiene.	
___	___	___	4. Move the medication cart to the outside of the patient's room or prepare for administration in the medication area.	
___	___	___	5. Unlock the medication cart or drawer. Enter pass code and scan employee identification, if required.	
___	___	___	6. **Prepare medication for one patient at a time.**	
___	___	___	7. Read the MAR and select the proper medication from the patient's medication drawer or unit stock.	
___	___	___	8. Compare the label with the MAR. Check expiration dates and perform calculations, if necessary. Scan the bar code on the package, if required.	
___	___	___	9. If necessary, withdraw medication from an ampule or vial as described in Skills 5-2 and 5-3.	
___	___	___	10. **Recheck the label with the MAR before taking it to the patient.**	
___	___	___	11. Lock the medication cart before leaving it.	
___	___	___	12. Transport medications and equipment to the patient's bedside carefully, and keep the medications in sight at all times.	
___	___	___	13. Perform hand hygiene.	

Excellent	Satisfactory	Needs Practice	SKILL 5-14 **Introducing Drugs Through a Medication or Drug Infusion Lock Using the Saline Flush (Intermittent Peripheral Venous Access Device)** *(Continued)*	
				Comments
——	——	——	14. **Identify the patient.** Usually, the patient should be identified using two methods. Compare information with the MAR or CMAR.	
——	——	——	a. Check the name and identification number on the patient's identification band.	
——	——	——	b. Ask the patient to state his or her name.	
——	——	——	c. If the patient cannot identify him or herself, verify the patient's identification with a staff member who knows the patient for the second source.	
——	——	——	15. Close the door to the room or pull the bedside curtain.	
——	——	——	16. Complete necessary assessments before administering medications. Check allergy bracelet or ask patient about allergies. Explain the purpose and action of the medication to the patient.	
——	——	——	17. Scan the patient's bar code on the identification band, if required.	
——	——	——	18. **Assess IV site for presence of inflammation or infiltration.**	
——	——	——	19. Put on clean gloves.	
——	——	——	20. Clean the access port of the medication lock with antimicrobial swab.	
——	——	——	21. Stabilize port with your nondominant hand and insert needleless device, syringe, or needle of syringe of normal saline into access port.	
——	——	——	22. Release the clamp on the extension tubing of the medication lock. Aspirate gently and check for blood return.	
——	——	——	23. Gently flush with normal saline by pushing slowly on the syringe plunger. Observe the insertion site while inserting the saline. Remove syringe.	
——	——	——	24. Insert needleless device or needle of syringe with medication into port and gently inject medication, using a watch to verify correct administration rate. **Do not force the injection if resistance is felt.**	
——	——	——	25. Remove medication syringe from port. Stabilize port with your nondominant hand and insert needleless device or needle of syringe of normal saline into port. Gently flush with normal saline by pushing slowly on the syringe plunger. To gain positive pressure, clamp the IV tubing as you are still flushing the last of the saline into the medication lock. Remove syringe.	

Excellent

Satisfactory

Needs Practice

SKILL 5-14

Introducing Drugs Through a Medication or Drug Infusion Lock Using the Saline Flush (Intermittent Peripheral Venous Access Device) *(Continued)*

Comments

Excellent	Satisfactory	Needs Practice		Comments
——	——	——	26. Do not recap the used needle. Engage the safety shield or needle guard, if present. Discard the needle and syringe in the appropriate receptacle.	
——	——	——	27. Remove gloves and perform hand hygiene.	
——	——	——	28. Evaluate patient's response to medication within appropriate time frame.	
——	——	——	29. Check medication lock site at least every 8 hours or according to facility policy.	

Skill Checklists to Accompany Taylor's Clinical Nursing Skills:
A Nursing Process Approach, 2nd edition

Name _____ Date _____

Unit _____ Position _____

Instructor/Evaluator: _____ Position _____

Excellent	Satisfactory	Needs Practice	SKILL 5-15 **Applying a Transdermal Patch**	
			Goal: The medication is delivered via the transdermal route.	**Comments**
____	____	____	1. Gather equipment. Check medication order against the original physician's order according to agency policy. Clarify any inconsistencies. Check the patient's chart for allergies.	
____	____	____	2. Know the actions, special nursing considerations, safe dose ranges, purpose of administration, and adverse effects of the medications to be administered. Consider the appropriateness of the medication for this patient.	
____	____	____	3. Perform hand hygiene.	
____	____	____	4. Move the medication cart to the outside of the patient's room or prepare for administration in the medication area.	
____	____	____	5. Unlock the medication cart or drawer. Enter pass code and scan employee identification, if required.	
____	____	____	6. **Prepare medications for one patient at a time.**	
____	____	____	7. Read the MAR and select the proper medication from the patient's medication drawer or unit stock.	
____	____	____	8. Compare the label with the MAR. Check expiration dates and perform calculations, if necessary. Scan the bar code on the package, if required.	
____	____	____	9. **When all medications for one patient have been prepared, recheck the label with the MAR before taking them to the patient. Lock the medication cart before leaving it.**	
____	____	____	10. Transport medications to the patient's bedside carefully, and keep the medications in sight at all times.	
____	____	____	11. **Ensure that the patient receives the medications at the correct time.**	
____	____	____	12. **Identify the patient.** Usually, the patient should be identified using two methods. Compare information with the MAR or CMAR.	
____	____	____	a. Check the name and identification number on the patient's identification band.	
____	____	____	b. Ask the patient to state his or her name.	

Excellent	Satisfactory	Needs Practice	

SKILL 5-15
Applying a Transdermal Patch *(Continued)*

Comments

—	—	—	c. If the patient cannot identify him or herself, verify the patient's identification with a staff member who knows the patient for the second source.	
—	—	—	13. **Complete necessary assessments before administering medications. Check allergy bracelet or ask patient about allergies. Explain the purpose and action of each medication to the patient.**	
—	—	—	14. Scan the patient's bar code on the identification band, if required.	
—	—	—	15. Perform hand hygiene and put on gloves.	
—	—	—	16. Assess patient's skin where patch is to be placed, looking for any signs of irritation or breakdown. Site should be clean, dry, and free of hair. Rotate application sites.	
—	—	—	17. **Remove any old transdermal patches from the patient's skin.** Fold the old patch in half with the adhesive sides sticking together and discard according to facility policy. Gently wash the area where the old patch was with soap and water.	
—	—	—	18. Remove the patch from its protective covering. Write your initials and the date and time of administration on the label side of the patch.	
—	—	—	19. Remove the covering on the patch without touching the medication surface. Apply the patch to the patient's skin. Use the palm of your hand to press firmly for about 10 seconds. Do not massage.	
—	—	—	20. Remove gloves and perform hand hygiene.	
—	—	—	21. Evaluate patient's response to medication within appropriate time frame.	

Skill Checklists to Accompany Taylor's Clinical Nursing Skills:
A Nursing Process Approach, 2nd edition

Name _____ Date _____

Unit _____ Position _____

Instructor/Evaluator: _____ Position _____

SKILL 5-16
Instilling Eye Drops

Excellent	Satisfactory	Needs Practice		Comments
			Goal: The medication is instilled successfully into the eye.	
____	____	____	1. Gather equipment. Check medication order against the original physician's order according to agency policy. Clarify any inconsistencies. Check the patient's chart for allergies.	
____	____	____	2. Know the actions, special nursing considerations, safe dose ranges, purpose of administration, and adverse effects of the medications to be administered. Consider the appropriateness of the medication for this patient.	
____	____	____	3. Perform hand hygiene.	
____	____	____	4. Move the medication cart to the outside of the patient's room or prepare for administration in the medication area.	
____	____	____	5. Unlock the medication cart or drawer. Enter pass code and scan employee identification, if required.	
____	____	____	6. **Prepare medications for one patient at a time.**	
____	____	____	7. Read the MAR and select the proper medication from the patient's medication drawer or unit stock.	
____	____	____	8. Compare the label with the MAR. Check expiration dates and perform calculations, if necessary. Scan the bar code on the package, if required.	
____	____	____	9. **When all medications for one patient have been prepared, recheck the label with the MAR before taking them to the patient. Lock the medication cart before leaving it.**	
____	____	____	10. Transport medications to the patient's bedside carefully, and keep the medications in sight at all times.	
____	____	____	11. **Ensure that the patient receives the medications at the correct time.**	
____	____	____	12. **Identify the patient.** Usually, the patient should be identified using two methods. Compare information with the MAR or CMAR.	
____	____	____	a. Check the name and identification number on the patient's identification band.	
____	____	____	b. Ask the patient to state his or her name.	

			SKILL 5-16 **Instilling Eye Drops** *(Continued)*	
Excellent	**Satisfactory**	**Needs Practice**		**Comments**
——	——	——	c. If the patient cannot identify him or herself, verify the patient's identification with a staff member who knows the patient for the second source.	
——	——	——	13. **Complete necessary assessments before administering medications. Check allergy bracelet or ask patient about allergies. Explain the purpose and action of each medication to the patient.**	
——	——	——	14. Scan the patient's bar code on the identification band, if required.	
——	——	——	15. Perform hand hygiene and put on gloves.	
——	——	——	16. Offer tissue to patient.	
——	——	——	17. **Cleanse the eyelids and eyelashes of any drainage with a washcloth, cotton balls, or gauze squares moistened with normal saline solution.** Use each area of the cleaning surface once, moving from the inner toward the outer canthus.	
——	——	——	18. Tilt the patient's head back slightly if sitting, or place the patient's head over a pillow if lying down. The head may be turned slightly to the affected side to prevent solution or tears from flowing toward the opposite eye.	
——	——	——	19. Remove cap from medication bottle, being careful to not touch the inner side of the cap.	
——	——	——	20. Invert the monodrip plastic container that is commonly used to instill eye drops. Have patient look up and focus on something on the ceiling.	
——	——	——	21. Place thumb or two fingers near margin of lower eyelid immediately below eyelashes, and exert pressure downward over bony prominence of cheek. Lower conjunctival sac is exposed as lower lid is pulled down.	
——	——	——	22. **Hold dropper close to eye, but avoid touching eyelids or lashes. Squeeze container and allow prescribed number of drops to fall in lower conjunctival sac.**	
——	——	——	23. Release lower lid after eye drops are instilled. Ask patient to close eyes gently.	
——	——	——	24. Apply gentle pressure over inner canthus to prevent eye drops from flowing into tear duct.	
——	——	——	25. Instruct patient not to rub affected eye.	
——	——	——	26. Remove gloves and perform hand hygiene.	
——	——	——	27. Assist patient to a comfortable position.	
——	——	——	28. Evaluate patient's response to medication within appropriate time frame.	

Skill Checklists to Accompany Taylor's Clinical Nursing Skills:
A Nursing Process Approach, 2nd edition

Name _____ Date _____

Unit _____ Position _____

Instructor/Evaluator: _____ Position _____

Excellent	Satisfactory	Needs Practice	SKILL 5-17 **Administering an Eye Irrigation**	Comments
			Goal: The eye is cleansed successfully.	
___	___	___	1. Gather equipment. Check the original physician's order for the irrigation according to agency policy. Clarify any inconsistencies. Check the patient's chart for allergies.	
___	___	___	2. **Identify the patient.** Usually, the patient should be identified using two methods. Compare information with the MAR or CMAR.	
___	___	___	a. Check the name and identification number on the patient's identification band.	
___	___	___	b. Ask the patient to state his or her name.	
___	___	___	c. If the patient cannot identify him or herself, verify the patient's identification with a staff member who knows the patient for the second source.	
___	___	___	3. Explain procedure to patient.	
___	___	___	4. Assemble equipment at patient's bedside.	
___	___	___	5. Perform hand hygiene.	
___	___	___	6. Have patient sit or lie with head tilted toward side of affected eye. Protect patient and bed with a waterproof pad.	
___	___	___	7. Put on disposable gloves. Clean lids and lashes with washcloth moistened with normal saline or the solution ordered for the irrigation. Wipe from inner canthus to outer canthus. Use a different corner of washcloth with each wipe.	
___	___	___	8. Place curved basin at cheek on side of affected eye to receive irrigating solution. If patient is able, ask him or her to support the basin.	
___	___	___	9. Expose lower conjunctival sac and hold upper lid open with your nondominant hand.	
___	___	___	10. Fill the irrigation syringe with the prescribed fluid. **Hold irrigation syringe about 2.5 cm (1″) from eye. Direct flow of solution from inner to outer canthus along conjunctival sac.**	

Administering an Eye Irrigation *(Continued)*

Excellent	Satisfactory	Needs Practice		Comments
——	——	——	11. Irrigate until the solution is clear or all the solution has been used. **Use only enough force to remove secretions gently from the conjunctiva. Avoid touching any part of the eye with the irrigating tip.**	
——	——	——	12. Pause irrigation and have patient close eye periodically during procedure.	
——	——	——	13. Dry periorbital area after irrigation with gauze sponge. Offer towel to patient if face and neck are wet.	
——	——	——	14. Remove gloves and perform hand hygiene.	
——	——	——	15. Assist the patient to a comfortable position.	
——	——	——	16. Evaluate patient's response to medication within appropriate time frame.	

Skill Checklists to Accompany Taylor's Clinical Nursing Skills:
A Nursing Process Approach, 2nd edition

Name _____   Date _____

Unit _____   Position _____

Instructor/Evaluator: _____   Position _____

Excellent	Satisfactory	Needs Practice	SKILL 5-18 **Instilling Eardrops**	Comments
			Goal: Drops are administered successfully.	
___	___	___	1. Gather equipment. Check medication order against the original physician's order according to agency policy. Clarify any inconsistencies. Check the patient's chart for allergies.	
___	___	___	2. Know the actions, special nursing considerations, safe dose ranges, purpose of administration, and adverse effects of the medication to be administered. Consider the appropriateness of the medication for this patient.	
___	___	___	3. Perform hand hygiene.	
___	___	___	4. Move the medication cart to the outside of the patient's room or prepare for administration in the medication area.	
___	___	___	5. Unlock the medication cart or drawer. Enter pass code and scan employee identification, if required.	
___	___	___	6. **Prepare medications for one patient at a time.**	
___	___	___	7. Read the MAR and select the proper medication from the patient's medication drawer or unit stock.	
___	___	___	8. Compare the label with the MAR. Check expiration dates and perform calculations, if necessary. Scan the bar code on the package, if required.	
___	___	___	9. **When all medications for one patient have been prepared, recheck the label with the MAR before taking them to the patient. Lock the medication cart before leaving it.**	
___	___	___	10. Transport medications to the patient's bedside carefully, and keep the medications in sight at all times.	
___	___	___	11. **Ensure that the patient receives the medications at the correct time.**	
___	___	___	12. **Identify the patient.** Usually, the patient should be identified using two methods. Compare information with the MAR or CMAR.	
___	___	___	a. Check the name and identification number on the patient's identification band.	
___	___	___	b. Ask the patient to state his or her name.	

SKILL 5-18

Instilling Eardrops *(Continued)*

Excellent	Satisfactory	Needs Practice		Comments
——	——	——	c. If the patient cannot identify him or herself, verify the patient's identification with a staff member who knows the patient for the second source.	
——	——	——	13. **Complete necessary assessments before administering medications. Check allergy bracelet or ask patient about allergies. Explain the purpose and action of each medication to the patient.**	
——	——	——	14. Scan the patient's bar code on the identification band, if required.	
——	——	——	15. Perform hand hygiene and put on gloves.	
——	——	——	16. Cleanse external ear of any drainage with cotton ball or washcloth moistened with normal saline.	
——	——	——	17. Place patient on his or her unaffected side in bed, or if ambulatory, have patient sit with head well tilted to the side so that affected ear is uppermost.	
——	——	——	18. Draw up the amount of solution needed in dropper. Do not return excess medication to stock bottle. A prepackaged monodrip plastic container may also be used.	
——	——	——	19. Straighten auditory canal by pulling cartilaginous portion of pinna up and back for an adult.	
——	——	——	20. Hold dropper in ear with its tip above auditory canal. Do not touch dropper to ear. For an infant or an irrational or confused patient, protect dropper with a piece of soft tubing to help prevent injury to ear.	
——	——	——	21. **Allow drops to fall on side of canal.**	
——	——	——	22. Release pinna after instilling drops, and have patient maintain the position to prevent escape of medication.	
——	——	——	23. Gently press on tragus a few times.	
——	——	——	24. If ordered, loosely insert a cotton ball into ear canal.	
——	——	——	25. Remove gloves and perform hand hygiene.	
——	——	——	26. Assist the patient to a comfortable position.	
——	——	——	27. Evaluate patient's response to medication within appropriate time frame.	

Skill Checklists to Accompany Taylor's Clinical Nursing Skills:
A Nursing Process Approach, 2nd edition

Name _____ Date _____

Unit _____ Position _____

Instructor/Evaluator: _____ Position _____

Excellent	Satisfactory	Needs Practice	SKILL 5-19 **Administering an Ear Irrigation**	
			Goal: The irrigation is administered successfully.	**Comments**
____	____	____	1. Gather equipment. Check the original physician's order for the irrigation according to agency policy. Clarify any inconsistencies. Check the patient's chart for allergies.	
____	____	____	2. **Identify the patient.** Usually, the patient should be identified using two methods. Compare information with the MAR or CMAR.	
____	____	____	a. Check the name and identification number on the patient's identification band.	
____	____	____	b. Ask the patient to state his or her name.	
____	____	____	c. If the patient cannot identify him or herself, verify the patient's identification with a staff member who knows the patient for the second source.	
____	____	____	3. Explain procedure to patient.	
____	____	____	4. Assemble equipment at patient's bedside.	
____	____	____	5. Perform hand hygiene and put on gloves.	
____	____	____	6. Have patient sit up or lie with head tilted toward side of affected ear. Protect patient and bed with a waterproof pad. Have patient support basin under the ear to receive the irrigating solution.	
____	____	____	7. Clean pinna and meatus of auditory canal as necessary with moistened cotton-tipped applicators dipped in warm tap water or the irrigating solution.	
____	____	____	8. Fill bulb syringe with warm solution. If an irrigating container is used, prime the tubing.	
____	____	____	9. Straighten auditory canal by pulling cartilaginous portion of pinna up and back for an adult.	
____	____	____	10. **Direct a steady, slow stream of solution against the roof of the auditory canal, using only enough force to remove secretions. Do not occlude the auditory canal with the irrigating nozzle. Allow solution to flow out unimpeded.**	
____	____	____	11. When irrigation is complete, place cotton ball loosely in auditory meatus and have patient lie on side of affected ear on a towel or absorbent pad.	

Administering an Ear Irrigation *(Continued)*

Excellent	Satisfactory	Needs Practice		Comments
——	——	——	12. Remove gloves and perform hand hygiene.	
——	——	——	13. Assist the patient to a comfortable position.	
——	——	——	14. Evaluate patient's response to the procedure. Return in 10 to 15 minutes and remove cotton ball and assess drainage.	

Skill Checklists to Accompany Taylor's Clinical Nursing Skills: A Nursing Process Approach, 2nd edition

Name _____ Date _____

Unit _____ Position _____

Instructor/Evaluator: _____ Position _____

Excellent	Satisfactory	Needs Practice	SKILL 5-20 **Instilling Nose Drops**	
			Goal: The medication is administered successfully into the nose.	**Comments**
___	___	___	1. Gather equipment. Check medication order against the original physician's order according to agency policy. Clarify any inconsistencies. Check the patient's chart for allergies.	
___	___	___	2. Know the actions, special nursing considerations, safe dose ranges, purpose of administration, and adverse effects of the medication to be administered. Consider the appropriateness of the medication for this patient.	
___	___	___	3. Perform hand hygiene.	
___	___	___	4. Move the medication cart to the outside of the patient's room or prepare for administration in the medication area.	
___	___	___	5. Unlock the medication cart or drawer. Enter pass code and scan employee identification, if required.	
___	___	___	6. **Prepare medications for one patient at a time.**	
___	___	___	7. Read the MAR and select the proper medication from the patient's medication drawer or unit stock.	
___	___	___	8. Compare the label with the MAR. Check expiration dates and perform calculations, if necessary. Scan the bar code on the package, if required.	
___	___	___	9. **When all medications for one patient have been prepared, recheck the label with the MAR before taking them to the patient. Lock the medication cart before leaving it.**	
___	___	___	10. Transport medications to the patient's bedside carefully, and keep the medications in sight at all times.	
___	___	___	11. **Ensure that the patient receives the medications at the correct time.**	
___	___	___	12. **Identify the patient.** Usually, the patient should be identified using two methods. Compare information with the MAR or CMAR.	
___	___	___	a. Check the name and identification number on the patient's identification band.	
___	___	___	b. Ask the patient to state his or her name.	

SKILL 5-20
Instilling Nose Drops *(Continued)*

Excellent	Satisfactory	Needs Practice		Comments
——	——	——	c. If the patient cannot identify him or herself, verify the patient's identification with a staff member who knows the patient for the second source.	
——	——	——	13. **Complete necessary assessments before administering medications. Check allergy bracelet or ask patient about allergies. Explain the purpose and action of each medication to the patient.**	
——	——	——	14. Scan the patient's bar code on the identification band, if required.	
——	——	——	15. Perform hand hygiene and put on gloves.	
——	——	——	16. **Provide patient with paper tissues and ask patient to blow his or her nose.**	
——	——	——	17. Have patient sit up with head tilted well back. If patient is lying down, tilt head back over a pillow.	
——	——	——	18. Draw sufficient solution into dropper for both nares. Do not return excess solution to a stock bottle.	
——	——	——	19. Ask the patient to breathe through the mouth. Hold tip of nose up and place dropper just above naris, about one third of an inch. Instill prescribed number of drops in one naris and then into the other. Protect dropper with a piece of soft tubing if patient is an infant or young child. Avoid touching naris with dropper.	
——	——	——	20. Have patient remain in position with head tilted back for a few minutes.	
——	——	——	21. Remove gloves and perform hand hygiene.	
——	——	——	22. Assist the patient to a comfortable position.	
——	——	——	23. Evaluate patient's response to the procedure and medication.	

Skill Checklists to Accompany Taylor's Clinical Nursing Skills:
A Nursing Process Approach, 2nd edition

Name _____ Date _____

Unit _____ Position _____

Instructor/Evaluator: _____ Position _____

SKILL 5-21
Administering a Vaginal Cream

Excellent	Satisfactory	Needs Practice		Comments
			Goal: The medication is administered successfully into the vagina.	
___	___	___	1. Gather equipment. Check medication order against the original physician's order according to agency policy. Clarify any inconsistencies. Check the patient's chart for allergies.	
___	___	___	2. Know the actions, special nursing considerations, safe dose ranges, purpose of administration, and adverse effects of the medication to be administered. Consider the appropriateness of the medication for this patient.	
___	___	___	3. Perform hand hygiene.	
___	___	___	4. Move the medication cart to the outside of the patient's room or prepare for administration in the medication area.	
___	___	___	5. Unlock the medication cart or drawer. Enter pass code and scan employee identification, if required.	
___	___	___	6. **Prepare medications for one patient at a time.**	
___	___	___	7. Read the MAR and select the proper medication from the patient's medication drawer or unit stock.	
___	___	___	8. Compare the label with the MAR. Check expiration dates and perform calculations, if necessary. Scan the bar code on the package, if required.	
___	___	___	9. **When all medications for one patient have been prepared, recheck the label with the MAR before taking them to the patient. Lock the medication cart before leaving it.**	
___	___	___	10. Transport medications to the patient's bedside carefully, and keep the medications in sight at all times.	
___	___	___	11. **Ensure that the patient receives the medications at the correct time.**	
___	___	___	12. **Identify the patient.** Usually, the patient should be identified using two methods. Compare information with the MAR or CMAR.	
___	___	___	a. Check the name and identification number on the patient's identification band.	
___	___	___	b. Ask the patient to state his or her name.	

SKILL 5-21
Administering a Vaginal Cream *(Continued)*

Excellent	Satisfactory	Needs Practice		Comments
___	___	___	c. If the patient cannot identify herself, verify the patient's identification with a staff member who knows the patient for the second source.	
___	___	___	13. **Complete necessary assessments before administering medications. Check allergy bracelet or ask patient about allergies. Explain the purpose and action of each medication to the patient.**	
___	___	___	14. Scan the patient's bar code on the identification band, if required.	
___	___	___	15. Perform hand hygiene and put on gloves.	
___	___	___	16. Ask the patient to void before inserting the medication.	
___	___	___	17. Position the patient so that she is lying on her back with the knees flexed. Maintain privacy with draping. Adequate light should be available to visualize the vaginal opening.	
___	___	___	18. **Spread labia with fingers, and clean area at vaginal orifice with washcloth and warm water, using a different corner of the washcloth with each stroke. Wipe from above orifice downward toward sacrum (front to back).**	
___	___	___	19. Replace your gloves.	
___	___	___	20. Fill vaginal applicator with prescribed amount of cream.	
___	___	___	21. Lubricate applicator with the lubricant, as necessary.	
___	___	___	22. Spread the labia with your nondominant hand and introduce applicator with your dominant hand gently, in a rolling manner, while directing it downward and backward.	
___	___	___	23. After applicator is properly positioned, labia may be allowed to fall in place if necessary to free the hand for manipulating plunger. Push plunger to its full length and then gently remove applicator with plunger depressed.	
___	___	___	24. Remove gloves and perform hand hygiene.	
___	___	___	25. **Ask patient to remain in supine position for 5 to 10 minutes after insertion.**	
___	___	___	26. Offer patient a perineal pad to collect drainage.	
___	___	___	27. Dispose of applicator in appropriate receptacle or clean nondisposable applicator according to manufacturer's directions.	
___	___	___	28. Evaluate patient's response to the procedure and medication.	

Skill Checklists to Accompany Taylor's Clinical Nursing Skills:
A Nursing Process Approach, 2nd edition

Name _____ Date _____

Unit _____ Position _____

Instructor/Evaluator: _____ Position _____

Excellent	Satisfactory	Needs Practice	SKILL 5-22 **Administering Medication via a Metered-Dose Inhaler (MDI)**	
			Goal: The patient receives the medication.	**Comments**
___	___	___	1. Gather equipment. Check each medication order against the original physician's order according to agency policy. Clarify any inconsistencies. Check the patient's chart for allergies.	
___	___	___	2. Know the actions, special nursing considerations, safe dose ranges, purpose of administration, and adverse effects of the medications to be administered. Consider the appropriateness of the medication for this patient.	
___	___	___	3. Perform hand hygiene.	
___	___	___	4. Move the medication cart to the outside of the patient's room or prepare for administration in the medication area.	
___	___	___	5. Unlock the medication cart or drawer. Enter pass code and scan employee identification, if required.	
___	___	___	6. **Prepare medications for one patient at a time.**	
___	___	___	7. Read the MAR and select the proper medication from the patient's medication drawer or unit stock.	
___	___	___	8. Compare the label with the MAR. Check expiration dates and perform calculations, if necessary. Scan the bar code on the package, if required.	
___	___	___	9. **When all medications for one patient have been prepared, recheck the label with the MAR before taking them to the patient. Lock the medication cart before leaving it.**	
___	___	___	10. Transport medications to the patient's bedside carefully, and keep the medications in sight at all times.	
___	___	___	11. **Ensure that the patient receives the medications at the correct time.**	
___	___	___	12. **Identify the patient.** Usually, the patient should be identified using two methods. Compare information with the MAR or CMAR.	
___	___	___	a. Check the name and identification number on the patient's identification band.	
___	___	___	b. Ask the patient to state his or her name.	

Excellent	Satisfactory	Needs Practice	SKILL 5-22 **Administering Medication via a Metered-Dose Inhaler (MDI)** *(Continued)*	Comments
——	——	——	c. If the patient cannot identify him or herself, verify the patient's identification with a staff member who knows the patient for the second source.	
——	——	——	13. **Complete necessary assessments before administering medications. Check allergy bracelet or ask patient about allergies.** Explain what you are going to do and the reason to the patient.	
——	——	——	14. Scan the patient's bar code on the identification band, if required.	
——	——	——	15. Perform hand hygiene.	
——	——	——	16. **Remove the mouthpiece cover from the MDI and the spacer.** Attach the MDI to the spacer.	
——	——	——	17. Shake the inhaler and spacer well.	
——	——	——	18. Have patient place the spacer's mouthpiece into mouth, grasping securely with teeth and lips. Have patient breathe normally through the spacer.	
——	——	——	19. Patient should depress the canister, releasing one puff into the spacer, then inhale slowly and deeply through the mouth.	
——	——	——	20. **Instruct patient to hold the breath for 5 to 10 seconds, or as long as possible, and then to exhale slowly through pursed lips.**	
——	——	——	21. **Wait 1 to 5 minutes, as prescribed, before administering the next puff.**	
——	——	——	22. After the prescribed amount of puffs has been administered, have patient remove the MDI from the spacer and replace the caps on both.	
——	——	——	23. **Reassess lung sounds, oxygenation saturation if ordered, and respirations.**	
——	——	——	24. Perform hand hygiene.	

Skill Checklists to Accompany Taylor's Clinical Nursing Skills:
A Nursing Process Approach, 2nd edition

Name _____ Date _____

Unit _____ Position _____

Instructor/Evaluator: _____ Position _____

SKILL 5-23

Administering Medication via a Small-Volume Nebulizer

Goal: The patient receives the medication.

Excellent	Satisfactory	Needs Practice		Comments
——	——	——	1. Gather equipment. Check each medication order against the original physician's order according to agency policy. Clarify any inconsistencies. Check the patient's chart for allergies.	
——	——	——	2. Know the actions, special nursing considerations, safe dose ranges, purpose of administration, and adverse effects of the medications to be administered. Consider the appropriateness of the medication for this patient.	
——	——	——	3. Perform hand hygiene.	
——	——	——	4. Move the medication cart to the outside of the patient's room or prepare for administration in the medication area.	
——	——	——	5. Unlock the medication cart or drawer. Enter pass code and scan employee identification, if required.	
——	——	——	6. **Prepare medications for one patient at a time.**	
——	——	——	7. Read the MAR and select the proper medication from the patient's medication drawer or unit stock.	
——	——	——	8. Compare the label with the MAR. Check expiration dates and perform calculations, if necessary. Scan the bar code on the package, if required.	
——	——	——	9. **When all medications for one patient have been prepared, recheck the label with the MAR before taking them to the patient. Lock the medication cart before leaving it.**	
——	——	——	10. Transport medications to the patient's bedside carefully, and keep the medications in sight at all times.	
——	——	——	11. **Ensure that the patient receives the medications at the correct time.**	
——	——	——	12. **Identify the patient.** Usually, the patient should be identified using two methods. Compare information with the MAR or CMAR.	
——	——	——	a. Check the name and identification number on the patient's identification band.	
——	——	——	b. Ask the patient to state his or her name.	

SKILL 5-23
Administering Medication via a
Small-Volume Nebulizer *(Continued)*

Excellent	Satisfactory	Needs Practice		Comments
——	——	——	c. If the patient cannot identify him or herself, verify the patient's identification with a staff member who knows the patient for the second source.	
——	——	——	13. **Complete necessary assessments before administering medications. Check allergy bracelet or ask patient about allergies.** Explain what you are going to do and the reason to the patient.	
——	——	——	14. Scan the patient's bar code on the identification band, if required.	
——	——	——	15. Perform hand hygiene.	
——	——	——	16. Remove the nebulizer cup from the device and open it. Place premeasured unit-dose medication in the bottom section of the cup or use a dropper to place concentrated dose of medication in cup and add prescribed diluent, if required.	
——	——	——	17. Screw the top portion of the nebulizer cup back in place and attach the cup to the nebulizer. Attach one end of tubing to the stem on the bottom of the nebulizer cuff and the other end to the air compressor or oxygen source.	
——	——	——	18. Turn on the air compressor or oxygen. Check that a fine medication mist is produced by opening the valve. Have patient place mouthpiece into mouth and grasp securely with teeth and lips.	
——	——	——	19. **Instruct patient to inhale slowly and deeply through the mouth. A nose clip may be necessary if patient is also breathing through nose. Hold each breath for a slight pause, before exhaling.**	
——	——	——	20. **Continue this inhalation technique until all medication in the nebulizer cup has been aerosolized (usually about 15 minutes). Once the fine mist decreases in amount, gently flick the sides of the nebulizer cup.**	
——	——	——	21. If desired, have the patient gargle with tap water after using nebulizer. Clean the nebulizer according to the manufacturer's directions.	
——	——	——	22. **Reassess lung sounds, oxygenation saturation if ordered, pulse, and respirations.**	
——	——	——	23. Perform hand hygiene.	

Name _____   Date _____

Unit _____   Position _____

Instructor/Evaluator: _____   Position _____

Excellent	Satisfactory	Needs Practice	SKILL 5-24 **Administering Medication via a Dry Powder Inhaler**	Comments
			Goal: The patient receives the medication.	
——	——	——	1. Gather equipment. Check each medication order against the original physician's order according to agency policy. Clarify any inconsistencies. Check the patient's chart for allergies.	
——	——	——	2. Know the actions, special nursing considerations, safe dose ranges, purpose of administration, and adverse effects of the medications to be administered. Consider the appropriateness of the medication for this patient.	
——	——	——	3. Perform hand hygiene.	
——	——	——	4. Move the medication cart to the outside of the patient's room or prepare for administration in the medication area.	
——	——	——	5. Unlock the medication cart or drawer. Enter pass code and scan employee identification, if required.	
——	——	——	6. **Prepare medications for one patient at a time.**	
——	——	——	7. Read the MAR and select the proper medication from the patient's medication drawer or unit stock.	
——	——	——	8. Compare the label with the MAR. Check expiration dates and perform calculations, if necessary. Scan the bar code on the package, if required.	
——	——	——	9. **When all medications for one patient have been prepared, recheck the label with the MAR before taking them to the patient. Lock the medication cart before leaving it.**	
——	——	——	10. Transport medications to the patient's bedside carefully, and keep the medications in sight at all times.	
——	——	——	11. **Ensure that the patient receives the medications at the correct time.**	
——	——	——	12. **Identify the patient.** Usually, the patient should be identified using two methods. Compare information with the MAR or CMAR.	
——	——	——	a. Check the name and identification number on the patient's identification band.	
——	——	——	b. Ask the patient to state his or her name.	

Administering Medication via a Dry Powder Inhaler *(Continued)*

Excellent	Satisfactory	Needs Practice		Comments
——	——	——	c. If the patient cannot identify him or herself, verify the patient's identification with a staff member who knows the patient for the second source.	
——	——	——	13. **Complete necessary assessments before administering medications. Check allergy bracelet or ask patient about allergies.** Explain what you are going to do and the reason to the patient.	
——	——	——	14. Scan the patient's bar code on the identification band, if required.	
——	——	——	15. Perform hand hygiene.	
——	——	——	16. **Remove the mouthpiece cover or remove from storage container. Load a dose into the device as directed by the manufacturer, if necessary. Alternately, activate the inhaler if necessary according to manufacturer's directions.**	
——	——	——	17. Have the patient breathe out slowly and completely, without breathing into the DPI.	
——	——	——	18. Patient should place his teeth over and seal his lips around the mouthpiece. Do not block opening with the tongue or teeth.	
——	——	——	19. Breathe in quickly and deeply through the mouth, more than 2 to 3 seconds.	
——	——	——	20. Remove inhaler from mouth. **Instruct patient to hold the breath for 5 to 10 seconds, or as long as possible, and then to exhale slowly through pursed lips.**	
——	——	——	21. **Wait 1 to 5 minutes, as prescribed, before administering the next puff.**	
——	——	——	22. After the prescribed amount of puffs has been administered, have patient replace the cap or storage container.	
——	——	——	23. **Reassess lung sounds, oxygenation saturation if ordered, and respirations.**	
——	——	——	24. Perform hand hygiene.	

Skill Checklists to Accompany Taylor's Clinical Nursing Skills:
A Nursing Process Approach, 2nd edition

Name _____ Date _____

Unit _____ Position _____

Instructor/Evaluator: _____ Position _____

Excellent	Satisfactory	Needs Practice	SKILL 5-25 **Administering Medications via a Gastric Tube**

Goal: The patient receives the medication via the tube and experiences the intended effect of the medication.   **Comments**

Excellent	Satisfactory	Needs Practice		Comments
——	——	——	1. Gather equipment. Check each medication order against the original physician's order according to agency policy. Clarify any inconsistencies. Check the patient's chart for allergies.	
——	——	——	2. Know the actions, special nursing considerations, safe dose ranges, purpose of administration, and adverse effects of the medications to be administered. Consider the appropriateness of the medication for this patient.	
——	——	——	3. Perform hand hygiene.	
——	——	——	4. Move the medication cart to the outside of the patient's room or prepare for administration in the medication area.	
——	——	——	5. Unlock the medication cart or drawer. Enter pass code and scan employee identification, if required.	
——	——	——	6. **Prepare medications for one patient at a time.**	
——	——	——	7. Read the MAR and select the proper medication from the patient's medication drawer or unit stock.	
——	——	——	8. Compare the label with the MAR. Check expiration dates and perform calculations, if necessary. Scan the bar code on the package, if required.	
——	——	——	9. Check to see if medications to be administered come in a liquid form. **If pills or capsules are to be given, check with pharmacy or drug reference to verify the ability to crush or open capsules.** Ensure that the tube is patent and irrigate as necessary.	
——	——	——	10. Prepare medication. *Pills:* Using a pill crusher, crush each pill one at a time. Dissolve the powder with water or other recommended liquid in a liquid medication cup, keeping each medication separate from the others. Keep the package label with the medication cup, for future comparison of information.	

Administering Medications via a Gastric Tube *(Continued)*

Excellent	Satisfactory	Needs Practice		Comments

Liquid: When pouring liquid medications in a multidose bottle, hold the bottle with the label against the palm. Use the appropriate measuring device when pouring liquids, and read the amount of medication at the bottom of the meniscus at eye level. Wipe the lip of the bottle with a paper towel.

11. **When all medications for one patient have been prepared, recheck the label with the MAR before taking them to the patient. Lock the medication cart before leaving it.**

12. Transport medications to the patient's bedside carefully, and keep the medications in sight at all times.

13. **Ensure that the patient receives the medications at the correct time.**

14. **Identify the patient.** Usually, the patient should be identified using two methods. Compare information with the MAR or CMAR.

    a. Check the name and identification number on the patient's identification band.

    b. Ask the patient to state his or her name.

    c. If the patient cannot identify him or herself, verify the patient's identification with a staff member who knows the patient for the second source.

15. **Complete necessary assessments before administering medications. Check allergy bracelet or ask patient about allergies.** Explain what you are going to do and the reason to the patient.

16. Scan the patient's bar code on the identification band, if required.

17. Assist the patient to the High Fowler's position, unless contraindicated.

18. Perform hand hygiene and put on gloves.

19. If patient is receiving continuous tube feedings, pause the tube feeding pump.

20. Pour the water into the irrigation container. Fold the gastric tube over on itself and pinch with fingers. Alternately, open port on gastric tube delegated to medication administration. If necessary, position stopcock to correct direction. Disconnect tubing for feeding or suction from gastric tube. Place cap on end of feeding tubing.

Excellent	Satisfactory	Needs Practice	SKILL 5-25 **Administering Medications via a Gastric Tube** *(Continued)*
			Comments
——	——	——	21. Insert tip of 60-mL syringe into tube. Release gastric tube. Pull plunger back using constant, gentle pressure to check for residual feeding and to check tube placement.
——	——	——	22. **Note the amount of any residual. Replace residual back into stomach.**
——	——	——	23. Fold gastric tube over and clamp with fingers. Remove 60-mL syringe. Remove the plunger of the syringe. Reinsert the syringe in the gastric tube without the plunger. Pour 30 mL of water into the syringe. **Unclamp the tube and allow the water to enter the stomach via gravity infusion.**
——	——	——	24. Administer the first dose of medication by pouring into the syringe. Follow with a 5- to 10-mL water flush between medication doses. Follow the last dose of medication with 30 to 60 mL of water flush.
——	——	——	25. Clamp the tube, remove the syringe, and replace the feeding tubing. If stopcock is used, position stopcock to correct direction. If tube medication port was used, cap port. Unclamp gastric tube and restart tube feeding, if appropriate for medications administered.
——	——	——	26. Remove gloves and perform hand hygiene.
——	——	——	27. Assist the patient to a comfortable position. If receiving a tube feeding, the head of the bed must remain elevated at least 30 degrees.
——	——	——	28. Evaluate patient's response to medication within appropriate time frame.

Skill Checklists to Accompany Taylor's Clinical Nursing Skills:
A Nursing Process Approach, 2nd edition

Name _____   Date _____

Unit _____   Position _____

Instructor/Evaluator: _____   Position _____

Excellent	Satisfactory	Needs Practice		
			SKILL 5-26 **Administering a Rectal Suppository**	
			Goal: The medication is administered successfully into the rectum.	**Comments**
——	——	——	1. Gather equipment. Check medication order against the original physician's order according to agency policy. Clarify any inconsistencies. Check the patient's chart for allergies.	
——	——	——	2. Know the actions, special nursing considerations, safe dose ranges, purpose of administration, and adverse effects of the medication to be administered. Consider the appropriateness of the medication for this patient.	
——	——	——	3. Perform hand hygiene.	
——	——	——	4. Move the medication cart to the outside of the patient's room or prepare for administration in the medication area.	
——	——	——	5. Unlock the medication cart or drawer. Enter pass code and scan employee identification, if required.	
——	——	——	6. **Prepare medications for one patient at a time.**	
——	——	——	7. Read the MAR and select the proper medication from the patient's medication drawer or unit stock.	
——	——	——	8. Compare the label with the MAR. Check expiration dates and perform calculations, if necessary. Scan the bar code on the package, if required.	
——	——	——	9. **When all medications for one patient have been prepared, recheck the label with the MAR before taking them to the patient. Lock the medication cart before leaving it.**	
——	——	——	10. Transport medications to the patient's bedside carefully, and keep the medications in sight at all times.	
——	——	——	11. **Ensure that the patient receives the medications at the correct time.**	
——	——	——	12. **Identify the patient.** Usually, the patient should be identified using two methods. Compare information with the MAR or CMAR.	
——	——	——	a. Check the name and identification number on the patient's identification band.	
——	——	——	b. Ask the patient to state his or her name.	

SKILL 5-26

Excellent	Satisfactory	Needs Practice	SKILL 5-26 **Administering a Rectal Suppository** *(Continued)*	Comments
——	——	——	c. If the patient cannot identify him or herself, verify the patient's identification with a staff member who knows the patient for the second source.	
——	——	——	**13. Complete necessary assessments before administering medications. Check allergy bracelet or ask patient about allergies. Explain the purpose and action of each medication to the patient.**	
——	——	——	14. Scan the patient's bar code on the identification band, if required.	
——	——	——	15. Perform hand hygiene and put on gloves.	
——	——	——	16. Assist the patient to his or her left side in a Sims' position. Drape accordingly to only expose the buttocks.	
——	——	——	17. Remove the suppository from its wrapper. Apply lubricant to the rounded end. Lubricate the index finger of your dominant hand.	
——	——	——	18. Separate the buttocks with your nondominant hand and instruct the patient to breathe slowly and deeply through his or her mouth while the suppository is being inserted.	
——	——	——	**19. Using your index finger, insert the suppository, round end first, along the rectal wall. Insert about 3″ to 4″.**	
——	——	——	20. Use toilet tissue to clean any stool or lubricant from around the anus. Release the buttocks. Encourage the patient to remain on his or her side for at least 5 minutes and retain the suppository for the appropriate amount of time for the specific medication.	
——	——	——	21. Remove gloves and perform hand hygiene.	
——	——	——	22. Evaluate patient's response to the procedure and medication.	

Skill Checklists to Accompany Taylor's Clinical Nursing Skills:
A Nursing Process Approach, 2nd edition

Name _____   Date _____

Unit _____   Position _____

Instructor/Evaluator: _____   Position _____

SKILL 6-1
Providing Preoperative Patient Care: Hospitalized Patient

Goal: The patient will proceed to surgery, be free from anxiety and fear, and demonstrate an understanding of the need for surgery and measures to minimize the postoperative risks associated with surgery.

Excellent	Satisfactory	Needs Practice		Comments
___	___	___	1. Check the patient's chart for the type of surgery and review the physician's orders. Review the nursing database, history, and physical examination. Check that the baseline data are recorded; report those that are abnormal.	
___	___	___	2. **Check that diagnostic testing has been completed and results are available; identify and report abnormal results.**	
___	___	___	3. Gather needed equipment and supplies.	
___	___	___	4. Perform hand hygiene.	
___	___	___	5. Identify the patient.	
___	___	___	6. Explore the psychological needs of the patient related to the surgery as well as the family.	
___	___	___	a. Establish the therapeutic relationship, encouraging the patient to verbalize concerns or fears.	
___	___	___	b. Use active learning skills, answering questions and clarifying any misinformation.	
___	___	___	c. Use touch, as appropriate, to convey genuine empathy.	
___	___	___	d. Offer to contact spiritual counselor (priest, minister, rabbi) to meet spiritual needs.	
___	___	___	7. **Identify learning needs of patient and family.** Ensure that the informed consent of the patient for the surgery has been signed, witnessed, and dated. Inquire if the patient has any questions regarding the surgical procedure. Check the patient's record to determine if an advance directive has been completed. If an advance directive has not been completed, discuss with the patient the possibility of completing as appropriate. If patient has had surgery before, ask about this experience.	
___	___	___	8. Provide teaching about deep-breathing exercises.	
___	___	___	a. Assist or ask the patient to sit up (semi-Fowler's position) and instruct the patient to place the palms of both hands along the lower anterior rib cage.	

Providing Preoperative Patient Care: Hospitalized Patient *(Continued)*

Excellent	Satisfactory	Needs Practice		Comments
___	___	___	b. Instruct the patient to exhale gently and completely.	
___	___	___	c. Instruct the patient to breathe in through the nose as deeply as possible and hold breath for 3 seconds.	
___	___	___	d. Instruct the patient to exhale through the mouth, pursing the lips like when whistling.	
___	___	___	e. Have the patient practice the breathing exercise three times. Instruct the patient that this exercise should be performed every 1 to 2 hours for the first 24 hours after surgery.	
___	___	___	9. Conduct teaching regarding coughing and splinting (providing support to the incision).	
___	___	___	a. Ask the patient to sit up (semi-Fowler's position) and apply a folded bath blanket or pillow against the part of the body where the incision will be (eg, abdomen or chest).	
___	___	___	b. Instruct the patient to inhale and exhale through the nose three times.	
___	___	___	c. Ask the patient to take a deep breath and hold it for 3 seconds and then cough out three short breaths.	
___	___	___	d. Ask the patient to take a breath through his/her mouth and strongly cough again two times.	
___	___	___	e. Instruct the patient that he/she should perform these actions every 2 hours when awake after surgery.	
___	___	___	10. Provide teaching regarding incentive spirometer.	
___	___	___	11. Provide teaching regarding leg exercises.	
___	___	___	a. Assist or ask the patient to sit up (semi-Fowler's position) and explain to patient that you will first demonstrate, and then coach him/her to exercise one leg at a time.	
___	___	___	b. Straighten the patient's knee, raise the foot, extend the lower leg and hold this position for a few seconds. Lower the entire leg. Practice this exercise with the other leg.	
___	___	___	c. Assist or ask the patient to point the toes of both legs toward the foot of the bed, then relax them. Next, flex or pull the toes toward the chin.	
___	___	___	d. Assist or ask the patient to keep legs extended and to make circles with both ankles, first circling to the left and then to the right. Instruct the patient to repeat these exercises three times.	

Excellent	Satisfactory	Needs Practice	SKILL 6-1 **Providing Preoperative Patient Care: Hospitalized Patient** (Continued)	Comments
___	___	___	12. Assist the patient in putting on antiembolism stockings and demonstrate how the pneumatic compression device operates.	
___	___	___	13. Provide teaching regarding turning in the bed.	
___	___	___	a. Instruct the patient to use a pillow or bath blanket to splint where the incision will be. Ask the patient to raise his or her left knee and reach across to grasp the right side rail of the bed when he/she is turning toward his or her right side. If patient is turning to his or her left side, he or she will bend the right knee and grasp the left side rail.	
___	___	___	b. When turning the patient onto his or her right side, ask the patient to push with bent left leg and pull on the right side rail. Explain to patient that the nurse will place a pillow behind his/her back to provide support, and that the call bell will be placed within easy reach.	
___	___	___	c. Explain to the patient that position change is recommended every 2 hours.	
___	___	___	14. Provide teaching about pain management.	
___	___	___	a. Discuss past experiences with pain and interventions that the patient has used to reduce pain.	
___	___	___	b. Discuss the availability of analgesic medication postoperatively.	
___	___	___	c. Explore the use of other alternative and nonpharmacologic methods to reduce pain, such as position change, massage, relaxation/diversion, guided imagery, and meditation.	
___	___	___	15. Review equipment.	
___	___	___	a. Show the patient various equipment, such as IV pumps, electronic blood pressure cuff, tubes, and surgical drains.	
___	___	___	16. Provide skin preparation.	
___	___	___	a. **Ask the patient to shower with the antiseptic solution. Remind the patient to carefully clean around the surgical site.**	
___	___	___	b. **For site-specific surgery such as a leg, ask the patient to mark the correct site with a marker.**	
___	___	___	17. Provide teaching about and follow dietary/fluid restrictions.	

Excellent	Satisfactory	Needs Practice	SKILL 6-1 **Providing Preoperative Patient Care:** **Hospitalized Patient** *(Continued)*	
				Comments
——	——	——	a. Explain to the patient that both food and fluid will be restricted before surgery to ensure that the stomach contains a minimal amount of gastric secretions. This restriction is important to reduce the risk of aspiration. Emphasize to the patient the importance of avoiding food and fluids during the prescribed time period, since failure to adhere may necessitate cancellation of the surgery.	
——	——	——	18. Provide intestinal preparation. In certain situations, the bowel will need to be prepared through the administering of enemas or laxatives to evacuate the bowel and to reduce the intestinal bacteria.	
——	——	——	a. As needed, provide explanation of the purpose of enemas or laxatives before surgery. If patient will be administering an enema, clarify the steps as needed.	
——	——	——	19. Check administration of regularly scheduled medications. Review with patient routine medications, OTC, and other herbal supplements that are taken regularly. Check the physician's orders and review with patient which meds he/she will be permitted to take the day of surgery.	
——	——	——	20. Perform hand hygiene.	

Skill Checklists to Accompany Taylor's Clinical Nursing Skills:
A Nursing Process Approach, 2nd edition

Name _____   Date _____

Unit _____   Position _____

Instructor/Evaluator: _____   Position _____

Excellent	Satisfactory	Needs Practice		Comments
			SKILL 6-2 **Providing Preoperative Patient Care: Hospitalized Patient (Day of Surgery)** **Goal:** The patient will proceed to surgery, be free from anxiety and fear, and demonstrate an understanding of the need for surgery and measures to minimize the postoperative risks associated with surgery.	
___ ___ ___			1. Identify the patient.	
___ ___ ___			2. Check that preoperative consent forms are signed, witnessed, and correct, that advance directives are in the medical record (as applicable), and that the patient's chart is in order.	
___ ___ ___			3. Gather the needed equipment and supplies.	
___ ___ ___			4. Perform hand hygiene.	
___ ___ ___			5. **Check vital signs.** Notify physician of any pertinent changes (ie, rise or drop in blood pressure, elevated temperature, cough, symptoms of infection).	
___ ___ ___			6. Provide hygiene and oral care. Assess for loose teeth. **Remind patient of food and fluid restrictions before surgery.**	
___ ___ ___			7. Instruct the patient to remove all personal clothing including underwear and put on a hospital gown.	
___ ___ ___			8. Ask patient to remove cosmetics, jewelry including body-piercing, nail polish, and prostheses (eg, contact lenses, false eyelashes, dentures, and so forth). Some facilities allow a wedding band to be left in place depending on the type of surgery, provided it is secured to the finger with tape.	
___ ___ ___			9. If possible, give valuables to family member or place valuables in appropriate area, such as the hospital safe, if this is not possible. They should not be placed in narcotics drawer.	
___ ___ ___			10. **Have patient empty bladder and bowel before surgery.**	
___ ___ ___			11. Attend to any special preoperative orders, such as starting an IV line.	
___ ___ ___			12. Complete preoperative checklist and record of patient's preoperative preparation.	
___ ___ ___			13. **Administer preoperative medication as prescribed by physician/anesthesia provider.**	

Providing Preoperative Patient Care: Hospitalized Patient (Day of Surgery) *(Continued)*

Excellent	Satisfactory	Needs Practice		Comments
___	___	___	14. Raise side rails of bed; place bed in lowest position. Instruct patient to remain in bed or on stretcher. If necessary, a safety belt may be used.	
___	___	___	15. Help move the patient from the bed to the transport stretcher if necessary. Reconfirm patient identification and ensure that all preoperative events and measures are documented.	
___	___	___	16. Tell the family of the patient where the patient will be taken after surgery and the location of the waiting area where the surgeon will come to explain the outcome of the surgery.	
___	___	___	17. After the patient leaves for the operating room, prepare the room and make a postoperative bed for the patient. Anticipate any necessary equipment based on the type of surgery and the patient's history.	
___	___	___	18. Perform hand hygiene.	

Skill Checklists to Accompany Taylor's Clinical Nursing Skills:
A Nursing Process Approach, 2nd edition

Name _____   Date _____

Unit _____   Position _____

Instructor/Evaluator: _____   Position _____

Excellent	Satisfactory	Needs Practice	SKILL 6-3 **Providing Postoperative Care When Patient Returns to Room**	Comments
			Goal: The patient will recover from the surgery, free of complications.	
			Immediate Care	
——	——	——	1. When patient returns from the PACU, obtain a report from the PACU nurse and review the operating room and PACU data.	
——	——	——	2. Perform hand hygiene.	
——	——	——	3. Identify the patient.	
——	——	——	4. **Place patient in safe position (semi- or high Fowler's or side-lying). Note level of consciousness.**	
——	——	——	5. **Obtain vital signs. Monitor and record vital signs frequently.** Assessment order may vary, but usual frequency includes taking vital signs every 15 minutes the first hour, every 30 minutes the next 2 hours, every hour for 4 hours, and finally every 4 hours.	
——	——	——	6. Provide for warmth, using heated blankets as necessary. Assess skin color and condition.	
——	——	——	7. **Check dressings for color, odor, presence of drains, and amount of drainage. Mark the drainage on the dressing by circulating the amount, and include the time. Assess under the patient for bleeding from the surgical site.**	
——	——	——	8. **Verify that all tubes and drains are patent and equipment is operative; note amount of drainage in collection device. If Foley catheter in place, note urinary output.**	
——	——	——	9. Maintain IV infusion at correct rate.	
——	——	——	10. Provide for a safe environment. Keep bed in low position with side rails up. Have call bell within patient's reach.	
——	——	——	11. Assess for and relieve pain by administering medications ordered by physician. If patient has been instructed in use of PCA for pain management, review use. Check record to verify if analgesic medication was administered in the PACU.	
——	——	——	12. Record assessments and interventions on chart.	

SKILL 6-3
Providing Postoperative Care When Patient Returns to Room *(Continued)*

Excellent	Satisfactory	Needs Practice		Comments

Ongoing Care

13. Promote optimal respiratory function.

    a. Assess respiratory rate, depth, quality, color, and capillary refill. Ask if any difficulty breathing.

    b. Assist with coughing and deep-breathing exercises.

    c. Assist with incentive spirometry.

    d. Assist with early ambulation.

    e. Provide frequent position change.

    f. Administer oxygen as ordered.

    g. Monitor pulse oximetry.

14. Promote optimal cardiovascular function:

    a. Assess apical rate, rhythm, and quality and compare to peripheral pulses, color, and blood pressure. Ask if the patient has any chest pains or shortness of breath.

    b. Provide frequent position changes.

    c. Assist with early ambulation.

    d. Apply antiembolism stockings or pneumatic compression devices, if ordered by physician.

    e. Provide leg and range-of-motion exercises if not contraindicated.

15. Promote optimal neurologic function:

    a. Assess level of consciousness, motor, and sensation.

    b. Determine the level of orientation to person, place, and time.

    c. Test motor ability by asking the patient to move each extremity.

    d. Evaluate sensation by asking the patient if he/she can feel your touch on an extremity.

16. **Promote optimal renal and urinary function and fluid and electrolyte status. Assess intake and output for urinary retention and serum electrolytes.**

    a. Promote voiding by offering bedpan at regular intervals, noting the frequency, amount, and if any burning or urgency symptoms.

    b. Monitor urinary catheter drainage if present.

    c. Measure intake and output.

Providing Postoperative Care When Patient Returns to Room *(Continued)*

Excellent	Satisfactory	Needs Practice		Comments
——	——	——	17. Promote optimal gastrointestinal function and meet nutritional needs:	
——	——	——	a. Assess abdomen for distention and firmness. Ask if patient feels nauseated, any vomiting, and if passing flatus.	
——	——	——	b. Auscultate for bowel sounds.	
——	——	——	c. Assist with diet progression.	
——	——	——	d. Encourage fluid intake.	
——	——	——	e. Monitor intake.	
——	——	——	f. Medicate for nausea and vomiting as ordered by physician.	
——	——	——	18. Promote optimal wound healing.	
——	——	——	a. Assess condition of wound for presence of drains and any drainage.	
——	——	——	b. Use surgical asepsis for dressing changes.	
——	——	——	c. Inspect all skin surfaces for beginning signs of pressure ulcer development and use pressure-relieving supports to minimize potential skin breakdown.	
——	——	——	19. Promote optimal comfort and relief from pain.	
——	——	——	a. Assess for pain (location and intensity using scale).	
——	——	——	b. Provide for rest and comfort.	
——	——	——	c. Administer pain medications as needed or other nonpharmacologic methods.	
——	——	——	20. Promote optimal meeting of psychosocial needs:	
——	——	——	a. Provide emotional support to patient and family as needed.	
——	——	——	b. Explain procedures and offer explanations regarding postoperative recovery as needed to both patient and family members.	

Skill Checklists to Accompany Taylor's Clinical Nursing Skills:
A Nursing Process Approach, 2nd edition

Name _____ Date _____

Unit _____ Position _____

Instructor/Evaluator: _____ Position _____

SKILL 6-4

Applying a Forced-Air Warming Device

Goal: The patient will return to and maintain a temperature of 36.5° to 37.5°C (97.7° to 99.5°F).

Excellent	Satisfactory	Needs Practice		Comments
___	___	___	1. Gather equipment. Check physician's order and explain procedure to patient.	
___	___	___	2. Perform hand hygiene.	
___	___	___	3. Identify the patient.	
___	___	___	4. **Assess patient's temperature, and document.**	
___	___	___	5. Plug forced-air warming device into electrical outlet. Place blanket over patient, with plastic side up. Keep air-hose inlet at foot of bed.	
___	___	___	6. Securely insert air hose into inlet. Place a lightweight fabric blanket over forced-air blanket. Turn machine on and adjust temperature of air to desired effect.	
___	___	___	7. **Monitor patient's temperature at least every 30 minutes while using the forced-air device. If rewarming a patient with hypothermia, do not raise temperature more than 1°C per hour to prevent a rapid vasodilation effect.**	
___	___	___	8. Discontinue use of forced-air device once patient's temperature is adequate and patient can maintain the temperature without assistance.	
___	___	___	9. Remove device and clean according to agency policy and manufacturer's instructions.	
___	___	___	10. Perform hand hygiene.	

Skill Checklists to Accompany Taylor's Clinical Nursing Skills:
A Nursing Process Approach, 2nd edition

Name _____ Date _____

Unit _____ Position _____

Instructor/Evaluator: _____ Position _____

Excellent	Satisfactory	Needs Practice	SKILL 7-1 **Giving a Bed Bath**	Comments
			Goal: The patient will be clean and fresh.	
——	——	——	1. Review chart for any limitations in physical activity. Identify the patient. Discuss procedure with patient and assess patient's ability to assist in the bathing process, as well as personal hygiene preferences.	
——	——	——	2. Bring necessary equipment to the bedside stand or overbed table. Remove sequential compression devices and antiembolism stockings from lower extremities according to agency protocol.	
——	——	——	3. Close curtains around bed and close door to room if possible. Adjust the room temperature if necessary.	
——	——	——	4. Offer patient bedpan or urinal.	
——	——	——	5. Perform hand hygiene.	
——	——	——	6. Raise bed to a comfortable working height.	
——	——	——	7. Lower side rail nearer to you and assist patient to side of bed where you will work. Have patient lie on his or her back.	
——	——	——	8. Loosen top covers and remove all except the top sheet. Place bath blanket over patient and then remove top sheet while patient holds bath blanket in place. If linen is to be reused, fold it over a chair. Place soiled linen in laundry bag. Take care to prevent linen from coming in contact with your clothing.	
——	——	——	9. Remove patient's gown and keep bath blanket in place. If patient has an IV line and is not wearing a gown with snap sleeves, remove gown from other arm first. **Lower the IV container and pass gown over the tubing and the container. Rehang the container and check the drip rate.**	
——	——	——	10. **Raise side rail.** Fill basin with a sufficient amount of comfortably warm water (110°–115°F). Change as necessary throughout the bath. Lower side rail closer to you when you return to the bedside to begin the bath.	
——	——	——	11. Put on gloves, if necessary. Fold the washcloth like a mitt on your hand so that there are no loose ends.	

Excellent	Satisfactory	Needs Practice	SKILL 7-1 **Giving a Bed Bath** *(Continued)*	Comments
――	――	――	12. Lay a towel across patient's chest and on top of bath blanket.	
――	――	――	13. **With no soap on the washcloth, wipe one eye from the inner part of the eye, near the nose, to the outer part. Rinse or turn the cloth before washing the other eye.**	
――	――	――	14. Bathe patient's face, neck, and ears, avoiding soap on the face if the patient prefers. Apply appropriate emollient.	
――	――	――	15. Expose patient's far arm and place towel lengthwise under it. Using firm strokes, wash arm and axilla, lifting the arm as necessary to access axillary region. Rinse, if necessary, and dry. Apply appropriate emollient.	
――	――	――	16. Place a folded towel on the bed next to patient's hand and put basin on it. Soak patient's hand in basin. Wash, rinse, if necessary, and dry hand. Apply appropriate emollient.	
――	――	――	17. Repeat Actions 15 and 16 for the arm nearer you. An option for the shorter nurse or one prone to back strain might be to bathe one side of the patient and move to the other side of the bed to complete the bath.	
――	――	――	18. Spread a towel across patient's chest. Lower bath blanket to patient's umbilical area. Wash, rinse, if necessary, and dry chest. Keep chest covered with towel between the wash and rinse. Pay special attention to skin folds under the breasts.	
――	――	――	19. Lower bath blanket to perineal area. Place a towel over patient's chest.	
――	――	――	20. Wash, rinse, if necessary, and dry abdomen. Carefully inspect and clean umbilical area and any abdominal folds or creases.	
――	――	――	21. Return bath blanket to original position and expose far leg. Place towel under far leg. Using firm strokes, wash, rinse, if necessary, and dry leg from ankle to knee and knee to groin. Apply appropriate emollient.	
――	――	――	22. Fold a towel near patient's foot area and place basin on it. Place foot in basin while supporting the ankle and heel in your hand and the leg on your arm. Wash, rinse, if necessary, and dry, paying particular attention to area between toes. Apply appropriate emollient.	
――	――	――	23. Repeat Actions 21 and 22 for the other leg and foot.	
――	――	――	24. Make sure patient is covered with bath blanket. Change water and washcloth at this point or earlier if necessary.	

			SKILL 7-1

Giving a Bed Bath *(Continued)*

Excellent	Satisfactory	Needs Practice		Comments
—	—	—	25. Assist patient to prone or side-lying position. Put on gloves, if not applied earlier. Position bath blanket and towel to expose only the back and buttocks.	
—	—	—	26. Wash, rinse, if necessary, and dry back and buttocks area. **Pay particular attention to cleansing between gluteal folds, and observe for any redness or skin breakdown in the sacral area.**	
—	—	—	27. If not contraindicated, give patient a backrub. Back massage may be given also after perineal care. Apply appropriate emollient and/or skin-barrier product.	
—	—	—	28. Raise the side rail. Refill basin with clean water. Discard washcloth and towel. Remove gloves and put on clean gloves.	
—	—	—	29. Clean perineal area or set up patient so that he or she can complete perineal self-care. If the patient is unable, lower the side rail and complete perineal care. Raise side rail, remove gloves, and perform hand hygiene.	
—	—	—	30. Help patient put on a clean gown and assist with the use of other personal toiletries, such as deodorant or cosmetics.	
—	—	—	31. Protect pillow with towel and groom patient's hair.	
—	—	—	32. Change bed linens, as described in Skills 7-9 and 7-10. Remove gloves and perform hand hygiene. Dispose of soiled linens according to agency policy.	

Name _____   Date _____

Unit _____   Position _____

Instructor/Evaluator: _____   Position _____

Excellent	Satisfactory	Needs Practice	SKILL 7-2 **Assisting the Patient With Oral Care**	
			Goal: The patient's mouth and teeth will be clean; the patient will exhibit a positive body image; and the patient will verbalize the importance of oral care.	**Comments**
____	____	____	1. Identify the patient. Explain procedure to patient.	
____	____	____	2. Perform hand hygiene. Put on disposable gloves if assisting with oral care.	
____	____	____	3. Assemble equipment on overbed table within patient's reach.	
____	____	____	4. Provide privacy for patient.	
____	____	____	5. Lower side rail and assist patient to sitting position if permitted, or turn patient onto side. Place towel across patient's chest. Raise bed to a comfortable working position.	
____	____	____	6. Encourage patient to brush own teeth, or assist if necessary.	
____	____	____	a. Moisten toothbrush and apply toothpaste to bristles.	
____	____	____	b. Place brush at a 45-degree angle to gum line and brush from gum line to crown of each tooth. Brush outer and inner surfaces. Brush back and forth across biting surface of each tooth.	
____	____	____	c. Brush tongue gently with toothbrush.	
____	____	____	d. Have patient rinse vigorously with water and spit into emesis basin. Repeat until clear. Suction may be used as an alternative for removal of fluid and secretions from mouth.	
____	____	____	7. Assist patient to floss teeth, if appropriate:	
____	____	____	a. Remove approximately 6″ of dental floss from container or use a plastic floss holder. Wrap the floss around the index fingers, keeping about 1″ to 1.5″ of floss taut between the fingers.	
____	____	____	b. Insert floss gently between teeth, moving it back and forth downward to the gums.	
____	____	____	c. Move the floss up and down, first on one side of a tooth and then on the side of the other tooth, until the surfaces are clean. Repeat in the spaces between all teeth.	
____	____	____	d. Instruct patient to rinse mouth well with water after flossing.	

Assisting the Patient With Oral Care *(Continued)*

Excellent	Satisfactory	Needs Practice		Comments
——	——	——	8. Offer mouthwash if patient prefers.	
——	——	——	9. Offer lip balm or petroleum jelly.	
——	——	——	10. Remove equipment. Remove gloves and discard. Raise side rail and lower bed. Assist patient to a position of comfort.	
——	——	——	11. Perform hand hygiene.	

*Skill Checklists to Accompany Taylor's Clinical Nursing Skills:
A Nursing Process Approach, 2nd edition*

Name _____ Date _____

Unit _____ Position _____

Instructor/Evaluator: _____ Position _____

SKILL 7-3
Providing Oral Care for the Dependent Patient

Goal: The patient's mouth and teeth will be clean.

Excellent	Satisfactory	Needs Practice		Comments
___	___	___	1. Identify the patient. Explain procedure to patient.	
___	___	___	2. Perform hand hygiene and put on disposable gloves.	
___	___	___	3. Assemble equipment on overbed table within reach.	
___	___	___	4. Provide privacy for patient. Adjust height of bed to a comfortable position. Lower one side rail and position patient on the side, with head tilted forward. Place towel across patient's chest and emesis basin in position under chin.	
___	___	___	5. Open patient's mouth and gently insert a padded tongue blade between back molars if necessary.	
___	___	___	6. If teeth are present, brush carefully with toothbrush and paste. Remove dentures if present and use a toothette or gauze-padded tongue blade moistened with water or dilute mouthwash solution to gently clean gums, mucous membranes, and tongue. Clean the dentures before replacing (see Skill 7-4).	
___	___	___	7. Use gauze-padded tongue blade or toothette dipped in mouthwash solution to rinse the oral cavity. If desired, insert the rubber tip of the irrigating syringe into patient's mouth and rinse gently with a small amount of water. Position patient's head to allow for return of water or use suction apparatus to remove the water from oral cavity	
___	___	___	8. Apply lubricant to patient's lips.	
___	___	___	9. Remove equipment and return patient to a position of comfort. Remove your gloves. Raise side rail and lower bed.	
___	___	___	10. Perform hand hygiene.	

Skill Checklists to Accompany Taylor's Clinical Nursing Skills:
A Nursing Process Approach, 2nd edition

Name _____   Date _____

Unit _____   Position _____

Instructor/Evaluator: _____   Position _____

SKILL 7-4

Providing Denture Care

Goal: The patient's mouth and dentures will be clean; the patient will exhibit a positive body image; and the patient will verbalize the importance of oral care.

Excellent	Satisfactory	Needs Practice		Comments
⎯	⎯	⎯	1. Identify patient. Explain procedure to patient.	
⎯	⎯	⎯	2. Perform hand hygiene. Put on disposable gloves.	
⎯	⎯	⎯	3. Assemble equipment on overbed table within reach.	
⎯	⎯	⎯	4. Provide privacy for patient.	
⎯	⎯	⎯	5. Lower side rail and assist patient to sitting position if permitted, or turn patient onto side. Place towel across patient's chest. Raise bed to a comfortable working position.	
⎯	⎯	⎯	6. Apply gentle pressure with 4 × 4 gauze to grasp upper denture plate and remove. Place it immediately in denture cup. Lift lower dentures with gauze, using slight rocking motion. Remove, and place in denture cup.	
⎯	⎯	⎯	7. Place paper towels or washcloth in sink while brushing. Using the toothbrush and paste, brush all surfaces gently but thoroughly. If patient prefers, add denture cleaner to cup with water and follow directions on preparation.	
⎯	⎯	⎯	8. Rinse thoroughly with water. Apply denture adhesive if appropriate.	
⎯	⎯	⎯	9. Use a toothbrush or toothette moistened with water or dilute mouthwash solution to gently clean gums, mucous membranes, and tongue. Offer mouthwash so patient can rinse mouth before replacing dentures, if desired.	
⎯	⎯	⎯	10. Insert upper denture in mouth and press firmly. Insert lower denture. Check that the dentures are securely in place and comfortable.	
⎯	⎯	⎯	11. If the patient desires, dentures can be stored in the denture cup in cold water, instead of returning to the mouth. Label the cup and place in the patient's bedside table.	
⎯	⎯	⎯	12. Remove gloves and perform hand hygiene.	

Skill Checklists to Accompany Taylor's Clinical Nursing Skills:
A Nursing Process Approach, 2nd edition

Name _____ Date _____

Unit _____ Position _____

Instructor/Evaluator: _____ Position _____

SKILL 7-5

Removing Contact Lenses

Excellent	Satisfactory	Needs Practice	**Goal:** The lenses are removed without trauma to the eye and stored safely.	Comments
——	——	——	1. Check the patient's identification band and ask the patient to state name, if appropriate.	
——	——	——	2. Explain what you are going to do.	
——	——	——	3. Close curtains around bed and close door to room if possible.	
——	——	——	4. Perform hand hygiene and put on clean gloves.	
——	——	——	5. Assist patient to supine position. Elevate bed. Lower side rail closest to you.	
——	——	——	6. If containers are not already labeled, do so now. Place 5 mL of normal saline in each container.	
——	——	——	7. Remove soft contact lens:	
——	——	——	a. Have the patient look forward. Retract the lower lid with one hand. Using the pad of the index finger of the other hand, move the lens down to the sclera.	
——	——	——	b. Using the pads of the thumb and index finger, grasp the lens with a gentle pinching motion and remove.	
——	——	——	8. Place the first lens in its designated cup in the storage case before removing the second lens.	
——	——	——	9. Repeat actions to remove other contact lens.	
——	——	——	10. If patient is awake and has glasses at bedside, offer patient glasses.	
——	——	——	11. Remove gloves. Perform hand hygiene.	

Skill Checklists to Accompany Taylor's Clinical Nursing Skills:
A Nursing Process Approach, 2nd edition

Name _____ Date _____

Unit _____ Position _____

Instructor/Evaluator: _____ Position _____

			SKILL 7-6 **Shampooing a Patient's Hair in Bed**	
Excellent	**Satisfactory**	**Needs Practice**	**Goal:** The patient's hair will be clean.	**Comments**
____	____	____	1. Identify the patient. Explain procedure to patient.	
____	____	____	2. Assemble equipment on overbed table within reach.	
____	____	____	3. Close the room door or curtain.	
____	____	____	4. Perform hand hygiene. **If you suspect there are any cuts of the scalp or blood in the hair, put on disposable gloves.** Lower head of bed.	
____	____	____	5. Remove pillow and place protective pad under patient's head and shoulders.	
____	____	____	6. **Fill the pitcher with warm water (43°–46°C [110°–115°F]).** Position the patient at the top of the bed, in a supine position. Have the patient lift his head and place shampoo board underneath patient's head. If necessary, pad the edge of the board with a small towel.	
____	____	____	7. Place bucket on floor underneath the drain of the shampoo board.	
____	____	____	8. If the patient is able, have him or her hold a folded washcloth at the forehead. Pour pitcher of warm water slowly over patient's head, making sure that all hair is saturated. Refill pitcher if needed.	
____	____	____	9. Apply a small amount of shampoo to patient's hair. **Massage deep into the scalp, avoiding any cuts, lesions, or sore spots.**	
____	____	____	10. Rinse with warm water (43°–46°C [110°–115°F]) until all shampoo is out of hair. Repeat shampoo if necessary.	
____	____	____	11. If patient has thick hair or requests it, apply a small amount of conditioner to hair and massage throughout. Avoid any cuts, lesions, or sore spots.	
____	____	____	12. If bucket is small, empty before rinsing hair. Rinse with warm water (43°–46°C [110°–115°F]) until all conditioner is out of hair.	
____	____	____	13. Remove shampoo board. Place towel around patient's hair.	

SKILL 7-6
Shampooing a Patient's Hair in Bed *(Continued)*

Excellent	Satisfactory	Needs Practice		Comments
——	——	——	14. Pat hair dry, avoiding any cuts, lesions, or sore spots. Remove protective padding but keep one dry protective pad under patient's hair.	
——	——	——	15. Gently brush hair, removing tangles as needed.	
——	——	——	16. Blow-dry hair on a cool setting if allowed and if patient wishes.	
——	——	——	17. Change patient's gown and remove protective pad. Replace pillow.	
——	——	——	18. Remove gloves. Perform hand hygiene.	

Skill Checklists to Accompany Taylor's Clinical Nursing Skills:
A Nursing Process Approach, 2nd edition

Name _____   Date _____

Unit _____   Position _____

Instructor/Evaluator: _____   Position _____

Excellent	Satisfactory	Needs Practice	SKILL 7-7 **Assisting the Patient to Shave**	
			Goal: The patient will be clean, without evidence of hair growth or trauma to the skin.	**Comments**
___	___	___	1. Identify patient. Explain procedure to patient.	
___	___	___	2. Assemble equipment on overbed table within reach.	
___	___	___	3. Close the room door or curtain.	
___	___	___	4. Perform hand hygiene and put on disposable gloves.	
___	___	___	5. Cover patient's chest with a towel or waterproof pad. Fill bath basin with warm (43°–46°C [110°–115°F]) water. Moisten the area to be shaved with a washcloth.	
___	___	___	6. Dispense shaving cream into palm of hand. Rub hands together, then apply to area to be shaved in a layer about 0.5″ thick.	
___	___	___	7. With one hand, pull the skin taut at the area to be shaved. Using a smooth stroke, begin shaving. *If shaving the face,* shave with the direction of hair growth in downward, short strokes. *If shaving a leg,* shave against the hair in upward, short strokes.	
___	___	___	8. Wash off residual shaving cream.	
___	___	___	9. If patient requests, apply aftershave or lotion to area shaved.	
___	___	___	10. Remove and discard gloves and perform hand hygiene.	

Name _____   Date _____

Unit _____   Position _____

Instructor/Evaluator: _____   Position _____

SKILL 7-8
Applying and Removing Antiembolism Stockings

Goal: The stockings will be applied and removed with minimal discomfort to patient.

Excellent	Satisfactory	Needs Practice		Comments
——	——	——	1. Check the patient's identification band and ask the patient to state name, if appropriate.	
——	——	——	2. Explain what you are going to do and the rationale for use of elastic stockings.	
——	——	——	3. Close curtains around bed and close door to room if possible.	
——	——	——	4. Perform hand hygiene.	
——	——	——	5. Assist patient to supine position. If patient has been sitting or walking, have him or her lie down with legs and feet well elevated for at least 15 minutes before applying stockings.	
——	——	——	6. Expose legs one at a time. Wash and dry legs, if necessary. Powder the leg lightly unless patient has a breathing problem, dry skin, or sensitivity to the powder. If the skin is dry, a lotion may be used. Powders and lotions are not recommended by some manufacturers; check the package material for manufacturer specifications.	
——	——	——	7. Stand at the foot of the bed. Place hand inside stocking and grasp heel area securely. Turn stocking inside-out to the heel area, leaving the foot inside the stocking leg.	
——	——	——	8. With the heel pocket down, ease the foot of stocking over foot and heel. Check that patient's heel is centered in heel pocket of stocking.	
——	——	——	9. Using your fingers and thumbs, carefully grasp edge of stocking and pull it up smoothly over ankle and calf, toward the knee. Make sure it is distributed evenly.	
——	——	——	10. Pull forward slightly on toe section. If the stocking has a toe window, make sure it is properly positioned. Adjust if necessary to ensure material is smooth.	
——	——	——	11. If the stockings are knee-length, make sure each stocking top is 1″–2″ below the patella. Make sure the stocking does not roll down.	
——	——	——	12. If applying thigh-length stocking, continue the application. Flex the patient's leg. Stretch the stocking over the knee.	

Applying and Removing
Antiembolism Stockings *(Continued)*

Excellent	Satisfactory	Needs Practice		Comments
——	——	——	13. Pull the stocking over the thigh until the top is 1–3 inches below the gluteal fold. Adjust the stocking as necessary to distribute the fabric evenly. Make sure the stocking does not roll down.	
——	——	——	14. Perform hand hygiene.	
			Removing Stockings	
——	——	——	15. To remove stocking, grasp top of stocking with your thumb and fingers and smoothly pull stocking off inside-out to heel. Support foot and ease stocking over it.	

Skill Checklists to Accompany Taylor's Clinical Nursing Skills:
A Nursing Process Approach, 2nd edition

Name _____   Date _____

Unit _____   Position _____

Instructor/Evaluator: _____   Position _____

Excellent	Satisfactory	Needs Practice	SKILL 7-9 **Making an Unoccupied Bed**	Comments
			Goal: The bed linens will be changed without injury to the nurse or patient.	
——	——	——	1. Assemble equipment and arrange on a bedside chair in the order in which items will be used.	
——	——	——	2. Perform hand hygiene.	
——	——	——	3. Adjust bed to high position and drop side rails.	
——	——	——	4. Disconnect call bell or any tubes from bed linens.	
——	——	——	5. Put on gloves if linens are soiled. Loosen all linen as you move around the bed, from the head of the bed on the far side to the head of the bed on the near side.	
——	——	——	6. Fold reusable linens, such as sheets, blankets, or spread, in place on the bed in fourths and hang them over a clean chair.	
——	——	——	7. **Snugly roll all the soiled linen inside the bottom sheet and place directly into the laundry hamper. Do not place on floor or furniture. Do not hold soiled linens against your uniform.**	
——	——	——	8. If possible, shift mattress up to head of bed. If mattress is soiled, clean and dry according to facility policy before applying new sheets.	
——	——	——	9. Remove your gloves. Place the bottom sheet with its center fold in the center of the bed. Open the sheet and fan-fold to the center.	
——	——	——	10. If using, place the drawsheet with its center fold in the center of the bed and positioned so it will be located under the patient's midsection. Open the drawsheet and fan-fold to the center of the mattress. If a protective pad is used, place it over the drawsheet in the proper area and open to the centerfold. Not all agencies use drawsheets routinely. The nurse may decide to use one.	
——	——	——	11. Pull the bottom sheet over the corners at the head and foot of the mattress. Tuck the drawsheet securely under the mattress.	

Making an Unoccupied Bed *(Continued)*

Excellent	Satisfactory	Needs Practice		Comments
___	___	___	12. Move to the other side of the bed to secure bottom linens. Pull the bottom sheet tightly and secure over the corners at the head and foot of the mattress. Pull the drawsheet tightly and tuck it securely under the mattress.	
___	___	___	13. Place the top sheet on the bed with its center fold in the center of the bed and with the hem even with the head of the mattress. Unfold the top sheet. Follow same procedure with top blanket or spread, placing the upper edge about 6″ below the top of the sheet.	
___	___	___	14. Tuck the top sheet and blanket under the foot of the bed on the near side. Miter the corners.	
___	___	___	15. Fold the upper 6″ of the top sheet down over the spread and make a cuff.	
___	___	___	16. Move to the other side of the bed and follow the same procedure for securing top sheets under the foot of the bed and making a cuff.	
___	___	___	17. Place the pillows on the bed. Open each pillowcase in the same manner as you opened other linens. Gather the pillowcase over one hand toward the closed end. Grasp the pillow with the hand inside the pillowcase. Keep a firm hold on the top of the pillow and pull the cover onto the pillow. Place the pillow at the head of the bed.	
___	___	___	18. Fan-fold or pie-fold the top linens.	
___	___	___	19. **Secure the signal device on the bed according to agency policy.**	
___	___	___	20. **Adjust bed to low position.**	
___	___	___	21. Dispose of soiled linen according to agency policy. Perform hand hygiene.	

Skill Checklists to Accompany Taylor's Clinical Nursing Skills:
A Nursing Process Approach, 2nd edition

Name _____   Date _____

Unit _____   Position _____

Instructor/Evaluator: _____   Position _____

SKILL 7-10

Making an Occupied Bed

Goal: The bed linens are applied without injury to the patient or nurse.

Excellent	Satisfactory	Needs Practice		Comments
----	----	----	1. Identify patient. Explain procedure to patient. Check chart for limitations on patient's physical activity.	
----	----	----	2. Perform hand hygiene.	
----	----	----	3. Assemble equipment and arrange on bedside chair in the order the items will be used.	
----	----	----	4. Close door or curtain.	
----	----	----	5. Adjust bed to high position. Lower side rail nearest you, leaving the opposite side rail up. Place bed in flat position unless contraindicated.	
----	----	----	6. Check bed linens for patient's personal items. **Disconnect the call bell or any tubes/drains from bed linens.**	
----	----	----	7. Put on gloves if linens are soiled. Place a bath blanket over patient. Have patient hold onto bath blanket while you reach under it and remove top linens. Leave top sheet in place if a bath blanket is not used. Fold linen that is to be reused over the back of a chair. Discard soiled linen in laundry bag or hamper. Keep soiled linen away from uniform.	
----	----	----	8. If possible and another person is available to assist, grasp mattress securely and shift it up to head of bed.	
----	----	----	9. Assist patient to turn toward opposite side of the bed, and reposition pillow under patient's head.	
----	----	----	10. Loosen all bottom linens from head, foot, and side of bed.	
----	----	----	11. Fan-fold soiled linens as close to patient as possible.	
----	----	----	12. Remove your gloves, if used. Use clean linen and make the near side of the bed. Place the bottom sheet with its center fold in the center of the bed. Open the sheet and fan-fold to the center, positioning it under the old linens. Pull the bottom sheet over the corners at the head and foot of the mattress.	

Making an Occupied Bed *(Continued)*

Excellent	Satisfactory	Needs Practice		Comments
____	____	____	13. If using, place the drawsheet with its center fold in the center of the bed and positioned so it will be located under the patient's midsection. Open the drawsheet and fan-fold to the center of the mattress. Tuck the drawsheet securely under the mattress. If a protective pad is used, place it over the drawsheet in the proper area and open to the centerfold. Not all agencies use drawsheets routinely. The nurse may decide to use one.	
____	____	____	14. Raise side rail. Assist patient to roll over the folded linen in the middle of the bed toward you. Reposition pillow and bath blanket or top sheet. Move to other side of the bed and lower side rail.	
____	____	____	15. Put on clean gloves, if linen is soiled. Loosen and remove all bottom linen. Place in linen bag or hamper. Hold soiled linen away from your uniform. Remove gloves, if used.	
____	____	____	16. Ease clean linen from under patient. Pull the bottom sheet taut and secure at the corners at the head and foot of the mattress. Pull the drawsheet tight and smooth. Tuck the drawsheet securely under the mattress.	
____	____	____	17. Assist patient to turn back to the center of bed. If pillowcase is soiled with blood or body fluids, put on unsterile gloves. Remove pillow and change pillowcase. Open each pillowcase in the same manner as you opened other linens. Gather the pillowcase over one hand toward the closed end. Grasp the pillow with the hand inside the pillowcase. Keep a firm hold on the top of the pillow and pull the cover onto the pillow. Place the pillow under the patient's head. Remove gloves, if worn.	
____	____	____	18. Apply top linen, sheet and blanket if desired, so that it is centered. Fold the top linens over at the patient's shoulders to make a cuff. Have patient hold onto top linen and remove the bath blanket from underneath.	
____	____	____	19. Secure top linens under foot of mattress and miter corners. Loosen top linens over patient's feet by grasping them in the area of the feet and pulling gently toward foot of bed.	
____	____	____	20. **Raise side rail. Lower bed height and adjust head of bed to a comfortable position. Reattach call bell.**	
____	____	____	21. Dispose of soiled linens according to agency policy. Perform hand hygiene.	

Skill Checklists to Accompany Taylor's Clinical Nursing Skills:
A Nursing Process Approach, 2nd edition

Name _____ Date _____

Unit _____ Position _____

Instructor/Evaluator: _____ Position _____

Excellent	Satisfactory	Needs Practice	SKILL 8-1 **Cleaning a Wound and Applying a Dry, Sterile Dressing**	Comments
			Goal: The wound is cleaned and protected with a dressing without contaminating the wound area, without causing trauma to the wound, and without causing the patient to experience pain or discomfort.	
——	——	——	1. Review the physician's order for wound care or the nursing plan of care related to wound care.	
——	——	——	2. Gather the necessary supplies.	
——	——	——	3. Identify the patient.	
——	——	——	4. Explain the procedure to the patient.	
			5. Assess the patient for possible need for nonpharmacologic pain-reducing interventions or analgesic medication before wound care dressing change. Administer appropriate analgesic, consulting physician's orders, and allow enough time for analgesic to achieve its effectiveness.	
——	——	——	6. Perform hand hygiene.	
——	——	——	7. Close the room door or curtains. Place the bed at an appropriate and comfortable working height.	
——	——	——	8. Place a waste receptacle or bag at a convenient location for use during the procedure.	
——	——	——	9. Assist the patient to a comfortable position that provides easy access to the wound area. Use the bath blanket to cover any exposed area other than the wound. If necessary, place the waterproof pad under the wound site.	
——	——	——	10. Check the position of drains, tubes, or other adjuncts before removing the dressing. Put on clean, disposable gloves and loosen tape on the old dressings. If necessary, use an adhesive remover to help get the tape off.	
——	——	——	11. Carefully remove the soiled dressings. If any part of the dressing sticks to the underlying skin, use small amounts of sterile saline to help loosen and remove. Do not reach over the wound.	
——	——	——	12. After removing the dressing, note the presence, amount, type, color, and odor of any drainage on the dressings. Place soiled dressings in the appropriate waste receptacle. Remove your gloves and dispose of them in an appropriate waste receptacle.	

Excellent

Satisfactory

Needs Practice

SKILL 8-1
Cleaning a Wound and Applying a Dry, Sterile Dressing *(Continued)*

				Comments
Excellent	Satisfactory	Needs Practice		
___	___	___	13. Inspect the wound site for size, appearance, and drainage. Assess if any pain is present. Check the sutures, Steri-Strips, staples, and drains or tubes. Note any problems to include in your documentation.	
___	___	___	14. **Using sterile technique, prepare a sterile work area and open the needed supplies.**	
___	___	___	15. Open the sterile cleaning solution. Depending on the amount of cleaning needed, the solution might be poured directly over gauze sponges over a container for small cleaning jobs, or into a basin for more complex or larger cleaning.	
___	___	___	16. Put on sterile gloves.	
___	___	___	17. Clean the wound. If needed, use sterile forceps to clean the area. **Clean the wound from top to bottom and from the center to the outside. Following this pattern, use a new gauze for each wipe, placing the used gauze in the waste receptacle. Do not touch any surface with the gloves or forceps.**	
___	___	___	18. **If a drain is in use, clean around the drain using a circular motion. Wipe from the center toward the outside. Use the gauze a single time and then dispose of it.**	
___	___	___	19. Once the wound is cleaned, dry the area using a gauze sponge in the same manner. Apply ointment or any other treatments if ordered.	
___	___	___	20. Apply a layer of dry sterile dressing over the wound. Forceps may be used to apply the dressing.	
___	___	___	21. Place a second layer of gauze over the wound site.	
___	___	___	22. Apply a Surgi-pad or ABD dressing over the gauze at the site as the outermost layer of the dressing.	
___	___	___	23. Remove and discard sterile gloves. Apply tape or tie tapes to secure the dressings.	
___	___	___	24. After securing the dressing, label dressing with date and time. Remove all remaining equipment, place the patient in a comfortable position. with side rails up and bed in the lowest position. Perform hand hygiene.	
___	___	___	25. Check all wound dressings every shift. More frequent checks may be needed if the wound is more complex or dressings become saturated quickly.	

Skill Checklists to Accompany Taylor's Clinical Nursing Skills:
A Nursing Process Approach, 2nd edition

Name _____   Date _____

Unit _____   Position _____

Instructor/Evaluator: _____   Position _____

Excellent	Satisfactory	Needs Practice	SKILL 8-2 **Applying a Saline-Moistened Dressing** **Goal:** The procedure is accomplished without contaminating the wound area, without causing trauma to the wound, and without causing the patient to experience pain or discomfort.	Comments
——	——	——	1. Review the physician's order and/or nursing plan of care for the application of a saline-moistened dressing.	
——	——	——	2. Gather the necessary supplies.	
——	——	——	3. Identify the patient.	
——	——	——	4. Explain the procedure to the patient.	
——	——	——	5. Assess the patient for possible need for non-pharmacologic pain-reducing interventions or analgesic medication before wound care dressing change. Administer appropriate analgesic, consulting physician's orders, and allow enough time for analgesic to achieve its effectiveness before beginning procedure.	
——	——	——	6. Perform hand hygiene.	
——	——	——	7. Close the room door or curtains. Place the bed at a comfortable working height.	
——	——	——	8. Place a waste receptacle or bag at a convenient location for use during procedure.	
——	——	——	9. Assist the patient to a comfortable position that provides easy access to the wound area. Position the patient so the irrigation solution will flow from the clean end of the wound toward the dirtier end, if wound irrigation is necessary (See Skill 8-4 for irrigation techniques). Expose the area and drape the patient with the bath blanket if needed. Put the waterproof pad under the wound area to protect the bed.	
——	——	——	10. Put on personal protective equipment as appropriate.	
——	——	——	11. Put on clean disposable gloves and gently remove the soiled dressings. If the dressing adheres to the underlying tissues, moisten it with saline to loosen it.	
——	——	——	12. After removing the dressing, note the presence, amount, type, color, and odor of any drainage on the dressings. Place soiled dressings in the appropriate waste receptacle.	

Excellent	Satisfactory	Needs Practice	SKILL 8-2 **Applying a Saline-Moistened Dressing** *(Continued)*	
				Comments
____	____	____	13. Assess the wound for appearance, stage, the presence of eschar, granulation tissue, epithelialization, undermining, tunneling, necrosis, sinus tract, and drainage. Assess the appearance of the surrounding tissue. Measure the wound.	
____	____	____	14. Remove your gloves and put them in the receptacle.	
____	____	____	15. Using sterile technique, open the supplies and dressings. Place the fine-mesh gauze into the basin and pour the ordered solution over the mesh to saturate it.	
____	____	____	16. Put on the sterile gloves.	
____	____	____	17. Clean the wound. If needed, use sterile forceps to clean the area. **Clean the wound from top to bottom and from the center to the outside. Following this pattern, use a new gauze for each wipe, placing the used gauze in the waste receptacle. Do not touch any surface with the gloves or forceps.** Irrigate the wound, if needed (see Skill 8-4).	
____	____	____	18. Dry the surrounding skin with sterile gauze dressings.	
____	____	____	19. Squeeze excess fluid from the gauze dressing. Unfold and fluff the dressing.	
____	____	____	20. Gently press to loosely pack the moistened gauze into the wound. If necessary, use the forceps or cotton-tipped applicators to press the gauze into all wound surfaces.	
____	____	____	21. Apply several dry, sterile gauze pads over the wet gauze.	
____	____	____	22. Place the ABD pad over the gauze.	
____	____	____	23. Remove and discard your sterile gloves. Apply a skin protectant to the surrounding skin if needed. Apply tape or tie tapes to secure the dressings.	
____	____	____	24. After securing the dressing, remove all remaining equipment, place the patient in a position of comfort, with side rails up and the bed in the lowest position, and perform hand hygiene.	
____	____	____	25. Check all wound dressings every shift. You might need to check more frequently if a wound is more complex or dressings become saturated more frequently.	

Skill Checklists to Accompany Taylor's Clinical Nursing Skills:
A Nursing Process Approach, 2nd edition

Name _____ Date _____

Unit _____ Position _____

Instructor/Evaluator: _____ Position _____

SKILL 8-3
Applying a Hydrocolloid Dressing

Goal: The procedure is accomplished without contaminating the wound area, without causing trauma to the wound, and without causing the patient to experience pain or discomfort.

Excellent	Satisfactory	Needs Practice		Comments
——	——	——	1. Review the physician's order and/or nursing plan of care for the application of a hydrocolloid dressing.	
——	——	——	2. Gather the necessary supplies.	
——	——	——	3. Identify the patient.	
——	——	——	4. Explain the procedure to the patient.	
——	——	——	5. Assess the patient for possible need for nonpharmacologic pain-reducing interventions or analgesic medication before wound care dressing change. Administer appropriate analgesic, consulting physician's orders, and allow enough time for analgesic to achieve its effectiveness before beginning procedure.	
——	——	——	6. Perform hand hygiene.	
——	——	——	7. Close the room door or curtains. Place the bed at a comfortable working height.	
——	——	——	8. Have the disposal bag or waste receptacle within easy reach.	
——	——	——	9. Assist the patient to a comfortable position that provides easy access to the wound area. Position the patient so the irrigation solution will flow from the cleanest to the dirtiest end of the wound, if necessary. Expose the area and drape the patient with the bath blanket if needed. Put the waterproof pad under the wound area to protect the bed.	
——	——	——	10. Put on personal protective equipment as appropriate.	
——	——	——	11. Put on clean disposable gloves and gently remove the soiled dressing. Discard it in the receptacle.	
——	——	——	12. Assess the wound for appearance, stage, granulation tissue, epithelialization, undermining, tunneling, necrosis, sinus tract, and drainage. Assess the appearance of the surrounding tissue. Measure the wound if needed.	
——	——	——	13. Remove your gloves and put them in the receptacle.	
——	——	——	14. Set up a sterile field and put on the sterile gloves if indicated.	

SKILL 8-3
Applying a Hydrocolloid Dressing *(Continued)*

Excellent	Satisfactory	Needs Practice		Comments
___	___	___	15. Clean the wound. If needed, use sterile forceps to clean the area. **Clean the wound from top to bottom and from the center to the outside. Following this pattern, use a new gauze for each wipe, placing the used gauze in the waste receptacle. Do not touch any surface with the gloves or forceps.** Irrigate the wound, if appropriate (see Skill 8-4).	
___	___	___	16. Dry the surrounding skin with sterile gauze dressings.	
___	___	___	17. Choose a clean, dry, presized dressing or cut one to size using sterile scissors. The dressing must be sized generously, allowing at least a 1″ margin of healthy skin around the wound to be covered with the dressing.	
___	___	___	18. Remove the release paper from the adherent side of the dressing. Apply the dressing to the wound without stretching the dressing. Smooth wrinkles as it is applied.	
___	___	___	19. Apply a skin protectant to the skin surrounding the wound if needed. If necessary, secure the dressing edges with tape. Dressings that are near the anus need to have the edges taped. Apply additional skin barrier to the areas to be covered with tape, if necessary.	
___	___	___	20. Remove and discard your sterile gloves.	
___	___	___	21. Remove all remaining equipment, place the patient in a position of comfort with side rails up and the bed in the lowest position, and perform hand hygiene.	
___	___	___	22. Check all wound dressings every shift to validate that they are intact.	

Skill Checklists to Accompany Taylor's Clinical Nursing Skills:
A Nursing Process Approach, 2nd edition

Name _____ Date _____

Unit _____ Position _____

Instructor/Evaluator: _____ Position _____

Excellent	Satisfactory	Needs Practice	SKILL 8-4 **Performing a Sterile Irrigation of a Wound**	Comments
			Goal: The wound is cleaned without contamination or trauma and without causing the patient to experience pain or discomfort.	
___	___	___	1. Review the physician's order for wound care or the nursing plan of care related to wound care.	
___	___	___	2. Gather the necessary supplies.	
___	___	___	3. Identify the patient.	
___	___	___	4. Explain the procedure to the patient.	
___	___	___	5. Assess the patient for possible need for nonpharmacologic pain-reducing interventions or analgesic medication before wound care dressing change. Administer appropriate analgesic, consulting physician's orders, and allow enough time for analgesic to achieve its effectiveness.	
___	___	___	6. Perform hand hygiene.	
___	___	___	7. Close the room door or curtains. Place the bed at a comfortable working height.	
___	___	___	8. Have the disposal bag or waste receptacle within easy reach prior to the irrigation for soiled dressing disposal.	
___	___	___	9. Assist the patient to a comfortable position that provides easy access to the wound area. **Position the patient so that the irrigation solution will flow from the clean to dirty end of the wound.** Expose the area and drape the patient with a bath blanket if needed. Put the waterproof pad under the wound area.	
___	___	___	10. Put on a gown, mask, and eye protection.	
___	___	___	11. Put on clean disposable gloves and remove the soiled dressings.	
___	___	___	12. Assess the wound for size, appearance, and drainage on the dressing. Assess the appearance of the surrounding tissue.	
___	___	___	13. Discard the dressings in the receptacle. Remove gloves and put them in the receptacle.	
___	___	___	14. **Using sterile technique, prepare a sterile field and add all the sterile supplies needed for the procedure to the field. Pour warmed sterile irrigating solution into the sterile container.**	
___	___	___	15. Put on sterile gloves.	

Performing a Sterile Irrigation of a Wound (Continued)

Excellent	Satisfactory	Needs Practice		Comments
——	——	——	16. Position the sterile basin below the wound to collect the irrigation fluid.	
——	——	——	17. Fill the irrigation syringe with solution. **Using your nondominant hand, gently apply pressure to the basin against the skin below the wound to form a seal with the skin.**	
——	——	——	18. **Gently direct a stream of solution into the wound. Keep the tip of the syringe at least 1″ above the upper tip of the wound. When using a catheter tip, insert it gently into the wound until it meets resistance. Gently flush all wound areas.**	
——	——	——	19. Watch for the solution to flow smoothly and evenly. When the solution from the wound flows out clear, discontinue irrigation.	
——	——	——	20. Dry the surrounding skin with a sterile gauze sponge.	
——	——	——	21. Apply a new sterile dressing to the wound (see Skill 8-1).	
——	——	——	22. Remove gloves and dispose of them properly. Apply a skin protectant to the surrounding skin if needed. Apply tie straps or tape as needed to secure the dressing. Remove other protective equipment and dispose in bedside waste receptacle container or bag.	
——	——	——	23. Return the bed to the lowest position while making the patient comfortable and raising the side rails as needed.	
——	——	——	24. Remove any remaining personal protective equipment and the waste receptacle out of the patient's room and dispose of it properly. If any irrigating solution remains in the bottle, recap the bottle and note on the bottle the date and time it was opened.	
——	——	——	25. Perform hand hygiene.	
——	——	——	26. Check all wound dressings every shift. You might need to check more frequently if a wound is more complex or dressings become saturated more frequently.	

Skill Checklists to Accompany Taylor's Clinical Nursing Skills:
A Nursing Process Approach, 2nd edition

Name _____ Date _____

Unit _____ Position _____

Instructor/Evaluator: _____ Position _____

Excellent	Satisfactory	Needs Practice	SKILL 8-5 **Collecting a Wound Culture**	Comments
			Goal: The culture is obtained without evidence of contamination, without exposing the patient to additional pathogens, and without causing discomfort for the patient.	
——	——	——	1. Review the physician's order for obtaining a wound culture.	
——	——	——	2. Gather the necessary supplies.	
——	——	——	3. Identify the patient.	
——	——	——	4. Explain the procedure to the patient.	
——	——	——	5. Perform hand hygiene.	
——	——	——	6. Close the room door or curtains. Place the bed at an appropriate and comfortable working height.	
——	——	——	7. Place an appropriate waste receptacle within easy reach for use during the procedure.	
——	——	——	8. Assist the patient to a comfortable position that provides easy access to the wound. If necessary, drape the patient with the bath blanket to expose only the wound area. Check the culture label again against the patient's identification bracelet.	
——	——	——	9. Put on the clean, disposable gloves to remove any dressings. Loosen the tape and old dressings. Do not reach over the wound. Remove the dressing and dispose of it in the receptacle. Assess the wound and the characteristics of any drainage. Remove gloves and dispose of them.	
——	——	——	10. Set up sterile field with supplies if necessary. Put on sterile gloves and clean the wound according to facility policies and procedures. Remove the sterile gloves.	
——	——	——	11. Put on clean gloves. Twist the cap to loosen the swab on the Culturette tube, or open the separate swab and remove the cap from the culture tube. **Keep the swab and inside of the culture tube sterile.**	
——	——	——	12. Put on a clean glove or new sterile glove, if necessary.	
——	——	——	13. **Carefully insert the swab into the wound and gently roll the swab to obtain a sample. Use another swab if collecting a specimen from another site.**	

Collecting a Wound Culture *(Continued)*

Excellent	Satisfactory	Needs Practice		Comments
——	——	——	14. Place the swab back in the culture tube. **Do not touch the outside of the tube with the swab.** Secure the cap. Some Culturette tubes have an ampule of medium at the bottom of the tube. It might be necessary to crush this ampule to activate. Follow the manufacturer's instructions for use.	
——	——	——	15. Remove gloves and discard them accordingly.	
——	——	——	16. Put on sterile gloves and replace the dressing as needed following the appropriate procedure.	
——	——	——	17. Remove gloves and perform hand hygiene. Remove any equipment and leave the patient comfortable, with the side rails up and the bed in the lowest position.	
——	——	——	18. Label the specimen according to your institution's guidelines and send it to the laboratory in a biohazard bag.	

Name _____   Date _____

Unit _____   Position _____

Instructor/Evaluator: _____   Position _____

Excellent	Satisfactory	Needs Practice	SKILL 8-6 **Applying Montgomery Straps**	Comments
			Goal: The patient's skin is free from irritation and injury.	
___	___	___	1. Review the physician's order for wound care or the nursing plan of care related to wound care.	
___	___	___	2. Gather the necessary supplies.	
___	___	___	3. Identify the patient.	
___	___	___	4. Explain the procedure to the patient.	
___	___	___	5. Assess the patient for possible need for nonpharmacologic pain-reducing interventions or analgesic medication before wound care dressing change. Administer appropriate analgesic, consulting physician's orders, and allow enough time for analgesic to achieve its effectiveness before beginning procedure.	
___	___	___	6. Perform hand hygiene.	
___	___	___	7. Close the room door or curtains. Place the bed at an appropriate and comfortable working height.	
___	___	___	8. Place a waste receptacle at a convenient location for use during the procedure.	
___	___	___	9. Assist the patient to a comfortable position that provides easy access to the wound area. Use a bath blanket to cover any exposed area other than the wound. If necessary, place a waterproof pad under the wound site.	
___	___	___	10. Perform wound care and a dressing change as outlined in Skill 8-1, as ordered.	
___	___	___	11. If ready-made straps are not available, cut four to six strips of tape long enough to extend about 6″ beyond the wound. The number of strips will depend on the size of the wound and dressing.	
___	___	___	12. Fold one end of each strip 2″ to 3″ back on itself, sticky sides together, to form a nonadhesive tab. Cut a small hole in the folded tab's center, close to the top edge. Make as many pairs of straps as necessary to secure the dressing.	
___	___	___	13. Put on clean gloves. Clean the skin on either side of the wound with the gauze, moistened with normal saline. Dry the skin.	

Excellent	Satisfactory	Needs Practice	SKILL 8-6 **Applying Montgomery Straps** *(Continued)*	
				Comments
——	——	——	14. **Apply a skin protectant to the skin where the straps will be placed.**	
——	——	——	15. Remove gloves.	
——	——	——	16. Apply the sticky side of each tape or strap to a skin barrier sheet. Apply the sheet directly to the skin near the dressing. Repeat for the other side.	
——	——	——	17. Thread a separate string through each pair of holes in the straps. Tie one end of the string in the hole. Fasten the other end with the opposing tie, like a shoelace. **Do not secure too tightly.** Repeat according to the number of straps needed. If commercially prepared straps are used, tie strings like a shoelace. Note date and time of application on strap.	
——	——	——	18. Return the bed to the lowest position while making the patient comfortable and raising the side rails as needed.	
——	——	——	19. Perform hand hygiene.	
——	——	——	20. Replace the ties and straps whenever they are soiled, or every 2 to 3 days.	

Skill Checklists to Accompany Taylor's Clinical Nursing Skills:
A Nursing Process Approach, 2nd edition

Name _____ Date _____

Unit _____ Position _____

Instructor/Evaluator: _____ Position _____

Excellent	Satisfactory	Needs Practice	SKILL 8-7 **Caring for a Penrose Drain**	
			Goal: The Penrose drain remains patent and intact.	**Comments**
____	____	____	1. Review the physician's order for drain and site care or the nursing plan of care related to drain care.	
____	____	____	2. Gather the necessary supplies.	
____	____	____	3. Identify the patient.	
____	____	____	4. Explain the procedure to the patient.	
____	____	____	5. Assess the patient for possible need for nonpharmalogic pain-reducing interventions or analgesic medication before wound care dressing change. Administer appropriate analgesic, consulting physician's orders, and allow enough time for analgesic to achieve its effectiveness.	
____	____	____	6. Perform hand hygiene.	
____	____	____	7. Close the room door or curtains. Place the bed at an appropriate and comfortable working height.	
____	____	____	8. Place a waste receptacle at a convenient location for use during the procedure.	
____	____	____	9. Assist the patient to a comfortable position that provides easy access to the drain area. Use the bath blanket to cover any exposed area other than the drain. If necessary, place the waterproof pad under the drain site.	
____	____	____	10. Check the position of the drain or drains before removing the dressing. Put on clean, disposable gloves and loosen tape on the old dressings. Use an adhesive remover to help get the tape off, if necessary.	
____	____	____	11. **Carefully remove the soiled dressings.** If any part of the dressing sticks to the underlying skin, use small amounts of sterile saline to help loosen and remove it. Do not reach over the drain site.	
____	____	____	12. After removing the dressing, note the presence, amount, type, color, and odor of any drainage on the dressings. Place soiled dressings in the appropriate waste receptacle. Remove gloves and dispose of them in the appropriate waste receptacle.	

SKILL 8-7
Caring for a Penrose Drain *(Continued)*

Excellent	Satisfactory	Needs Practice		Comments
——	——	——	13. Inspect the drain site for appearance and drainage. Assess if any pain is present. **Closely observe the safety pin in the drain.** Include any problems noted in documentation.	
——	——	——	14. If the pin or drain is crusted, replace the pin with a new sterile pin. Take care not to dislodge the drain.	
——	——	——	15. Using sterile technique, prepare a sterile work area and open the needed supplies.	
——	——	——	16. Open the sterile cleaning solution. Pour the cleansing solution into the basin. Add the gauze sponges.	
——	——	——	17. Put on sterile gloves.	
——	——	——	18. Cleanse the drain site with the cleaning solution. Use the forceps and the moistened gauze or cotton-tipped applicators. **Start at the drain insertion site, moving in a circular motion toward the periphery. Use each gauze sponge or applicator only once. Discard and use new gauze if additional cleansing is needed.**	
——	——	——	19. Dry the skin with a new gauze pad. Place the presplit drain sponge under the drain. Place several gauze pads around the drain site. Apply gauze pads over the drain.	
——	——	——	20. Apply ABD pads over the gauze. Remove gloves and dispose of them.	
——	——	——	21. Tape the ABD pads securely to the patient's skin.	
——	——	——	22. After securing the dressing, remove all remaining equipment, place the patient in a position of comfort, with side rails up and bed in the lowest position, and perform hand hygiene.	
——	——	——	23. Record the procedure, wound assessment, and the patient's reaction to the procedure according to institution's guidelines.	
——	——	——	24. Check all dressings every shift. More frequent checking may be needed if a wound is more complex or dressings become saturated more frequently.	

Skill Checklists to Accompany Taylor's Clinical Nursing Skills:
A Nursing Process Approach, 2nd edition

Name _____   Date _____

Unit _____   Position _____

Instructor/Evaluator: _____   Position _____

Excellent	Satisfactory	Needs Practice	SKILL 8-8 **Caring for a T-Tube Drain**	
			Goal: The drain remains patent and intact.	**Comments**
——	——	——	1. Review the physician's order for drain and site care or the nursing plan of care related to drain care.	
——	——	——	2. Gather the necessary supplies.	
——	——	——	3. Identify the patient.	
——	——	——	4. Explain the procedure to the patient.	
——	——	——	5. Assess the patient for possible need for nonpharmacologic pain-reducing interventions or analgesic medication before wound care dressing change. Administer appropriate analgesic, consulting physician's orders, and allow enough time for analgesic to achieve its effectiveness.	
——	——	——	6. Perform hand hygiene.	
——	——	——	7. Close the room door or curtains. Place the bed at an appropriate and comfortable working height.	
——	——	——	8. Place a waste receptacle at a convenient location for use during the procedure.	
——	——	——	9. Assist the patient to a comfortable position that provides easy access to the drain area. Use the bath blanket to cover any exposed area other than the drain. Place the waterproof pad under the drain site.	
			Emptying Drainage	
——	——	——	10. Put on clean gloves.	
——	——	——	11. Using sterile technique, open a gauze pad, making a sterile field with the outer wrapper.	
——	——	——	12. Place the graduated collection container under the outlet valve of the drainage bag. **Without contaminating the outlet valve, pull the cap off and empty the bag's contents completely into the container; use the gauze to wipe the valve, and reseal the outlet valve.**	
——	——	——	13. Carefully measure and record the character, color, and amount of the drainage. Discard the drainage according to facility policy.	
——	——	——	14. Remove gloves and perform hand hygiene.	

SKILL 8-8

Caring for a T-Tube Drain *(Continued)*

Excellent	Satisfactory	Needs Practice		Comments

Cleaning the Drain Site

____ ____ ____ 15. Put on clean gloves. Check the position of the drain or drains before removing the dressing. Loosen the tape on the old dressings. If necessary, use an adhesive remover to help get the tape off.

____ ____ ____ 16. Carefully remove the soiled dressings. If any part of the dressing sticks to the underlying skin, use small amounts of sterile saline to help loosen and remove. Do not reach over the drain site.

____ ____ ____ 17. After removing the dressing, note the presence, amount, type, color, and odor of any drainage on the dressings. Place soiled dressings in the appropriate waste receptacle. Remove gloves and dispose of in appropriate waste receptacle.

____ ____ ____ 18. Inspect the drain site for appearance and drainage. Assess if any pain is present. Note any problems to include in your documentation.

____ ____ ____ 19. Using sterile technique, prepare a sterile work area and open the needed supplies.

____ ____ ____ 20. Open the sterile cleaning solution. Pour the cleansing solution into the basin. Add the gauze sponges.

____ ____ ____ 21. Put on sterile gloves.

____ ____ ____ 22. Cleanse the drain site with the cleaning solution. Use the forceps and the moistened gauze or cotton-tipped applicators. **Start at the drain insertion site, moving in a circular motion toward the periphery. Use each gauze sponge only once. Discard and use new gauze if additional cleansing is needed.**

____ ____ ____ 23. Allow the area to dry or dry with a new sterile gauze.

____ ____ ____ 24. Place the drain sponge under the drain. Place several gauze pads around the drain site. Apply gauze pads over the drain. Alternatively, place the transparent dressing over the tube and dressings.

____ ____ ____ 25. Secure the dressings with tape as needed. **Be careful not to kink the tubing.**

Excellent	Satisfactory	Needs Practice		Comments
			SKILL 8-8 **Caring for a T-Tube Drain** *(Continued)*	
——	——	——	26. After securing the dressing, remove all remaining equipment. Apply skin protectant to the surrounding skin if needed. Place the patient in a position of comfort, with side rails up and bed in the lowest position, and perform hand hygiene.	
——	——	——	27. Check all dressings every shift. More frequent checking may be needed if a wound is more complex or dressings become saturated quickly.	

Skill Checklists to Accompany Taylor's Clinical Nursing Skills:
A Nursing Process Approach, 2nd edition

Name _____   Date _____

Unit _____   Position _____

Instructor/Evaluator: _____   Position _____

SKILL 8-9
Caring for a Jackson-Pratt Drain

Goal: The drain is patent and intact.

Excellent	Satisfactory	Needs Practice		Comments
——	——	——	1. Review the physician's order for drain and site care or the nursing plan of care related to drain care.	
——	——	——	2. Gather the necessary supplies.	
——	——	——	3. Identify the patient.	
——	——	——	4. Assess the patient for possible need for nonpharmacologic pain-reducing interventions or analgesic medication before wound care dressing change. Administer appropriate analgesic, consulting physician's orders, and allow enough time for analgesic to achieve its effectiveness.	
——	——	——	5. Perform hand hygiene.	
——	——	——	6. Close the room door or curtains. Place the bed at an appropriate and comfortable working height.	
——	——	——	7. Assist the patient to a comfortable position that provides easy access to the drain area. Use the bath blanket to cover any exposed area other than the drain. Place the waterproof pad under the drain site.	
——	——	——	8. Put on clean gloves; put on mask or face shield if indicated.	
——	——	——	9. Place the graduated collection container under the outlet valve of the drain. Without contaminating the outlet valve, pull the cap off. The chamber will expand completely as it draws in air. **Empty the chamber's contents completely into the container. Use the alcohol pad to clean the chamber's spout and cap. Fully compress the chamber with one hand and replace the plug with your other hand.**	
——	——	——	10. Check the patency of the equipment. Make sure the tubing is free from twists and kinks.	
——	——	——	11. Secure the Jackson-Pratt drain to the patient's gown below the wound with a safety pin, making sure that there is no tension on the tubing.	
——	——	——	12. Carefully measure and record the character, color, and amount of the drainage. Discard the drainage according to facility policy.	

Excellent	Satisfactory	Needs Practice	SKILL 8-9 **Caring for a Jackson-Pratt Drain** *(Continued)*	Comments
——	——	——	13. If the drain site has a dressing, redress the site as outlined in Skill 8-3.	
——	——	——	14. If the drain site is open to air, observe the sutures that secure the drain to the skin. Look for signs of pulling, tearing, swelling, or infection of the surrounding skin.	
——	——	——	15. Gently clean the sutures with the gauze pad soaked in normal saline. Dry with a new gauze pad. Apply skin protectant to the surrounding skin if needed.	
——	——	——	16. Remove gloves and all remaining equipment, place the patient in a position of comfort, with side rails up and bed in the lowest position, and perform hand hygiene.	

Skill Checklists to Accompany Taylor's Clinical Nursing Skills:
A Nursing Process Approach, 2nd edition

Name _____ Date _____

Unit _____ Position _____

Instructor/Evaluator: _____ Position _____

SKILL 8-10

Caring for a Hemovac Drain

Excellent	Satisfactory	Needs Practice	**Goal:** The drain is patent and intact.	Comments
——	——	——	1. Review the physician's order for drain and site care or the nursing plan of care related to drain care.	
——	——	——	2. Gather the necessary supplies.	
——	——	——	3. Identify the patient.	
——	——	——	4. Explain the procedure to the patient.	
——	——	——	5. Assess the patient for possible need for nonpharmacologic pain-reducing interventions or analgesic medication before wound care dressing change. Administer appropriate analgesic, consulting physician's orders, and allow enough time for analgesic to achieve its effectiveness.	
——	——	——	6. Perform hand hygiene.	
——	——	——	7. Close the room door or curtains. Place the bed at an appropriate and comfortable working height.	
——	——	——	8. Assist the patient to a comfortable position that provides easy access to the drain area. Use the bath blanket to cover any exposed area other than the drain. Place the waterproof pad under the drain site.	
——	——	——	9. Put on clean gloves and other personal protective equipment, such as mask or face shield, as necessary.	
——	——	——	10. Place the graduated collection container under the pouring spout of the drain. Without contaminating the outlet valve, uncap the valve. The chamber will expand completely as it draws in air. Empty the chamber's contents completely into the container. Use the alcohol pad to clean the chamber's spout and cap. **Fully compress the chamber by pushing the top and bottom together with your hands. Keep the device tightly compressed while you reinsert the plug.**	
——	——	——	11. Check the patency of the equipment. Make sure the tubing is free from twists and kinks.	
——	——	——	12. Secure the Hemovac drain to the patient's gown below the wound with pins, making sure that there is no tension on the tubing.	

SKILL 8-10
Caring for a Hemovac Drain *(Continued)*

Excellent	Satisfactory	Needs Practice		Comments
___	___	___	13. Carefully measure and record the character, color, and amount of the drainage. Discard the drainage according to facility policy.	
___	___	___	14. If the drain site has a dressing, redress the site as outlined in Skill 8-3. Assess the patient for possible need for pain/analgesic medication prior to dressing change	
___	___	___	15. If the drain site is open to air, observe the sutures that secure the drain to the skin. Look for signs of pulling, tearing, swelling, or infection of the surrounding skin.	
___	___	___	16. Gently clean the sutures with the gauze pad soaked in normal saline. Dry with a new gauze pad.	
___	___	___	17. Remove gloves and all remaining equipment, place the patient in a position of comfort, with side rails up and bed in the lowest position, and perform hand hygiene.	

Skill Checklists to Accompany Taylor's Clinical Nursing Skills:
A Nursing Process Approach, 2nd edition

Name _____ Date _____

Unit _____ Position _____

Instructor/Evaluator: _____ Position _____

Excellent	Satisfactory	Needs Practice	SKILL 8-11 **Applying a Wound Vacuum-Assisted Closure**	Comments
			Goal: The therapy is accomplished without contaminating the wound area, without causing trauma to the wound, and without causing the patient to experience pain or discomfort.	
——	——	——	1. Review the physician's order for the application of wound VAC therapy, including the ordered setting for the negative pressure.	
——	——	——	2. Gather the necessary supplies.	
——	——	——	3. Identify the patient.	
——	——	——	4. Explain the procedure.	
——	——	——	5. Assess the patient for possible need for nonpharmacologic pain-reducing interventions or analgesic medication before wound care dressing change. Administer appropriate analgesic, consulting physician's orders, and allow enough time for analgesic to achieve its effectiveness before beginning procedure.	
——	——	——	6. Perform hand hygiene.	
——	——	——	7. Close the room door or curtains. Place the bed in a comfortable working height.	
——	——	——	8. Assist the patient to a comfortable position that provides easy access to the wound area. Position the patient so the irrigation solution will flow from the clean end of the wound toward the dirty end. Expose the area and drape the patient with a bath blanket if needed. Put a waterproof pad under the wound area.	
——	——	——	9. Have the disposal bag or waste receptacle within easy reach for use during the procedure.	
——	——	——	10. Assemble the VAC device according to the manufacturer's instructions. Set the negative pressure according to the physician's order (25–200 mm Hg).	
——	——	——	11. Using sterile technique, prepare a sterile field and add all the sterile supplies needed for the procedure to the field. Pour warmed, sterile irrigating solution into the sterile container.	
——	——	——	12. Put on a gown, mask, and eye protection.	
——	——	——	13. Put on clean disposable gloves and remove the soiled dressings.	

Excellent	Satisfactory	Needs Practice	SKILL 8-11 **Applying a Wound Vacuum-Assisted Closure** *(Continued)*	Comments
——	——	——	14. Assess the wound for appearance and drainage. Assess the appearance of the surrounding tissue.	
——	——	——	15. Discard the dressings in the receptacle. Remove your gloves and put them in the receptacle.	
——	——	——	16. Put on sterile gloves. Using sterile technique, irrigate the wound (see Skill 8-4).	
——	——	——	17. Clean the area around the skin with normal saline. Dry the surrounding skin with a sterile gauze sponge.	
——	——	——	18. **Wipe intact skin around the wound with a skin-protectant wipe and allow it to dry well.**	
——	——	——	19. Remove gloves if they become contaminated and discard them into the receptacle.	
——	——	——	20. Put on a new pair of sterile gloves. **Using sterile scissors, cut the foam to the shape and measurement of the wound.** More than one piece of foam may be necessary if the first piece is cut too small. **Carefully place the foam in the wound.**	
——	——	——	21. **Place the fenestrated tubing into the center of the foam. There should be foam between the tubing and the base of the wound and foam over top of the tubing.**	
——	——	——	22. **Cover the foam and tubing with the transparent occlusive air-permeable dressing, leaving at least a 2″ margin on the intact skin around the wound.**	
——	——	——	23. Connect the free end of the fenestrated tubing to the tubing that is connected to the evacuation canister.	
——	——	——	24. Remove and discard gloves. Turn on the vacuum unit. **Observe the shrinking of the transparent dressing to the foam and skin.**	
——	——	——	25. Lower the bed and make sure the patient is comfortable.	
——	——	——	26. Perform hand hygiene.	
——	——	——	27. Dispose of used supplies and equipment according to facility policy.	
——	——	——	28. Check all wound dressings every shift.	

Skill Checklists to Accompany Taylor's Clinical Nursing Skills:
A Nursing Process Approach, 2nd edition

Name _____   Date _____

Unit _____   Position _____

Instructor/Evaluator: _____   Position _____

SKILL 8-12
Removing Sutures

Goal: The sutures are removed without contaminating the incisional area by maintaining sterile technique, without causing trauma to the wound, and without causing the patient to experience pain or discomfort.

Excellent	Satisfactory	Needs Practice		Comments
——	——	——	1. Review the physician's order for suture removal.	
——	——	——	2. Gather the necessary supplies.	
——	——	——	3. Identify the patient.	
——	——	——	4. Explain the procedure to the patient. Describe the sensation as a pulling or slightly uncomfortable experience.	
——	——	——	5. Perform hand hygiene.	
——	——	——	6. Close the room door or curtains. Place the bed at an appropriate and comfortable working height.	
——	——	——	7. Assist the patient to a comfortable position that provides easy access to the wound area. Use the bath blanket to cover any exposed area other than the wound.	
——	——	——	8. Put on clean gloves. Remove and dispose of any dressings on the surgical incision. Remove gloves and put on sterile gloves. Inspect the incision area.	
——	——	——	9. Clean the incision using the wound cleanser and gauze, according to facility policies and procedures.	
——	——	——	10. **Using the sterile forceps, grasp the knot of the first suture and gently lift the knot up off the skin.**	
——	——	——	11. Using the sterile scissors, cut one side of the suture below the knot, close to the skin. **Grasp the knot with the forceps and pull the cut suture through the skin. Avoid pulling the visible portion of the suture through the underlying tissue.**	
——	——	——	12. Remove every other suture to be sure the wound edges are healed. If they are, remove the remaining sutures as ordered. Dispose of sutures in a biohazard bag.	
——	——	——	13. Apply Steri-Strips if ordered. If necessary, prepare skin with tincture of benzoin before applying Steri-Strips.	
——	——	——	14. Reapply the dressing, depending on the physician's orders and facility policy.	
——	——	——	15. Remove gloves and perform hand hygiene.	

Skill Checklists to Accompany Taylor's Clinical Nursing Skills:
A Nursing Process Approach, 2nd edition

Name _____   Date _____

Unit _____   Position _____

Instructor/Evaluator: _____   Position _____

Excellent	Satisfactory	Needs Practice	SKILL 8-13 **Removing Surgical Staples** **Goal:** The staples are removed without contaminating the incision area, without causing trauma to the wound, and without causing the patient to experience pain or discomfort.	Comments
___	___	___	1. Review the physician's order for staple removal.	
___	___	___	2. Gather the necessary supplies.	
___	___	___	3. Identify the patient. Explain the procedure to the patient. Describe the sensation as a pulling or slightly uncomfortable experience.	
___	___	___	4. Perform hand hygiene.	
___	___	___	5. Close the room door or curtains. Place the bed at an appropriate and comfortable working height.	
___	___	___	6. Assist the patient to a comfortable position that provides easy access to the wound area. Use the bath blanket to cover any exposed area other than the wound.	
___	___	___	7. Put on gloves. Remove and dispose of any dressings on the surgical incision using proper technique. Remove gloves and put on a new pair.	
___	___	___	8. Clean the incision using the wound cleanser and gauze, according to facility policies and procedures.	
___	___	___	9. **Position the sterile staple remover under the staple to be removed. Firmly close the staple remover. The staple will bend in the middle and the edges will pull up out of the skin.**	
___	___	___	10. Remove every other staple to be sure the wound edges are healed. If they are, remove the remaining staples as ordered. Dispose of staples in the sharps container.	
___	___	___	11. Apply Steri-Strips according to facility policy or physician's order. Prepare skin with tincture of benzoin if indicated.	
___	___	___	12. Reapply the dressing, depending on the physician's orders and facility policy.	
___	___	___	13. Remove gloves and perform hand hygiene.	

Skill Checklists to Accompany Taylor's Clinical Nursing Skills:
A Nursing Process Approach, 2nd edition

Name _____ Date _____

Unit _____ Position _____

Instructor/Evaluator: _____ Position _____

SKILL 8-14

Applying an External Heating Device: Aquathermia Pad and Hot Water Bag

Goal: The patient experiences increased comfort; the patient experiences decreased muscle spasms; the patient exhibits improved wound healing; the patient demonstrates a reduction in inflammation; and the patient remains free of injury.

Excellent	Satisfactory	Needs Practice		Comments
____	____	____	1. Review the physician's order for the application of heat therapy, including frequency, type of therapy, body area to be treated, and length of time for the application.	
____	____	____	2. Gather the necessary supplies.	
____	____	____	3. Identify the patient.	
____	____	____	4. Explain the procedure.	
____	____	____	5. Assess the condition of the skin where the heat is to be applied.	
____	____	____	6. Perform hand hygiene.	
____	____	____	7. Close the room door or curtains. Place the bed at a comfortable working height.	
____	____	____	8. Assist the patient to a comfortable position that provides easy access to the area to be treated. Expose the area and drape the patient with a bath blanket if needed. Put a waterproof pad under the wound area to protect the bed, if necessary.	
____	____	____	9. Check that the water is at the appropriate level. Fill the control unit two-thirds full with distilled water, or to the fill mark, if necessary. Check the temperature setting on the unit to ensure it is within the safe range	
____	____	____	10. Check for leaks and tilt the unit in several directions.	
____	____	____	11. Plug in the unit and warm the pad before use. Cover the pad with an absorbent cloth. Apply the heat source to the prescribed area. Secure with gauze bandage or tape.	
____	____	____	12. **Assess the condition of the skin and the patient's response to the heat at frequent intervals, according to facility policy. Do not exceed the prescribed length of time for the application of heat.**	
____	____	____	13. Remove after the prescribed amount of time. Perform hand hygiene.	

Skill Checklists to Accompany Taylor's Clinical Nursing Skills: A Nursing Process Approach, 2nd edition

Name _____   Date _____

Unit _____   Position _____

Instructor/Evaluator: _____   Position _____

SKILL 8-15
Applying a Warm Sterile Compress to an Open Wound

Goal: The patient shows signs such as decreased inflammation, decreased muscle spasms, or decreased pain that indicate problems have been relieved.

Excellent	Satisfactory	Needs Practice		Comments
____	____	____	1. Review the physician's order.	
____	____	____	2. Gather the necessary supplies.	
____	____	____	3. Identify the patient.	
____	____	____	4. Explain the procedure.	
____	____	____	5. Assess the patient for possible need for nonpharmacologic pain-reducing interventions or analgesic medication before wound care dressing change. Administer appropriate analgesic, consulting physician's orders, and allow enough time for analgesic to achieve its effectiveness before beginning procedure.	
____	____	____	6. Perform hand hygiene.	
____	____	____	7. Close the room door or curtains. Place the bed at a comfortable working height.	
____	____	____	8. Assist the patient to a comfortable position that provides easy access to the wound area. Expose the area and drape the patient with a bath blanket if needed. Put the waterproof pad under the wound area.	
____	____	____	9. Have the disposal bag or waste receptacle within easy reach for use during the procedure.	
____	____	____	10. Prepare the external heating pad or Aquathermia pad if one is being used.	
____	____	____	11. Using sterile technique, prepare a working field and open all sterile packaging, dressings, and the warmed solution. Pour the solution into the sterile container and drop the sterile gauze for the compress into the solution.	
____	____	____	12. Put on clean disposable gloves and remove any old dressing in place. Discard the old dressing in the appropriate receptacle. Remove your gloves and discard them.	
____	____	____	13. Assess wound site and surrounding tissues. Look for inflammation, drainage, skin color, ecchymosis, and odor.	
____	____	____	14. Put on sterile gloves, following proper procedure.	

SKILL 8-15

Applying a Warm Sterile Compress
to an Open Wound (Continued)

Excellent	Satisfactory	Needs Practice		Comments
——	——	——	15. Retrieve the sterile compress from the warmed solution, squeezing out any excess moisture. Apply the compress by gently and carefully molding it around the wound site. Ask patient if the application feels too hot.	
——	——	——	16. **Cover the site with a single layer of gauze and with a clean dry bath towel;** secure in place if necessary.	
——	——	——	17. Place the Aquathermia or heating device, if used, over the towel.	
——	——	——	18. Remove sterile gloves and discard them appropriately. Perform hand hygiene.	
——	——	——	19. **Monitor the time the compress is in place to prevent burns or skin damage. Monitor the condition of the patient's skin and the patient's response at frequent intervals.**	
——	——	——	20. After the prescribed time for the treatment (up to 30 minutes), remove the external heating device (if used) and put on sterile gloves.	
——	——	——	21. Carefully remove the compress while assessing the skin condition around the wound site and observing the patient's response to the heat application. Note any wound changes.	
——	——	——	22. Apply a new dry sterile dressing to the wound, following proper procedure.	
——	——	——	23. Remove gloves. Place the patient in a comfortable position. Lower the bed. Dispose of any other supplies appropriately.	
——	——	——	24. Perform hand hygiene.	

Skill Checklists to Accompany Taylor's Clinical Nursing Skills: A Nursing Process Approach, 2nd edition

Name _____   Date _____

Unit _____   Position _____

Instructor/Evaluator: _____   Position _____

SKILL 8-16

Assisting With a Sitz Bath

Excellent	Satisfactory	Needs Practice	**Goal:** The patient will state an increase in comfort.	Comments
——	——	——	1. Identify the patient.	
——	——	——	2. Explain what you are going to do.	
——	——	——	3. Close curtains around bed and close door to room if possible.	
——	——	——	4. Perform hand hygiene and put on clean gloves.	
——	——	——	5. Assemble equipment in bathroom.	
——	——	——	6. Raise lid of toilet. Place bowl of sitz bath, with drainage ports to rear and infusion port in front, in the toilet. Fill bowl of sitz bath about halfway full with tepid to warm water (37°–46°C [98°–115°F]).	
——	——	——	7. Clamp tubing on bag. Fill bag with same temperature water as mentioned above. Hang bag above patient's shoulder height on hook or IV pole.	
——	——	——	8. Assist patient to sit on toilet and provide any extra draping if needed. Insert tubing into infusion port of sitz bath. Slowly unclamp tubing and allow sitz bath to fill.	
——	——	——	9. Clamp tubing once sitz bath is full. Instruct patient to open clamp when water in bowl becomes cool. **Ensure that call bell is within reach. Instruct patient to call if she feels light-headed or dizzy or has any problems. Instruct patient not to try standing without assistance.**	
——	——	——	10. When patient is finished (in about 15–20 minutes), help patient stand and gently pat perineal area dry. Assist patient to bed or chair. Ensure that call bell is within reach.	
——	——	——	11. Empty and disinfect sitz bath bowl according to agency policy. Remove gloves and perform hand hygiene.	

Skill Checklists to Accompany Taylor's Clinical Nursing Skills:
A Nursing Process Approach, 2nd edition

Name _____ Date _____

Unit _____ Position _____

Instructor/Evaluator: _____ Position _____

Excellent	Satisfactory	Needs Practice	SKILL 8-17 **Using a Cooling Blanket**	
			Goal: The patient maintains a normal body temperature.	**Comments**
——	——	——	1. Review the physician's order for the application of the hypothermia blanket. Obtain consent for the therapy per facility policy.	
——	——	——	2. Gather the necessary supplies.	
——	——	——	3. Identify the patient. Determine if the patient has had any previous adverse reaction to hypothermia therapy.	
——	——	——	4. Explain the procedure.	
——	——	——	5. Assess the patient's vital signs, neurologic status, peripheral circulation, and skin integrity.	
——	——	——	6. Perform hand hygiene.	
——	——	——	7. Close the room door or curtains. Place the bed at a comfortable working height.	
——	——	——	8. Make sure the patient's gown has cloth ties, not snaps or pins.	
——	——	——	9. Apply lanolin or a mixture of lanolin and cold cream to the patient's skin where it will be in contact with the blanket.	
——	——	——	10. Turn on the blanket and make sure the cooling light is on. Verify that the temperature limits are set within the desired safety range.	
——	——	——	11. Cover the hypothermia blanket with a thin sheet or bath blanket.	
——	——	——	12. Position the blanket under the patient so that the top edge of the pad is aligned with the patient's neck.	
——	——	——	13. Put on gloves. Lubricate the rectal probe and insert it into the patient's rectum unless contraindicated. Or tuck the skin probe deep into the patient's axilla and tape it in place. For patients who are comatose or anesthetized, use an esophageal probe. Attach the probe to the control panel for the blanket.	
——	——	——	14. Wrap the patient's hands and feet in gauze if ordered, or if the patient desires. **For male patients, elevate the scrotum off the cooling blanket with towels.**	
——	——	——	15. Recheck the thermometer and settings on the control panel.	

Excellent	Satisfactory	Needs Practice	SKILL 8-17 **Using a Cooling Blanket** *(Continued)*	Comments
—	—	—	16. Remove gloves and perform hand hygiene.	
—	—	—	17. **Turn and position the patient regularly (every 30 minutes to 1 hour).** Keep linens free from condensation. Reapply cream as needed. Observe the patient's skin for change in color, changes in lips and nail beds, edema, pain, and sensory impairment.	
—	—	—	18. **Monitor vital signs and perform a neurologic assessment per facility policy, usually every 15 minutes, until the body temperature is stable.**	
—	—	—	19. Observe for signs of shivering, including verbalized sensations, facial muscle twitching, hyperventilation, or twitching of extremities.	
—	—	—	20. Assess the patient's level of comfort.	
—	—	—	21. Turn off blanket according to facility policy, usually when the patient's body temperature reaches 1° above the desired temperature. Continue to monitor the patient's temperature until it stabilizes.	
—	—	—	22. Document assessments, vital signs, and time of initiation of therapy. Document the control settings, the duration of treatment, and the patient's response.	

Skill Checklists to Accompany Taylor's Clinical Nursing Skills:
A Nursing Process Approach, 2nd edition

Name _____   Date _____

Unit _____   Position _____

Instructor/Evaluator: _____   Position _____

Excellent	Satisfactory	Needs Practice	SKILL 8-18 **Applying Cold Therapy**	Comments
			Goal: The patient experiences increased comfort; the patient experiences decreased muscle spasms; the patient experiences decreased inflammation; and the patient does not show signs of bleeding or hematoma at the treatment site.	
____	____	____	1. Review the physician's order for the application of cold therapy, including frequency, type of therapy, body area to be treated, and length of time for the application.	
____	____	____	2. Gather the necessary supplies.	
____	____	____	3. Identify the patient. Determine if the patient has had any previous adverse reaction to cold therapy.	
____	____	____	4. Explain the procedure.	
____	____	____	5. Assess the condition of the skin where the ice is to be applied.	
____	____	____	6. Perform hand hygiene.	
____	____	____	7. Close the room door or curtains. Place the bed at a comfortable working height.	
____	____	____	8. Assist the patient to a comfortable position that provides easy access to the area to be treated. Expose the area and drape the patient with a bath blanket if needed. Put the waterproof pad under the wound area, if necessary.	
____	____	____	9. Prepare device: Fill the bag, collar, or glove about three-fourths full with ice. **Remove any excess air from the device.** Securely fasten the end of the bag or collar; tie the glove closed, checking for holes and leakage of water. Prepare commercially prepared ice pack if appropriate.	
____	____	____	10. **Cover the device with a towel or washcloth.** (If the device has a cloth exterior, this is not necessary.)	
____	____	____	11. Put on gloves. Position cooling device on top of dressing and lightly secure in place as needed.	
____	____	____	12. **Remove the ice and assess the site for redness after 30 seconds. Ask the patient about the presence of burning sensations.**	
____	____	____	13. Replace the device snugly against the site if no problems are evident. Secure it in place with gauze wrap or tape.	

SKILL 8-18

Applying Cold Therapy *(Continued)*

Excellent	Satisfactory	Needs Practice		Comments
⎯	⎯	⎯	14. Reassess the treatment area every 5 minutes or according to facility policy.	
⎯	⎯	⎯	15. **After 20 minutes or the prescribed amount of time, remove the ice and dry the skin.**	
⎯	⎯	⎯	16. Apply a new dressing to site, if necessary.	
⎯	⎯	⎯	17. Perform hand hygiene.	

Skill Checklists to Accompany Taylor's Clinical Nursing Skills: A Nursing Process Approach, 2nd edition

Name _____   Date _____

Unit _____   Position _____

Instructor/Evaluator: _____   Position _____

			SKILL 9-1	

Assisting a Patient With Turning in Bed

Excellent	Satisfactory	Needs Practice	**Goal:** The activity takes place without injury to patient or nurse.	Comments
____	____	____	1. Review the physician's orders and nursing plan of care for patient activity. Identify any movement limitations and the ability of the patient to assist with turning. Consult patient-handling algorithm, if available, to plan appropriate approach to moving the patient.	
____	____	____	2. Gather any positioning aids or supports, if necessary.	
____	____	____	3. Identify the patient. Explain the procedure to the patient.	
____	____	____	4. Perform hand hygiene and put on gloves, if necessary.	
____	____	____	5. Close the room door or curtains. Place the bed at an appropriate and comfortable working height.	
____	____	____	6. Adjust the head of the bed to a flat position or as low as the patient can tolerate. Place pillows, wedges, or any other supports to be used for positioning within easy reach.	
____	____	____	7. Lower the side rail nearest you if it has been raised. If not already in place, position a friction-reducing sheet or drawsheet under the patient.	
____	____	____	8. Using the friction-reducing sheet or drawsheet, move the patient to the edge of the bed, opposite the side to which he or she will be turned. Raise side rail and move to the opposite side of the bed.	
____	____	____	9. Stand on the side of the bed toward which the patient is turning. Lower the side rail nearest you.	
____	____	____	10. **Place the patient's arms across his or her chest and cross his or her far leg over the leg nearest you.**	
____	____	____	11. Stand opposite the patient's center with your feet spread about shoulder width and with one foot ahead of the other. **Tighten your gluteal and abdominal muscles and flex your knees. Use your leg muscles to do the pulling.**	
____	____	____	12. If available, activate the bed mechanism to inflate the side of the bed opposite from where you are standing.	

Assisting a Patient With Turning in Bed *(Continued)*

Excellent	Satisfactory	Needs Practice		Comments
——	——	——	13. Position your hands on the patient's far shoulder and hip, and roll the patient toward you. Or, you may use the friction-reducing sheet or draw sheet to gently pull the patient over on his or her side.	
——	——	——	14. Use a pillow or other support behind the patient's back. Pull the shoulder blade forward and out from under the patient.	
——	——	——	15. Make the patient comfortable and position in proper alignment, using pillows or other supports under the leg and arm as needed. Readjust the pillow under the patient's head. Elevate the head of the bed as needed for comfort.	
——	——	——	16. Place the bed in the lowest position, with the side rails up. Make sure the call bell and other necessary items are within easy reach.	
——	——	——	17. Perform hand hygiene.	

Skill Checklists to Accompany Taylor's Clinical Nursing Skills:
A Nursing Process Approach, 2nd edition

Name _____ Date _____

Unit _____ Position _____

Instructor/Evaluator: _____ Position _____

Excellent	Satisfactory	Needs Practice	SKILL 9-2 **Providing Range-of-Motion Exercises**	
			Goal: The patient maintains joint mobility.	**Comments**
——	——	——	1. Review the physician's orders and nursing plan of care for patient activity. Identify any movement limitations.	
——	——	——	2. Identify the patient. Explain the procedure to the patient.	
——	——	——	3. Perform hand hygiene and put on gloves, if necessary.	
——	——	——	4. Close the room door or curtains. Place the bed at an appropriate and comfortable working height. Adjust the head of the bed to a flat position or as low as the patient can tolerate.	
——	——	——	5. Stand on the side of the bed where the joints are to be exercised. Lower side rail on that side, if in place. Uncover only the limb to be used during the exercise.	
——	——	——	6. Perform the exercises slowly and gently, providing support by holding the areas proximal and distal to the joint. Repeat each exercise two to five times, moving each joint in a smooth and rhythmic manner. **Stop movement if the patient complains of pain or if you meet resistance.**	
——	——	——	7. **While performing the exercises, begin at the head and move down one side of the body at a time.**	
——	——	——	8. Move the chin down to rest on the chest. Return the head to a normal upright position. Tilt the head as far as possible toward each shoulder.	
——	——	——	9. Move the head from side to side, bringing the chin toward each shoulder.	
——	——	——	10. Start with the arm at the patient's side and lift the arm forward to above the head. Return the arm to the starting position at the side of the body.	
——	——	——	11. With the arm back at the patient's side, move the arm laterally to an upright position above the head, and then return to the original position. Move the arm across the body as far as possible.	
——	——	——	12. Raise the arm at the side until the upper arm is in line with the shoulder. Bend the elbow at a 90-degree angle and move the forearm upward and downward, then return the arm to the side.	

Excellent	Satisfactory	Needs Practice		Comments
——	——	——	13. Bend the elbow and move the lower arm and hand upward toward the shoulder. Return the lower arm and hand to the original position while straightening the elbow.	
——	——	——	14. Rotate the lower arm and hand so the palm is up. Rotate the lower arm and hand so the palm of the hand is down.	
——	——	——	15. Move the hand downward toward the inner aspect of the forearm. Return the hand to a neutral position even with the forearm. Then move the dorsal portion of the hand backward as far as possible.	
——	——	——	16. Bend the fingers to make a fist, and then straighten them out. Spread the fingers apart and return them back together. Touch the thumb to each finger on the hand.	
——	——	——	17. Extend the leg and lift it upward. Return the leg to the original position beside the other leg.	
——	——	——	18. Lift the leg laterally away from the patient's body. Return the leg back toward the other leg and try to extend it beyond the midline.	
——	——	——	19. Turn the foot and leg toward the other leg to rotate it internally. Turn the foot and leg outward away from the other leg to rotate it externally.	
——	——	——	20. Bend the leg and bring the heel toward the back of the leg. Return the leg to a straight position.	
——	——	——	21. At the ankle, move the foot up and back until the toes are upright. Move the foot with the toes pointing downward.	
——	——	——	22. Turn the sole of the foot toward the midline. Turn the sole of the foot outward.	
——	——	——	23. Curl the toes downward, and then straighten them out. Spread the toes apart and bring them together.	
——	——	——	24. Repeat these exercises on the other side of the body. Encourage the patient to do as many of these exercises by himself or herself as possible.	
——	——	——	25. When finished, make sure the patient is comfortable, with the side rails up and the bed in the lowest position.	
——	——	——	26. Remove gloves if used and perform hand hygiene.	

Skill Checklists to Accompany Taylor's Clinical Nursing Skills:
A Nursing Process Approach, 2nd edition

Name _____ Date _____

Unit _____ Position _____

Instructor/Evaluator: _____ Position _____

SKILL 9-3

Moving a Patient Up in Bed With the Assistance of Another Nurse

Goal: The patient remains free from injury and maintains proper body alignment.

Excellent	Satisfactory	Needs Practice		Comments

1. Review the medical record and nursing plan of care for conditions that may influence the patient's ability to move or to be positioned. Assess for tubes, intravenous lines, incisions, or equipment that may alter the positioning procedure. Identify any movement limitations. Consult patient handling algorithm, if available, to plan appropriate approach to moving the patient.

2. Identify the patient. Explain the procedure to the patient.

3. Perform hand hygiene and put on gloves, if necessary.

4. Close the room door or curtains. Place the bed at an appropriate and comfortable working height. Adjust the head of the bed to a flat position or as low as the patient can tolerate. Placing the bed in slight Trendelenburg position aids movement, if the patient is able to tolerate it.

5. Remove all pillows from under the patient. Leave one at the head of the bed, leaning upright against the headboard.

6. Position at least one nurse on either side of the bed, and lower both side rails.

7. If a friction-reducing sheet or drawsheet is not in place under the patient, place one under the patient's midsection.

8. Ask the patient (if able) to bend his or her legs and put his or her feet flat on the bed to assist with the movement.

9. **Have the patient fold the arms across the chest. Have the patient (if able) lift the head with chin on chest.**

10. Position yourself at the patient's midsection with your feet spread shoulder width apart and one foot slightly in front of the other.

11. If available on bed, engage mechanism to make the bed surface firmer for repositioning.

12. **Fold or bunch the drawsheet close to the patient before grasping it securely and preparing to move the patient.**

13. Flex your knees and hips. Tighten your abdominal and gluteal muscles and keep your back straight.

Moving a Patient Up in Bed With the Assistance of Another Nurse *(Continued)*

Excellent	Satisfactory	Needs Practice		Comments
——	——	——	14. Shift your weight back and forth from your back leg to your front leg and count to three. On the count of three, move the patient up in bed. If possible, the patient can assist with the move by pushing with the legs. Repeat the process if necessary to get the patient to the right position.	
——	——	——	15. Assist the patient to a comfortable position and readjust the pillows and supports as needed. Return bed surface to normal position, if necessary. Raise the side rails. Place the bed in the lowest position.	
——	——	——	16. Remove gloves if used and perform hand hygiene.	

Skill Checklists to Accompany Taylor's Clinical Nursing Skills:
A Nursing Process Approach, 2nd edition

Name _____ Date _____

Unit _____ Position _____

Instructor/Evaluator: _____ Position _____

			SKILL 9-4	
Excellent	**Satisfactory**	**Needs Practice**	**Transferring a Patient From the Bed to a Stretcher**	
			Goal: The patient is transferred without injury to patient or nurse.	**Comments**
___	___	___	1. Review the medical record and nursing plan of care for conditions that may influence the patient's ability to move or to be positioned. Assess for tubes, IV lines, incisions, or equipment that may alter the positioning procedure. Identify any movement limitations. Consult patient-handling algorithm, if available, to plan appropriate approach to moving the patient.	
___	___	___	2. Identify the patient. Explain the procedure to the patient.	
___	___	___	3. Perform hand hygiene and put on gloves, if necessary.	
___	___	___	4. Close the room door or curtains. Adjust the head of the bed to a flat position or as low as the patient can tolerate. Raise the bed to a height 1/2″ higher than the transport stretcher. Lower the side rails, if in place.	
___	___	___	5. Place the bath blanket over the patient and remove the top covers from underneath.	
___	___	___	6. If a friction-reducing sheet or drawsheet is not in place under the patient, place one under the patient's midsection. Have patient fold arms against chest and move chin to chest. Use the drawsheet to move the patient to the side of the bed where the stretcher will be placed.	
___	___	___	7. Position the stretcher next to and parallel to the bed. **Lock the wheels on the stretcher and the bed.**	
___	___	___	8. Remove the pillow from the bed and place it on the stretcher. The two nurses should stand on the stretcher side of the bed. The third nurse should stand on the side of the bed without the stretcher.	
___	___	___	9. Position the transfer board or other lateral-assist device under the patient. Use the drawsheet to roll the patient away from the stretcher. Slide the transfer board across the space between the stretcher and the bed, partially under the patient. Roll the patient onto his back, so he is partially on transfer board.	

Excellent	Satisfactory	Needs Practice		Comments

SKILL 9-4

Transferring a Patient From the Bed to a Stretcher *(Continued)*

Excellent	Satisfactory	Needs Practice		Comments
____	____	____	10. The nurse on the side of the bed without the stretcher should kneel on the bed, with his or her knee at the upper torso closer to the patient than the other knee. Fold or bunch the drawsheet close to the patient before grasping it securely in preparation for the transfer.	
____	____	____	11. Have one of the nurses on the stretcher side of the bed reach across the stretcher and grasp the drawsheet at the head and chest areas of the patient. If the transfer device used has long handles, each nurse should grasp two of the handles.	
____	____	____	12. Have the other nurse reach across the stretcher and grasp the drawsheet at the patient's waist and thigh area.	
____	____	____	13. **At a signal given by one of the nurses, have the nurses standing on the stretcher side of the bed pull the sheet. At the same time, the nurse (or nurses) kneeling on the bed should lift the drawsheet, transferring the patient's weight toward the transfer board, and pushing the patient from the bed to the stretcher.**	
____	____	____	14. Once the patient is transferred to the stretcher, remove the transfer board, and secure the patient until the side rails are raised. Raise the side rails. Ensure the patient's comfort. Cover the patient with blanket and remove the bath blanket from underneath. Leave the friction-reducing sheet or drawsheet in place for the return transfer.	
____	____	____	15. Remove gloves (if used) and perform hand hygiene.	

Skill Checklists to Accompany Taylor's Clinical Nursing Skills:
A Nursing Process Approach, 2nd edition

Name _____ Date _____

Unit _____ Position _____

Instructor/Evaluator: _____ Position _____

Excellent	Satisfactory	Needs Practice	SKILL 9-5 **Transferring a Patient From the Bed to a Chair**	Comments
			Goal: The transfer is accomplished without injury to patient or nurse and the patient remains free of any complications of immobility.	
——	——	——	1. Review the medical record and nursing plan of care for conditions that may influence the patient's ability to move or to be positioned. Assess for tubes, IV lines, incisions, or equipment that may alter the positioning procedure. Identify any movement limitations. Consult patient-handling algorithm, if available, to plan appropriate approach to moving the patient.	
——	——	——	2. Identify the patient. Explain the procedure to the patient.	
——	——	——	3. Perform hand hygiene and put on gloves, if necessary.	
——	——	——	4. If needed, move equipment to make room for the chair. Close the door or draw the curtains.	
——	——	——	5. Place the bed in the lowest position. Raise the head of the bed to a sitting position, or as high as the patient can tolerate.	
——	——	——	6. **Make sure the bed brakes are locked. Put the chair next to the bed, facing the foot of the bed. If available, lock the brakes of the chair. If the chair does not have brakes, brace the chair against a secure object.**	
——	——	——	7. Encourage the patient to make use of a stand-assist aid, either free-standing or attached to the side of the bed, if available, to move to the side of the bed and to a side-lying position, facing the side of the bed the patient will sit on.	
——	——	——	8. Lower the side rail if necessary and stand near the patient's hips. Stand with your legs shoulder width apart with one foot near the head of the bed, slightly in front of the other foot.	
——	——	——	9. Encourage the patient to make use of the stand-assist device. Assist the patient to sit up on the side of the bed; ask the patient to swing his or her legs over the side of the bed. At the same time, pivot on your back leg to lift the patient's trunk and shoulders. **Keep your back straight; avoid twisting.**	

Excellent	Satisfactory	Needs Practice	SKILL 9-5 **Transferring a Patient From the Bed to a Chair** *(Continued)*	
				Comments
——	——	——	10. Stand in front of the patient, and assess for any balance problems or complaints of dizziness. Allow legs to dangle a few minutes before continuing.	
——	——	——	11. Assist the patient to put on a robe and nonskid footwear.	
——	——	——	12. Wrap the gait belt around the patient's waist, based on assessed need and facility policy.	
——	——	——	13. Stand facing the patient. Spread your feet about shoulder width apart and flex your hips and knees.	
——	——	——	14. Ask the patient to slide his or her buttocks to the edge of the bed until the feet touch the floor. Position yourself as close as possible to the patient, with your foot positioned on the outside of the patient's foot. If a second staff person is assisting, have him/her assume a similar position.	
——	——	——	15. Encourage the patient to make use of the stand-assist device. If necessary, have second staff person grasp gait belt on opposite side. Using the gait belt, assist the patient to stand. Rock back and forth while counting to three. **On the count of three, use your legs (not your back) to help raise the patient to a standing position. If indicated, brace your front knee against the patient's weak extremity as he or she stands.** Assess the patient's balance and leg strength. If the patient is weak or unsteady, return the patient to bed.	
——	——	——	16. Pivot on your back foot and assist the patient to turn until the patient feels the chair against his or her legs.	
——	——	——	17. Ask the patient to use an arm to steady himself or herself on the arm of the chair while slowly lowering to a sitting position. **Continue to brace the patient's knees with your knees and hold the gait belt. Flex your hips and knees when helping the patient sit in the chair.**	
——	——	——	18. Assess the patient's alignment in the chair. Remove gait belt, if desired. Depending on patient comfort, it could be left in place to use when returning to bed. Cover with a blanket if needed. Place the call bell close.	
——	——	——	19. Remove gloves if used and perform hand hygiene.	

Skill Checklists to Accompany Taylor's Clinical Nursing Skills:
A Nursing Process Approach, 2nd edition

Name _____ Date _____

Unit _____ Position _____

Instructor/Evaluator: _____ Position _____

Excellent	Satisfactory	Needs Practice	SKILL 9-6 **Transferring a Patient Using a Powered Full Body Sling Lift**	Comments
			Goal: The transfer is accomplished without injury to patient or nurse and the patient is free of any complications of immobility.	
―	―	―	1. Review the medical record and nursing plan of care for conditions that may influence the patient's ability to move or to be positioned. Assess for tubes, IV lines, incisions, or equipment that may alter the positioning procedure. Identify any movement limitations.	
―	―	―	2. Identify the patient. Explain the procedure to the patient.	
―	―	―	3. Perform hand hygiene and put on gloves, if necessary.	
―	―	―	4. If needed, move the equipment to make room for the chair. Close the door or draw the curtains.	
―	―	―	5. Adjust the bed to a comfortable working height. **Lock the bed brakes.**	
―	―	―	6. Lower the side rail, if in use, on the side of the bed you are working. If the sling is for use with more than one patient, place a cover or pad on the sling. Place the sling evenly under the patient. Roll the patient to one side and place half of the sling with the sheet or pad on it under the patient from shoulders to midthigh. Raise the rail and move to the other side. Lower the rail, if necessary. Roll the patient to the other side and pull the sling under the patient. Raise the side rail.	
―	―	―	7. Bring the chair to the side of the bed. **Lock the wheels, if present.**	
―	―	―	8. Lower the side rail on the chair side of the bed. **Roll the base of the lift under the side of the bed nearest to the chair. Center the frame over the patient. Lock the wheels of the lift.**	
―	―	―	9. Using the base-adjustment lever, widen the stance of the base.	
―	―	―	10. Lower the arms close enough to attach the sling to the frame.	

Excellent	Satisfactory	Needs Practice		Comments

SKILL 9-6
Transferring a Patient Using a Powered Full Body Sling Lift *(Continued)*

___ ___ ___			11. Place the strap or chain hooks through the holes of the sling. Short straps attach behind the patient's back and long straps attach at the other end. Check the patient to make sure the hooks are not pressing into the skin. Some lifts have straps on the sling that attach to hooks on the frame. Check the manufacturer's instructions for each lift.
___ ___ ___			12. Check all equipment, lines, and drains attached to the patient so that they are not interfering with the device. Have the patient fold his or her arms across the chest.
___ ___ ___			13. With a person standing on each side of the lift, tell the patient that he or she will be lifted from the bed. Support injured limbs as necessary. Engage the pump to raise the patient about 6″ above the bed.
___ ___ ___			14. Unlock the wheels of the lift. **Carefully wheel the patient straight back and away from the bed.** Support the patient's limbs as needed.
___ ___ ___			15. Position the patient over the chair with the base of the lift straddling the chair. Lock the wheels of the lift.
___ ___ ___			16. Gently lower the patient to the chair until the hooks or straps are slightly loosened from the sling or frame. Guide the patient into the chair with your hands as the sling lowers.
___ ___ ___			17. Disconnect the hooks or strap from the frame. Keep the sling in place under the patient.
___ ___ ___			18. Adjust the patient's position, using pillows if necessary. Check the patient's alignment in the chair. Cover the patient with a blanket if necessary. Place the call bell within reach. When it is time for the patient to return to bed, reattach the hooks or straps and reverse the steps.
___ ___ ___			19. Remove gloves, if used, and perform hand hygiene.

Skill Checklists to Accompany Taylor's Clinical Nursing Skills:
A Nursing Process Approach, 2nd edition

Name _____   Date _____

Unit _____   Position _____

Instructor/Evaluator: _____   Position _____

Excellent	Satisfactory	Needs Practice	SKILL 9-7 **Assisting a Patient With Ambulation**	
			Goal: The patient ambulates safely, without falls or injury.	**Comments**
——	——	——	1. Review the medical record and nursing plan of care for conditions that may influence the patient's ability to move and ambulate. Assess for tubes, IV lines, incisions, or equipment that may alter the procedure for ambulation. Identify any movement limitations.	
——	——	——	2. Identify the patient. Explain the procedure to the patient. Ask the patient to report any feelings of dizziness, weakness, or shortness of breath while walking. Decide how far to walk.	
——	——	——	3. Perform hand hygiene.	
——	——	——	4. Place the bed in the lowest position.	
——	——	——	5. Encourage the patient to make use of a stand-assist aid, either free-standing or attached to the side of the bed, if available, to move to the side of the bed.	
——	——	——	6. Assist the patient to the side of the bed, if necessary. Have the patient sit on the side of the bed for several minutes and assess for dizziness or lightheadedness. Have the patient stay sitting until he or she feels secure.	
——	——	——	7. Assist the patient to put on footwear and a robe, if desired.	
——	——	——	8. Wrap the gait belt around the patient's waist, based on assessed need and facility policy.	
——	——	——	9. Encourage the patient to make use of the stand-assist device. Assist the patient to stand, using the gait belt if necessary. Assess the patient's balance and leg strength. If the patient is weak or unsteady, return the patient to bed or assist to a chair.	
——	——	——	10. If you are the only nurse assisting, position yourself to the side and slightly behind the patient. Support the patient by the waist or transfer belt.	

Excellent	Satisfactory	Needs Practice	SKILL 9-7 **Assisting a Patient With Ambulation** *(Continued)*	Comments
			When two nurses assist, position yourself to the side and slightly behind the patient, supporting the patient by the waist or gait belt. Have the other nurse carry or manage equipment or provide additional support from the other side.	
			Alternatively, when two nurses assist, stand at the patient's sides (one nurse on each side) with near hands grasping the gait belt and far hands holding the patient's lower arm or hand.	
___	___	___	11. Take several steps forward with the patient. **Continue to assess the patient's strength and balance.** Remind patient to stand erect.	
___	___	___	12. Continue with ambulation for the planned distance and time. Return the patient to the bed or chair based on the patient's tolerance and condition.	
___	___	___	13. Remove gait belt. Perform hand hygiene.	

Skill Checklists to Accompany Taylor's Clinical Nursing Skills:
A Nursing Process Approach, 2nd edition

Name _____   Date _____

Unit _____   Position _____

Instructor/Evaluator: _____   Position _____

SKILL 9-8

Assisting a Patient With Ambulation Using a Walker

Goal: The patient ambulates safely with the walker and is free from falls or injury.

Excellent	Satisfactory	Needs Practice		Comments
—	—	—	1. Review the medical record and nursing plan of care for conditions that may influence the patient's ability to move and ambulate, and for specific instructions for ambulation such as distance. Assess for tubes, IV lines, incisions, or equipment that may alter the procedure for ambulation. Assess the patient's knowledge and previous experience regarding the use of a walker. Identify any movement limitations.	
—	—	—	2. Identify the patient. Explain the procedure to the patient. Tell the patient to report any feelings of dizziness, weakness, or shortness of breath while walking. Decide how far to walk.	
—	—	—	3. Perform hand hygiene.	
—	—	—	4. Place the bed in the lowest position.	
—	—	—	5. Encourage the patient to make use of a stand-assist aid, either free standing or attached to the side of the bed, if available, to move to the side of the bed.	
—	—	—	6. Assist the patient to the side of the bed, if necessary. Have the patient sit on the side of the bed. Assess for dizziness or lightheadedness. Have the patient stay sitting until he or she feels secure.	
—	—	—	7. Assist the patient to put on footwear and a robe, if desired.	
—	—	—	8. Wrap the gait belt around the patient's waist, based on assessed need and facility policy.	
—	—	—	9. **Place the walker directly in front of the patient.** Ask the patient to push himself or herself off the bed or chair, make use of the stand-assist device, or assist the patient to stand. Once the patient is standing, have him or her hold the walker's hand grips firmly and equally. Stand slightly behind the patient, on one side.	

Excellent	Satisfactory	Needs Practice	SKILL 9-8 **Assisting a Patient With Ambulation** **Using a Walker** *(Continued)*	
				Comments
——	——	——	10. Have the patient move the walker forward 6″ to 8″ and set it down, making sure all four feet of the walker stay on the floor. Then, tell the patient to step forward with either foot into the walker, supporting himself or herself on his or her arms. Follow through with the other leg. **If one leg is weaker or impaired, have the patient step forward with the involved leg and follow with the uninvolved leg, again supporting himself or herself on his or her arms.**	
——	——	——	11. Move the walker forward again, and continue the same pattern. Continue with ambulation for the planned distance and time. Return the patient to the bed or chair based on the patient's tolerance and condition, ensuring that the patient is comfortable and call light is within reach.	
——	——	——	12. Remove gait belt. Perform hand hygiene.	

Skill Checklists to Accompany Taylor's Clinical Nursing Skills:
A Nursing Process Approach, 2nd edition

Name _____ Date _____

Unit _____ Position _____

Instructor/Evaluator: _____ Position _____

Excellent	Satisfactory	Needs Practice	SKILL 9-9 **Assisting a Patient With Ambulation Using Crutches**	Comments
			Goal: The patient ambulates safely without experiencing falls or injury.	
‒‒	‒‒	‒‒	1. Review the medical record and nursing plan of care for conditions that may influence the patient's ability to move and ambulate. Assess for tubes, IV lines, incisions, or equipment that may alter the procedure for ambulation. Assess the patient's knowledge and previous experience regarding the use of crutches. Determine that the appropriate size crutch has been obtained.	
‒‒	‒‒	‒‒	2. Identify the patient. Explain the procedure to the patient. Tell the patient to report any feelings of dizziness, weakness, or shortness of breath while walking. Decide how far to walk.	
‒‒	‒‒	‒‒	3. Perform hand hygiene.	
‒‒	‒‒	‒‒	4. Encourage the patient to make use of the stand-assist device, if available. Assist the patient to stand erect, face forward in the tripod position. This means the patient holds the crutches 6″ in front of and 6″ to the side of each foot.	
‒‒	‒‒	‒‒	5. For the four-point gait:	
‒‒	‒‒	‒‒	a. Have the patient move the right crutch forward 6″ and then move the left foot forward to the level of the right crutch.	
‒‒	‒‒	‒‒	b. Then have the patient move the left crutch forward 6″ and then move the right foot forward to the level of the left crutch.	
‒‒	‒‒	‒‒	6. For the three-point gait:	
‒‒	‒‒	‒‒	a. Have the patient move the affected leg and both crutches forward about 6″.	
‒‒	‒‒	‒‒	b. Have the patient move the stronger leg forward to the level of the crutches.	
‒‒	‒‒	‒‒	7. For the two-point gait:	
‒‒	‒‒	‒‒	a. Have the patient move the left crutch and the right foot forward about 6″ at the same time.	
‒‒	‒‒	‒‒	b. Have the patient move the right crutch and left leg forward to the level of the left crutch at the same time.	

Assisting a Patient With Ambulation Using Crutches *(Continued)*

Excellent	Satisfactory	Needs Practice		Comments

Excellent	Satisfactory	Needs Practice	
____	____	____	8. For the swing-to gait:
____	____	____	a. Have the patient move both crutches forward about 6″.
____	____	____	b. Have the patient lift the legs and swing them to the crutches, supporting his or her body weight on the crutches.
____	____	____	9. For the swing-through gait:
____	____	____	a. Have the patient move both crutches forward about 6″.
____	____	____	b. Have the patient lift the legs and swing through and ahead of the crutches, supporting his or her weight on the crutches.
____	____	____	10. **Continue with ambulation for the planned distance and time. Return the patient to the bed or chair based on the patient's tolerance and condition, ensuring that the patient is comfortable and that the call light is within reach.**
____	____	____	11. Perform hand hygiene.

Skill Checklists to Accompany Taylor's Clinical Nursing Skills:
A Nursing Process Approach, 2nd edition

Name _____ Date _____

Unit _____ Position _____

Instructor/Evaluator: _____ Position _____

Excellent	Satisfactory	Needs Practice	SKILL 9-10 **Assisting a Patient With Ambulation Using a Cane**
			Goal: The patient ambulates safely without falls or injury. **Comments**
___	___	___	1. Review the medical record and nursing plan of care for conditions that may influence the patient's ability to move and ambulate. Assess for tubes, IV lines, incisions, or equipment that may alter the procedure for ambulation. Assess the patient's knowledge and previous experience regarding the use of a cane. Identify any movement limitations.
___	___	___	2. Identify the patient. Explain the procedure to the patient. Tell the patient to report any feelings of dizziness, weakness, or shortness of breath while walking. Decide how far to walk.
___	___	___	3. Perform hand hygiene.
___	___	___	4. Encourage the patient to make use of a stand-assist aid, either free standing or attached to the side of the bed, if available, to move to and sit on the side of the bed.
___	___	___	5. Wrap the gait belt around the patient's waist, based on assessed need and facility policy.
___	___	___	6. Encourage the patient to make use of the stand-assist device to stand with weight evenly distributed between the feet and the cane.
___	___	___	7. Have the patient hold the cane on his or her stronger side, close to the body.
___	___	___	8. Tell the patient to advance the cane 4″ to 12″ (10–30 cm) and then, while supporting his or her weight on the stronger leg and the cane, advance the weaker foot forward, parallel with the cane.
___	___	___	9. While supporting his or her weight on the weaker leg and the cane, have the patient advance the stronger leg forward ahead of the cane (heel slightly beyond the tip of the cane).
___	___	___	10. Tell the patient to move the weaker leg forward until it is even with the stronger leg, and then advance the cane again.

Excellent	Satisfactory	Needs Practice		Comments

SKILL 9-10

Assisting a Patient With Ambulation Using a Cane *(Continued)*

Excellent	Satisfactory	Needs Practice		Comments
⎯	⎯	⎯	11. Continue with ambulation for the planned distance and time. Return the patient to the bed or chair based on the patient's tolerance and condition, ensuring the patient's comfort and that call light is within reach.	
⎯	⎯	⎯	12. Perform hand hygiene.	

Skill Checklists to Accompany Taylor's Clinical Nursing Skills:
A Nursing Process Approach, 2nd edition

Name _____ Date _____

Unit _____ Position _____

Instructor/Evaluator: _____ Position _____

Excellent	Satisfactory	Needs Practice	SKILL 9-11 **Applying Pneumatic Compression Devices**	Comments
			Goal: The patient maintains adequate circulation in extremities and is free from symptoms of neurovascular compromise.	
——	——	——	1. Review the medical record and nursing plan of care for conditions that may contraindicate the use of the PCD.	
——	——	——	2. Identify the patient. Explain the procedure to the patient.	
——	——	——	3. Perform hand hygiene.	
——	——	——	4. Close the room door or curtains. Place the bed at an appropriate and comfortable working height.	
——	——	——	5. Hang the compression pump on the foot of the bed and plug it into an electrical outlet. Attach the connecting tubing to the pump.	
——	——	——	6. Remove the compression sleeves from the package and unfold them. Lay the unfolded sleeves on the bed with the cotton lining facing up. Take note of the markings indicating the correct placement for the ankle and popliteal areas.	
——	——	——	7. Apply antiembolism stockings if ordered. Place a sleeve under the patient's leg with the tubing toward the heel. Each one fits either leg. For total leg sleeves, place the behind-the-knee opening at the popliteal space to prevent pressure there. For knee-high sleeves, make sure the back of the ankle is over the ankle marking.	
——	——	——	8. Wrap the sleeve snugly around the patient's leg so that two fingers fit between the leg and the sleeve. Secure the sleeve with the Velcro fasteners. Repeat for the second leg, if bilateral therapy is ordered. Connect each sleeve to the tubing, following manufacturer's recommendations.	
——	——	——	9. Set the pump to the prescribed maximum pressure (usually 35–55 mm Hg). Make sure the tubing is free from kinks. Check that the patient can move about without interrupting the airflow. Turn on the pump. Initiate cooling setting, if available.	
——	——	——	10. Observe the patient and the device during the first cycle. Check the audible alarms. Check the sleeves and pump at least once per shift or per facility policy.	
——	——	——	11. Place the bed in the lowest position. Make sure the call bell and other necessary items are within easy reach.	

Excellent	Satisfactory	Needs Practice		Comments
			SKILL 9-11 **Applying Pneumatic Compression Devices** *(Continued)*	
____	____	____	12. Perform hand hygiene.	
____	____	____	13. Assess the extremities for peripheral pulses, edema, changes in sensation, and movement. Remove the sleeves and assess and document skin integrity every 8 hours.	

Skill Checklists to Accompany Taylor's Clinical Nursing Skills:
A Nursing Process Approach, 2nd edition

Name _____ Date _____

Unit _____ Position _____

Instructor/Evaluator: _____ Position _____

SKILL 9-12
Applying a Continuous Passive Motion Device

Excellent	Satisfactory	Needs Practice	**Goal:** The patient experiences increased joint mobility.	Comments
___	___	___	1. Review the medical record and nursing plan of care for the appropriate degrees of flexion and extension, the cycle rate, and the length of time the CPM is to be used.	
___	___	___	2. Identify the patient. Explain the procedure to the patient.	
___	___	___	3. Obtain equipment. Apply the soft goods to the CPM device.	
___	___	___	4. Perform hand hygiene, and put on gloves if indicated.	
___	___	___	5. Close the room door or curtains. Place the bed at an appropriate and comfortable working height.	
___	___	___	6. Using the tape measure, determine the distance between the gluteal crease and the popliteal space.	
___	___	___	7. Measure the leg from the knee to 1/4" beyond the bottom of the foot.	
___	___	___	8. Position the patient in the middle of the bed. The affected extremity should be in a slightly abducted position.	
___	___	___	9. Support the affected extremity and elevate it, placing it in the padded CPM device.	
___	___	___	10. Make sure the knee is at the hinged joint of the CPM device.	
___	___	___	11. Adjust the footplate to maintain the patient's foot in a neutral position. Assess the patient's position to make sure the leg is not internally or externally rotated.	
___	___	___	12. Apply the restraining straps under the CPM device and around the leg. **Check that two fingers fit between the strap and the leg.**	
___	___	___	13. Explain the use of the STOP/GO button to the patient. Set the controls to the prescribed levels of flexion and extension and cycles per minute. Turn on the power to the CPM.	
___	___	___	14. Set the device to ON and start the therapy by pressing the GO button. Observe the patient and the device during the first cycle. Determine the angle of flexion when the device reaches its greatest height using the goniometer. Compare with prescribed degree.	

Excellent	Satisfactory	Needs Practice		Comments
			SKILL 9-12 **Applying a Continuous Passive** **Motion Device** *(Continued)*	
___	___	___	15. Check the patient's level of comfort and perform skin and neurovascular assessment at least every 8 hours or per facility policy.	
___	___	___	16. Place the bed in the lowest position, with the side rails up. Make sure the call bell and other necessary items are within easy reach.	
___	___	___	17. Remove gloves, if used, and perform hand hygiene.	

Skill Checklists to Accompany Taylor's Clinical Nursing Skills:
A Nursing Process Approach, 2nd edition

Name _____ Date _____

Unit _____ Position _____

Instructor/Evaluator: _____ Position _____

Excellent	Satisfactory	Needs Practice	SKILL 9-13 **Applying a Sling**	Comments
			Goal: The arm is immobilized, and the patient maintains muscle strength and joint range of motion.	
⎯⎯	⎯⎯	⎯⎯	1. Review the medical record and nursing plan of care to determine the need for the use of a sling.	
⎯⎯	⎯⎯	⎯⎯	2. Identify the patient. Explain the procedure to the patient.	
⎯⎯	⎯⎯	⎯⎯	3. Perform hand hygiene.	
⎯⎯	⎯⎯	⎯⎯	4. Close the room door or curtains. Place the bed at an appropriate and comfortable working height, if necessary.	
⎯⎯	⎯⎯	⎯⎯	5. Assist the patient to a sitting position. Place the patient's forearm across the chest with the elbow flexed and the palm against the chest. Measure the sleeve length, if indicated.	
⎯⎯	⎯⎯	⎯⎯	6. Enclose the arm in the sling, making sure the elbow fits into the corner of the fabric. Run the strap up the patient's back and across the shoulder opposite the injury, then down the chest to the fastener on the end of the sling.	
⎯⎯	⎯⎯	⎯⎯	7. Place the ABD pad under the strap, between the strap and the patient's neck. Ensure that the sling and forearm are slightly elevated and at a right angle to the body.	
⎯⎯	⎯⎯	⎯⎯	8. Place the bed in the lowest position, with the side rails up. Make sure the call bell and other necessary items are within easy reach.	
⎯⎯	⎯⎯	⎯⎯	9. Perform hand hygiene.	
⎯⎯	⎯⎯	⎯⎯	10. Check the patient's level of comfort, arm positioning, and neurovascular status of the affected limb every 4 hours or according to facility policy. Assess the axillary and cervical skin frequently for irritation or breakdown.	

Skill Checklists to Accompany Taylor's Clinical Nursing Skills:
A Nursing Process Approach, 2nd edition

Name _____ Date _____

Unit _____ Position _____

Instructor/Evaluator: _____ Position _____

SKILL 9-14
Applying a Figure-Eight Bandage

Goal: The bandage is applied correctly without injury or complications.

Excellent	Satisfactory	Needs Practice		Comments
___	___	___	1. Review the medical record and nursing plan of care to determine the need for a figure-eight bandage.	
___	___	___	2. Identify the patient. Explain the procedure to the patient.	
___	___	___	3. Perform hand hygiene and put on gloves if contact with drainage is possible.	
___	___	___	4. Close the room door or curtains. Place the bed at an appropriate and comfortable working height.	
___	___	___	5. Assist the patient to a comfortable position, with the affected body part in a normal functioning position.	
___	___	___	6. Hold the bandage roll with the roll facing upward in one hand while holding the free end of the roll in the other hand. Make sure to hold the bandage roll so it is close to the affected body part.	
___	___	___	7. Wrap the bandage around the limb twice, below the joint, to anchor it.	
___	___	___	8. Use alternating ascending and descending turns to form a figure eight. Overlap each turn of the bandage by one-half to two-thirds the width of the strip.	
___	___	___	9. **Unroll the bandage as you wrap, not before wrapping.**	
___	___	___	10. **Wrap firmly, but not tightly.** Assess the patient's comfort as you wrap. If the patient reports tingling, itching, numbness, or pain, loosen the bandage.	
___	___	___	11. After the area is covered, wrap the bandage around the limb twice, above the joint, to anchor it. Secure the end of the bandage with tape, pins, or self-closures. Avoid metal clips.	
___	___	___	12. Remove your gloves, if worn, and discard them. Place the bed in the lowest position, with the side rails up. Make sure the call bell and other necessary items are within easy reach.	
___	___	___	13. Assess the distal circulation after the bandage is in place.	
___	___	___	14. **Elevate the wrapped extremity for 15 to 30 minutes after application of the bandage.**	

Applying a Figure-Eight Bandage *(Continued)*

Excellent	Satisfactory	Needs Practice		Comments
⎯	⎯	⎯	15. Lift the distal end of the bandage and assess the skin for color, temperature, and integrity. Assess for pain and perform a neurovascular assessment of the affected extremity after applying the bandage and at least every 4 hours, or per facility policy.	
⎯	⎯	⎯	16. Perform hand hygiene.	

Skill Checklists to Accompany Taylor's Clinical Nursing Skills:
A Nursing Process Approach, 2nd edition

Name _____ Date _____

Unit _____ Position _____

Instructor/Evaluator: _____ Position _____

			SKILL 9-15	

SKILL 9-15
Assisting With Cast Application

Goal: The cast is applied without interfering with neurovascular function and healing occurs.

Excellent	Satisfactory	Needs Practice		Comments
——	——	——	1. Review the medical record and medical orders to determine the need for the cast.	
——	——	——	2. Identify the patient. Explain the procedure to the patient and verify area to be casted.	
——	——	——	3. Perform a pain assessment and assess for muscle spasm. Administer prescribed medications in sufficient time to allow for the full effect of the analgesic and/or muscle relaxant.	
——	——	——	4. Perform hand hygiene and put on gloves, if necessary.	
——	——	——	5. Close the room door or curtains. Place the bed at an appropriate and comfortable working height, if necessary.	
——	——	——	6. Position the patient as needed, depending on the type of cast being applied and the location of the injury. Support the extremity or body part to be casted.	
——	——	——	7. Drape the patient with the waterproof pads.	
——	——	——	8. Cleanse and dry the affected body part.	
——	——	——	9. Position and maintain the affected body part in the position indicated by the physician as the stockinette, sheet wadding, and padding is applied. The stockinette should extend beyond the ends of the cast. As the wadding is applied, check for wrinkles.	
——	——	——	10. Continue to position and maintain the affected body part in the position indicated by the physician or advanced practice professional as the casting material is applied. Assist with finishing by folding the stockinette or other padding down over the outer edge of the cast.	
——	——	——	11. **Support the cast during hardening.** Handle hardening plaster casts with the palms of hands, not fingers. Support the cast on a firm, smooth surface. Do not rest it on a hard surface or sharp edges. Avoid placing pressure on the cast.	
——	——	——	12. **Elevate the injured limb above heart level with pillow or bath blankets as ordered, making sure pressure is evenly distributed under the cast.**	

SKILL 9-15
Assisting With Cast Application *(Continued)*

Excellent	Satisfactory	Needs Practice		Comments
——	——	——	13. Remove gloves and dispose of them properly; place the bed in the lowest position, if necessary.	
——	——	——	14. Obtain x-rays as ordered.	
——	——	——	15. **Instruct the patient to report pain, odor, drainage, changes in sensation, abnormal sensation, or the inability to move fingers or toes of the affected extremity.**	
——	——	——	16. Leave the cast uncovered and exposed to the air. Reposition the patient every 2 hours. Depending on facility policy, a fan may be used to dry the cast.	
——	——	——	17. Perform hand hygiene.	

Skill Checklists to Accompany Taylor's Clinical Nursing Skills: A Nursing Process Approach, 2nd edition

Name _____ Date _____

Unit _____ Position _____

Instructor/Evaluator: _____ Position _____

Excellent	Satisfactory	Needs Practice	SKILL 9-16 **Caring for a Cast**	Comments
			Goal: The cast remains intact and the patient does not experience neurovascular compromise.	
____	____	____	1. Review the medical record and the nursing plan of care to determine the need for cast care and care for the affected body part.	
____	____	____	2. Identify the patient. Explain the procedure to the patient.	
____	____	____	3. Perform hand hygiene and put on gloves, if necessary.	
____	____	____	4. Close the room door or curtains. Place the bed at an appropriate and comfortable working height, if necessary.	
____	____	____	5. If a plaster cast was applied, handle the casted extremity or body area with the palms of your hands for the first 24 to 36 hours, until the cast is fully dry.	
____	____	____	6. If the cast is on an extremity, elevate the affected area on pillows covered with waterproof pads. **Maintain the normal curvatures and angles of the cast.**	
____	____	____	7. Keep cast (plaster) uncovered until fully dry.	
____	____	____	8. Wash excess antiseptic or antimicrobial agents, such as povidone–iodine (Betadine), or residual casting material from the exposed skin. Dry thoroughly.	
____	____	____	9. Assess the condition of the cast. Be alert for cracks, dents, or the presence of drainage from the cast. Perform skin and neurovascular assessment according to facility policy, as often as every 1 to 2 hours. **Check for pain, edema, inability to move body parts distal to the cast, pallor, pulses, and abnormal sensations. If the cast is on an extremity, compare it to the uncasted extremity.**	
____	____	____	10. **If breakthrough bleeding or drainage is noted on the cast, mark the area on the cast. Indicate the date and time next to the area.** Follow physician orders or facility policy regarding the amount of drainage that needs to be reported to the physician.	
____	____	____	11. Assess for signs of infection. Monitor the patient's temperature. Assess for a foul odor from the cast, increased pain, or extreme warmth over an area of the cast.	
____	____	____	12. Reposition the patient every 2 hours. Provide back and skin care frequently. Encourage range of motion for unaffected joints. Encourage the patient to cough and deep breathe.	

Excellent	Satisfactory	Needs Practice	SKILL 9-16 **Caring for a Cast** *(Continued)*	Comments
——	——	——	13. Instruct the patient to report pain, odor, drainage, changes in sensation, abnormal sensation, or the inability to move fingers or toes of the affected extremity.	
——	——	——	14. Remove gloves and dispose of them appropriately; place the bed in the lowest position, if necessary.	
——	——	——	15. Perform hand hygiene.	

Skill Checklists to Accompany Taylor's Clinical Nursing Skills:
A Nursing Process Approach, 2nd edition

Name _____   Date _____

Unit _____   Position _____

Instructor/Evaluator: _____   Position _____

Excellent	Satisfactory	Needs Practice	SKILL 9-17 **Applying Skin Traction and Caring for a Patient in Skin Traction** **Goal:** The traction is maintained with the appropriate counterbalance and the patient is free from complications of immobility.	Comments
___	___	___	1. Review the medical record and the nursing plan of care to determine the type of traction being used and care for the affected body part.	
___	___	___	2. Identify the patient. Explain the procedure to the patient, emphasizing the importance of maintaining counterbalance, alignment, and position.	
___	___	___	3. Perform a pain assessment and assess for muscle spasm. Administer prescribed medications in sufficient time to allow for the full effect of the analgesic and/or muscle relaxant.	
___	___	___	4. Perform hand hygiene.	
___	___	___	5. Close the room door or curtains. Place the bed at an appropriate and comfortable working height.	
			Applying Skin Traction	
___	___	___	6. Ensure the traction apparatus is attached securely to the bed. Assess the traction setup.	
___	___	___	7. Check that the ropes move freely through the pulleys. Check that all knots are tight and are positioned away from the pulleys. Pulleys should be free from the linens.	
___	___	___	8. Place the patient in a supine position with the foot of the bed elevated slightly. The patient's head should be near the head of the bed and in alignment	
___	___	___	9. Cleanse the affected area. Place the elastic hose on the affected limb.	
___	___	___	10. Place the traction boot over the patient's leg. Be sure the patient's heel is in the heel of the boot. Secure the boot with the straps.	

Excellent	Satisfactory	Needs Practice		Comments

Applying Skin Traction and Caring for a Patient in Skin Traction *(Continued)*

___ ___ ___ 11. Attach the traction cord to the footplate of the boot. Pass the rope over the pulley fastened at the end of the bed. Attach the weight to the hook on the rope, usually 5 to 10 pounds for an adult. Gently let go of the weight. **The weight should hang freely, not touching the bed or the floor.**

___ ___ ___ 12. Check the patient's alignment with the traction.

___ ___ ___ 13. Check the boot for placement and alignment. **Make sure the line of pull is parallel to the bed and not angled downward.**

___ ___ ___ 14. Place the bed in the lowest position that still allows the weight to hang freely.

___ ___ ___ 15. Perform hand hygiene.

Caring for a Patient With Skin Traction

___ ___ ___ 16. Perform a skin-traction assessment per facility policy. This assessment includes checking the traction equipment, examining the affected body part, maintaining proper body alignment, and performing a skin assessment and a neurovascular assessment.

___ ___ ___ 17. Remove the straps every 4 hours per the physician's order or facility policy. Check bony prominences for skin breakdown, abrasions, and pressure areas. Remove the boot per physician's order or facility policy every 8 hours. Put on gloves and wash, rinse, and thoroughly dry the skin.

___ ___ ___ 18. Assess the extremity distal to the traction for edema, and assess peripheral pulses. Assess the temperature, color, and capillary refill, and compare with the unaffected limb. Check for pain, inability to move body parts distal to the traction, pallor, and abnormal sensations. Assess for indicators of deep-vein thrombosis, including calf tenderness, swelling, and a positive Homans' sign.

___ ___ ___ 19. Replace the traction and remove gloves and dispose of them appropriately.

___ ___ ___ 20. Check the boot for placement and alignment. **Make sure the line of pull is parallel to the bed and not angled downward.**

___ ___ ___ 21. **Ensure the patient is positioned in the center of the bed, with the affected leg aligned with the trunk of the patient's body.**

___ ___ ___ 22. Examine the weights and pulley system. **Weights should hang freely, off the floor and bed. Knots should be secure. Ropes should move freely through the pulleys. The pulleys should not be constrained by knots.**

Excellent	Satisfactory	Needs Practice	SKILL 9-17 **Applying Skin Traction and Caring for a Patient in Skin Traction** *(Continued)*	
				Comments
——	——	——	23. Perform range-of-motion exercises on all unaffected joint areas, unless contraindicated. Encourage the patient to cough and deep breathe every 2 hours.	
——	——	——	24. Raise the side rails. Place the bed in the lowest position that still allows the weight to hang freely.	
——	——	——	25. Perform hand hygiene.	

Skill Checklists to Accompany Taylor's Clinical Nursing Skills:
A Nursing Process Approach, 2nd edition

Name _____   Date _____

Unit _____   Position _____

Instructor/Evaluator: _____   Position _____

Excellent	Satisfactory	Needs Practice	SKILL 9-18 **Caring for a Patient in Skeletal Traction**	Comments
			Goal: The traction is maintained appropriately and the patient is free from complications of immobility and infection.	
___	___	___	1. Review the medical record and the nursing plan of care to determine the type of traction being used and the prescribed care.	
___	___	___	2. Identify the patient. Explain the procedure to the patient, emphasizing the importance of maintaining counterbalance, alignment, and position.	
___	___	___	3. Perform a pain assessment and assess for muscle spasm. Administer prescribed medications in sufficient time to allow for the full effect of the analgesic and/or muscle relaxant.	
___	___	___	4. Perform hand hygiene.	
___	___	___	5. Close the room door or curtains. Place the bed at an appropriate and comfortable working height.	
___	___	___	6. Ensure the traction apparatus is attached securely to the bed. Assess the traction setup, including application of the ordered amount of weight. **Be sure that the weights hang freely, not touching the bed or the floor.**	
___	___	___	7. Check that the ropes move freely through the pulleys. Check that all knots are tight and are positioned away from the pulleys. Pulleys should be free from the linens.	
___	___	___	8. Check the alignment of the patient's body as prescribed.	
___	___	___	9. Perform a skin assessment. Pay attention to pressure points, including the ischial tuberosity, popliteal space, Achilles tendon, sacrum, and heel.	
___	___	___	10. Perform a neurovascular assessment. Assess the extremity distal to the traction for edema and peripheral pulses. Assess the temperature and color and compare with the unaffected limb. Check for pain, inability to move body parts distal to the traction, pallor, and abnormal sensations. Assess for indicators of deep-vein thrombosis, including calf tenderness, swelling, and a positive Homans' sign.	
___	___	___	11. Assess the site at and around the pins for redness, edema, and odor. Assess for skin tenting, prolonged or purulent drainage, elevated body temperature, elevated pin site temperature, and bowing or bending of the pins.	

Excellent	Satisfactory	Needs Practice	SKILL 9-18 **Caring for a Patient in Skeletal Traction** *(Continued)*	Comments
——	——	——	12. Provide pin site care.	
——	——	——	a. Using sterile technique, open the applicator package and pour the cleansing agent into the sterile container.	
——	——	——	b. Put on the sterile gloves.	
——	——	——	c. Place the applicators into the solution.	
——	——	——	**d. Clean the pin site starting at the insertion area and working outward, away from the pin site.**	
——	——	——	**e. Use each applicator once. Use a new applicator for each pin site.**	
——	——	——	13. Depending on physician order and facility policy, apply the antimicrobial ointment to pin sites and apply a dressing.	
——	——	——	14. Remove gloves. Perform hand hygiene.	
——	——	——	15. Perform range-of-motion exercises on all joint areas, unless contraindicated. Encourage the patient to cough and deep breathe every 2 hours.	
——	——	——	16. Perform hand hygiene.	

Name _____   Date _____

Unit _____   Position _____

Instructor/Evaluator: _____   Position _____

SKILL 9-19

Caring for a Patient With an External Fixation Device

Goal: The patient shows no evidence of complication such as infection, contractures, venous stasis, thrombus formation, or skin breakdown.

Excellent	Satisfactory	Needs Practice		Comments
――	――	――	1. Review the medical record and the nursing plan of care to determine the type of device being used and prescribed care.	
――	――	――	2. Identify the patient. Explain the procedure to the patient. Assure the patient that there will be little pain after the fixation device is in place. Reinforce that the patient will be able to adjust to the device and will be able to move about with the device, allowing him or her to resume normal activities more quickly.	
――	――	――	3. After the fixation device is in place, **apply ice to the surgical site as ordered or per facility policy. Elevate the affected body part if appropriate.**	
――	――	――	4. Perform a pain assessment and assess for muscle spasm. Administer prescribed medications in sufficient time to allow for the full effect of the analgesic and/or muscle relaxant.	
――	――	――	5. Administer analgesics as ordered before exercising or mobilizing the affected body part.	
――	――	――	6. Perform neurovascular assessments per facility policy or physician's order, usually every 2 to 4 hours for 24 hours, then every 4 to 8 hours. Assess the affected body part for color, motion, sensation, edema, capillary refill, and pulses. If appropriate, compare with the unaffected side. Assess for pain not relieved by analgesics, burning, tingling, and numbness.	
――	――	――	7. Perform hand hygiene.	
――	――	――	8. Close the room door or curtains. Place the bed at an appropriate and comfortable working height.	
――	――	――	9. Assess the pin site for redness, tenting of the skin, prolonged or purulent drainage, swelling, and bowing, bending, or loosening of the pins. Monitor body temperature.	
――	――	――	10. Perform pin site care.	
――	――	――	a. Using sterile technique, open the applicator package and pour the cleansing agent into the sterile container.	

Excellent	Satisfactory	Needs Practice	SKILL 9-19 **Caring for a Patient With an External Fixation Device** *(Continued)*	
				Comments
⎯	⎯	⎯	b. Put on the sterile gloves.	
⎯	⎯	⎯	c. Place the applicators into the solution.	
⎯	⎯	⎯	d. **Clean the pin site starting at the insertion area and working outward, away from the pin site.**	
⎯	⎯	⎯	e. **Use each applicator once. Use a new applicator for each pin site.**	
⎯	⎯	⎯	11. Depending on physician order and facility policy, apply the antimicrobial ointment to pin sites and apply a dressing.	
⎯	⎯	⎯	12. Remove gloves. Perform hand hygiene.	

Skill Checklists to Accompany Taylor's Clinical Nursing Skills:
A Nursing Process Approach, 2nd edition

Name _____   Date _____

Unit _____   Position _____

Instructor/Evaluator: _____   Position _____

Excellent	Satisfactory	Needs Practice	SKILL 10-1 **Promoting Patient Comfort**	Comments
			Goal: The patient experiences relief from discomfort and/or pain without adverse effect.	
——	——	——	1. Identify the patient. Discuss pain with the patient, acknowledging that the patient's pain exists. Explain how pain medications and other pain management therapies work together to provide pain relief. Allow the patient to help choose interventions for pain relief.	
——	——	——	2. Perform hand hygiene. Put on nonsterile gloves, if necessary.	
——	——	——	3. Assess the patient's pain, using an appropriate assessment tool and measurement scale.	
——	——	——	4. Provide pharmacologic interventions, if indicated and ordered.	
——	——	——	5. Adjust the patient's environment to promote comfort.	
——	——	——	a. Adjust and maintain the room temperature per the patient's preference.	
——	——	——	b. Reduce harsh lighting, but provide adequate lighting per the patient's preference.	
——	——	——	c. Reduce harsh and unnecessary noise. Avoid carrying out conversations immediately outside the patient's room.	
——	——	——	d. Close room door and/or curtain whenever possible.	
——	——	——	e. Provide good ventilation in the patient's room. Reduce unpleasant odors by promptly emptying bedpans, urinals, and emesis basins after use. Remove trash and laundry promptly.	
——	——	——	6. Prevent unnecessary interruptions and coordinate patient activities to group activities together. Allow for and plan rest periods without disturbance.	
——	——	——	7. Assist the patient to change position frequently. Assist the patient to a comfortable position, maintaining good alignment and supporting extremities as needed. Raise the head of the bed as appropriate.	

Excellent	Satisfactory	Needs Practice		Comments
			SKILL 10-1 **Promoting Patient Comfort** *(Continued)*	

Excellent	Satisfactory	Needs Practice		Comments
——	——	——	8. Provide oral hygiene as often as necessary to keep the mouth and mucous membranes clean and moist, as often as every 1 or 2 hours if necessary. This is especially important for patients who cannot drink or are not permitted fluids by mouth.	
——	——	——	9. Ensure the availability of appropriate fluids for drinking, unless contraindicated. Make sure the patient's water pitcher is filled and within reach. Make other fluids of the patient's choice available.	
——	——	——	10. Remove physical situations that may cause discomfort.	
——	——	——	a. Change soiled and/or wet dressings; replace soiled and/or wet bed linens.	
——	——	——	b. Smooth wrinkles in bed linens.	
——	——	——	c. Ensure patient is not lying or sitting on tubes, tubing, wires, or other equipment.	
——	——	——	11. Assist the patient as necessary with ambulation, active range-of-motion exercises, and/or passive range-of-motion exercises as appropriate.	
——	——	——	12. Assess the patient's spirituality needs related to the pain experience. Ask the patient if he/she would like a spiritual counselor to visit.	
——	——	——	13. Consider the use of distraction. Distraction requires the patient to focus on something other than the pain.	
——	——	——	a. Have the patient recall a pleasant experience or focus attention on an enjoyable experience.	
——	——	——	b. Offer age/developmentally appropriate games, toys, books, audiobooks, access to television and/or videos, or other items of interest to the patient.	
——	——	——	c. Encourage the patient to hold or stroke a loved person, pet, or toy.	
——	——	——	d. Offer access to music the patient prefers. Turn on the music when pain begins, or before anticipated painful stimuli. The patient can close his/her eyes and concentrate on listening. Raising or lowering the volume as pain increases or decreases can be helpful.	
——	——	——	14. Consider the use of guided imagery.	
——	——	——	a. Help the patient to identify a scene or experience that the patient describes as happy, pleasant, or peaceful.	

Excellent	Satisfactory	Needs Practice		Comments

Excellent	Satisfactory	Needs Practice		Comments
——	——	——	b. Encourage the patient to begin with several minutes of focused breathing, relaxation, or meditation. (Refer to specific information in steps 14 and 16.)	
——	——	——	c. Help the patient concentrate on the peaceful, pleasant image.	
——	——	——	d. If indicated, read a description of the identified scene or experience, using a soothing, soft voice.	
——	——	——	e. Encourage the patient to concentrate on the details of the image, such as its sight, sounds, smells, tastes, and touch.	
——	——	——	15. Consider the use of relaxation activities, such as deep breathing.	
——	——	——	a. Have the patient sit or recline comfortably and place hands on stomach. Close the eyes.	
——	——	——	b. Ask the patient to mentally count to maintain a comfortable rate and rhythm. Have the patient inhale slowly and deeply while letting the abdomen expand as much as possible. Have the patient hold his/her breath for a few seconds.	
——	——	——	c. Tell the patient to exhale slowly through mouth, blowing through puckered lips. Have the patient continue to count to maintain comfortable rate and rhythm, concentrating on the rise and fall of abdomen.	
——	——	——	d. When the patient's abdomen feels empty, have the patient begin again with a deep inhalation.	
——	——	——	e. Encourage patient to practice at least twice a day, for 10 minutes, and then use as needed to assist with pain management.	
——	——	——	16. Consider the use of relaxation activities, such as progressive muscle relaxation.	
——	——	——	a. Assist the patient to a comfortable position.	
——	——	——	b. Direct the patient to focus on a particular muscle group. Start with the muscles of the jaw, then repeat with the neck muscles, shoulder muscles, upper and lower arm, hand, abdominal, buttocks, thigh, lower leg, and foot muscles.	

Excellent	Satisfactory	Needs Practice		Comments

SKILL 10-1
Promoting Patient Comfort *(Continued)*

Excellent	Satisfactory	Needs Practice		Comments
——	——	——	c. Ask the patient to tighten the muscle group and note the sensation that the tightened muscles produce. After 5 to 7 seconds, tell the patient to relax the muscles all at once and concentrate on the sensation of the relaxed state, noting the difference in feeling in the muscles when contracted and relaxed.	
——	——	——	d. Have the patient continue to tighten–hold–relax each muscle group until entire body has been covered.	
——	——	——	e. Encourage patient to practice at least twice a day, for 10 minutes, and then use as needed to assist with pain management.	
——	——	——	17. Consider the use of cutaneous stimulation, such as the intermittent application of heat or cold, or both.	
——	——	——	18. Consider the use of cutaneous stimulation, such as massage. (See Skill 10-2.)	
——	——	——	19. Discuss the potential for use of cutaneous stimulation such as TENS with the patient and primary care provider. (See Skill 10-3.)	
——	——	——	20. Remove gloves, if worn, and perform hand hygiene.	
——	——	——	21. Evaluate the patient's response to interventions. Reassess level of discomfort or pain using original assessment tools. Reassess and alter plan of care as appropriate.	

Skill Checklists to Accompany Taylor's Clinical Nursing Skills:
A Nursing Process Approach, 2nd edition

Name _____ Date _____

Unit _____ Position _____

Instructor/Evaluator: _____ Position _____

Excellent	Satisfactory	Needs Practice	SKILL 10-2 **Giving a Back Massage**	
			Goal: The patient reports increased comfort and/or decreased pain and the patient is relaxed.	**Comments**
____	____	____	1. Identify the patient. Offer a back massage to the patient and explain the procedure.	
____	____	____	2. Perform hand hygiene and put on nonsterile gloves, if indicated.	
____	____	____	3. Close room door and/or curtain.	
____	____	____	4. Assess the patient's pain, using an appropriate assessment tool and measurement scale.	
____	____	____	5. Raise the bed to a comfortable working height and lower the side rail nearest you.	
____	____	____	6. Assist the patient to a comfortable position, preferably the prone or side-lying position. Remove the covers and move the patient's gown just enough to expose the patient's back from the shoulders to sacral area. Drape the patient as needed with the bath blanket.	
____	____	____	7. **Warm the lubricant or lotion in the palm of your hand, or place the container in small basin of warm water.**	
____	____	____	8. Using light gliding strokes (*effleurage*), apply lotion to patient's shoulders, back, and sacral area.	
____	____	____	9. Place your hands beside each other at the base of the patient's spine and stroke upward to the shoulders and back downward to the buttocks in slow, continuous strokes. Continue for several minutes.	
____	____	____	10. Massage the patient's shoulder, entire back, areas over iliac crests, and sacrum with circular stroking motions. **Keep your hands in contact with the patient's skin.** Continue for several minutes, applying additional lotion as necessary.	
____	____	____	11. Knead the patient's skin by gently alternating grasping and compression motions (*pétrissage*).	
____	____	____	12. Complete the massage with additional long stroking movements that eventually become lighter in pressure.	
____	____	____	13. During massage, observe the patient's skin for reddened or open areas. **Pay particular attention to the skin over bony prominences.**	

Excellent	Satisfactory	Needs Practice		Comments
___	___	___	14. Use the towel to pat the patient dry and to remove excess lotion. Apply powder if the patient requests it.	
___	___	___	15. Reposition patient gown and covers. Raise side rail and lower bed. Assist patient to a position of comfort.	
___	___	___	16. Remove gloves, if worn, and perform hand hygiene.	
___	___	___	17. Evaluate the patient's response to interventions. Reassess level of discomfort or pain using original assessment tools. Reassess and alter plan of care as appropriate.	

Skill Checklists to Accompany Taylor's Clinical Nursing Skills:
A Nursing Process Approach, 2nd edition

Name _____   Date _____

Unit _____   Position _____

Instructor/Evaluator: _____   Position _____

SKILL 10-3
Applying a TENS Unit

Goal: The patient will verbalize decreased discomfort and pain, without experiencing any injury or skin irritation or breakdown.

Excellent	Satisfactory	Needs Practice		Comments
——	——	——	1. Identify the patient, show the patient the device, and explain the function of the device and the reason for its use.	
——	——	——	2. Perform hand hygiene.	
——	——	——	3. Assess the patient's pain, using an appropriate assessment tool and measurement scale.	
——	——	——	4. Inspect the area where the electrodes are to be placed. Clean the patient's skin, using skin cleanser and water. Dry the area thoroughly.	
——	——	——	5. Remove the adhesive backing from the electrodes and apply them to the specified location. **If the electrodes are not pregelled, apply a small amount of electrode gel to the bottom of each electrode.** If the electrodes are not self-adhering, tape them in place.	
——	——	——	6. **Check the placement of the electrodes; leave at least a 2″ (5 cm) space (about the width of one electrode) between them.**	
——	——	——	7. **Check the controls on the TENS unit to make sure that they are off.** Connect the wires to the electrodes (if not already attached) and plug them into the unit.	
——	——	——	8. Turn on the unit and adjust the intensity setting to the lowest intensity and determine if the patient can feel a tingling, burning, or buzzing sensation. Then adjust the intensity to the prescribed amount or the setting most comfortable for the patient. Secure the unit to the patient.	
——	——	——	9. Set the pulse width (duration of the each pulsation) as indicated or recommended.	
——	——	——	10. Assess the patient's pain level during therapy.	
——	——	——	a. If intermittent use is ordered, turn the unit off after the specified duration of treatment and remove the electrodes. Provide skin care to the area.	

Excellent	Satisfactory	Needs Practice	SKILL 10-3 **Applying a TENS Unit** *(Continued)*	Comments
___	___	___	b. If continuous therapy is ordered, periodically remove the electrodes from the skin (after turning the unit off) to inspect the area and clean the skin, according to facility policy. Reapply electrodes and continue therapy. Change electrodes according to manufacturer's directions.	
___	___	___	11. When therapy is discontinued, turn the unit off and remove the electrodes. Clean the patient's skin. Clean the unit and replace the batteries.	
___	___	___	12. Perform hand hygiene.	

Skill Checklists to Accompany Taylor's Clinical Nursing Skills:
A Nursing Process Approach, 2nd edition

Name _____   Date _____

Unit _____   Position _____

Instructor/Evaluator: _____   Position _____

SKILL 10-4

Caring for a Patient Receiving PCA Pump Therapy

Excellent	Satisfactory	Needs Practice	**Goal:** The patient reports increased comfort and/or decreased pain, without adverse effect, oversedation, and respiratory depression.	Comments
――	――	――	1. Gather equipment. Check the medication order against the original physician's order according to agency policy. Clarify any inconsistencies. Check the patient's chart for allergies.	
――	――	――	2. Know the actions, special nursing considerations, safe dose ranges, purpose of administration, and adverse effects of the medications to be administered. Consider the appropriateness of the medication for this patient.	
――	――	――	3. Prepare the medication syringe for administration.	
――	――	――	4. Identify the patient, show the patient the device, and explain the function of the device and reason for use. Explain the purpose and action of the medication to the patient.	
――	――	――	5. Plug the PCA device into the electrical outlet, if necessary. Check status of battery power, if appropriate.	
――	――	――	6. Close the door to the room or pull the bedside curtain.	
――	――	――	7. Complete necessary assessments before administering medication. Check allergy bracelet or ask patient about allergies. Assess the patient's pain, using an appropriate assessment tool and measurement scale.	
――	――	――	8. Perform hand hygiene and put on gloves, if indicated.	
――	――	――	9. **Check the label on the prefilled drug syringe with the medication record and patient identification.** Obtain verification of information from second nurse, according to facility policy.	
――	――	――	10. If using a bar code administration system, scan the patient's bar code on the identification band, if required.	
――	――	――	11. Connect tubing to prefilled syringe and place the syringe into the PCA device. **Prime the tubing.**	

SKILL 10-4

Caring for a Patient Receiving PCA Pump Therapy *(Continued)*

Excellent	Satisfactory	Needs Practice		Comments
——	——	——	12. Set the PCA device to administer the loading dose, if ordered, and then program the device based on the medical order for infusion dosage and lockout interval. Obtain verification of information from second nurse, according to facility policy.	
——	——	——	13. Using antimicrobial swab, clean connection port on intravenous infusion line or other site access, based on route of administration. Connect the PCA tubing to the patient's intravenous infusion line or appropriate access site, based on the specific site used. Secure the site per facility policy and procedure. Initiate the therapy by activating the appropriate button on the pump.	
——	——	——	14. Instruct the patient to press the button each time he or she needs relief from pain.	
——	——	——	15. Assess the patient's pain at least every 1 to 2 hours. Monitor vital signs, especially respiratory status, including oxygen saturation. Assess the patient's sedation score.	
——	——	——	16. Assess the infusion site periodically, according to facility policy and nursing judgment. Assess the patient's use of the medication, noting number of attempts and number of doses delivered. Replace the drug syringe when it is empty.	
——	——	——	17. Make sure the patient control (dosing button) is within the patient's reach. Remove gloves, if worn, and perform hand hygiene.	

Skill Checklists to Accompany Taylor's Clinical Nursing Skills:
A Nursing Process Approach, 2nd edition

Name _____   Date _____

Unit _____   Position _____

Instructor/Evaluator: _____   Position _____

Excellent	Satisfactory	Needs Practice	SKILL 10-5 **Caring for a Patient Receiving Epidural Analgesia** **Goal:** The patient reports increased comfort and/or decreased pain, without adverse effect, over sedation, and respiratory depression.	Comments
——	——	——	1. Check the medication order against the original medical order according to agency policy. Clarify any inconsistencies. Check the patient's chart for allergies.	
——	——	——	2. Know the actions, special nursing considerations, safe dose ranges, purpose of administration, and adverse effects of the medications to be administered. Consider the appropriateness of the medication for this patient.	
——	——	——	3. Identify the patient, show the patient the device, and explain the function of the device and reason for use. Explain the purpose and action of the medication to the patient.	
——	——	——	4. Close the door to the room or pull the bedside curtain.	
——	——	——	5. Perform hand hygiene. Put on nonsterile gloves, if indicated.	
——	——	——	6. Complete necessary assessments before administering medication. Check allergy bracelet or ask patient about allergies. Assess the patient's pain, using an appropriate assessment tool and measurement scale.	
——	——	——	7. **Have an ampule of 0.4-mg naloxone (Narcan) and a syringe at the bedside.**	
——	——	——	8. After the catheter has been inserted and the infusion initiated by the anesthesiologist or radiologist, **check the label on the medication container and rate of infusion with the medication record and patient identification.** Obtain verification of information from second nurse, according to facility policy.	
——	——	——	9. Tape all connection sites. Label the bag, tubing, and pump apparatus "For Epidural Infusion Only." **Do not administer any other narcotics or adjuvant drugs without the approval of the clinician responsible for the epidural injection.**	
——	——	——	10. Assess the exit site and apply a transparent dressing over the catheter insertion site, if not already in place. Monitor the infusion rate according to facility policy.	

Caring for a Patient Receiving Epidural Analgesia *(Continued)*

Excellent	Satisfactory	Needs Practice		Comments
——	——	——	11. Assess and record sedation level and respiratory status every hour for the first 24 hours, then at 4-hour intervals (or according to agency policy). **Notify the physician if the sedation rating is 3 or 4, the respiratory depth decreases, or the respiratory rate falls below 8 breaths per minute.**	
——	——	——	12. Keep the head of bed elevated 30 degrees unless contraindicated.	
——	——	——	13. Assess the patient's level of pain and the effectiveness of pain relief.	
——	——	——	14. Monitor urinary output and assess for bladder distention.	
——	——	——	15. Assess motor strength every 4 hours.	
——	——	——	16. Monitor for adverse effects (pruritus, nausea, and vomiting).	
——	——	——	17. Assess for signs of infection at the insertion site.	
——	——	——	18. Change the dressing over the catheter exit site every 24 to 48 hours or as needed per agency policy using aseptic technique. Change the infusion tubing every 48 hours or as specified by agency policy.	
——	——	——	19. Remove gloves, if worn, and perform hand hygiene.	

Skill Checklists to Accompany Taylor's Clinical Nursing Skills:
A Nursing Process Approach, 2nd edition

Name _____   Date _____

Unit _____   Position _____

Instructor/Evaluator: _____   Position _____

Excellent	Satisfactory	Needs Practice	SKILL 11-1 **Assisting With Patient Feeding**	Comments
			Goal: The patient consumes 50 to 60% of the contents of the meal tray.	
——	——	——	1. Check the physician's order for the type of diet.	
——	——	——	2. Identify the patient.	
——	——	——	3. Explain procedure to patient.	
——	——	——	4. Perform hand hygiene.	
——	——	——	5. Assess level of consciousness, for any physical limitations, decreased hearing or visual acuity. If patient uses a hearing aid or wears glasses or dentures, provide as needed. Ask if the patient has any cultural or religious preferences and food likes and dislikes, if possible.	
——	——	——	6. Pull the patient's bedside curtain. Assess the abdomen. Ask the patient if he/she has any nausea. Ask the patient if he/she has any difficulty swallowing. Assess the patient for nausea or pain and administer an antiemetic or analgesic as needed.	
——	——	——	7. Offer to assist the patient with any elimination needs.	
——	——	——	8. Provide hand hygiene and mouth care as needed.	
——	——	——	9. Remove any bedpans or undesirable equipment and odors if possible from the vicinity where meal will be eaten.	
——	——	——	10. Open the patient's bedside curtain. Assist or position the patient in a high Fowler's or sitting position. Position the bed in the low position.	
——	——	——	11. Place protective covering or towel over the patient if desired.	
——	——	——	12. Check tray to make sure that it is the correct tray before serving. Place tray on the overbed table so patient can see food if able. Ensure that hot foods are hot and cold foods are cold. Use caution with hot beverages, allowing sufficient time for cooling if needed. Ask the patient for his/her preference related to what foods are desired first. Cut food into small pieces as needed. Observe swallowing ability throughout the meal.	

SKILL 11-1
Assisting With Patient Feeding *(Continued)*

Excellent	Satisfactory	Needs Practice		Comments
___	___	___	13. If possible, sit facing the patient while feeding is taking place. It patient is able, encourage to hold finger foods and feed self as much as possible. Converse with patient during the meal as appropriate. Play relaxation music if patient desires.	
___	___	___	14. Allow enough time for the patient to adequately chew and swallow the food. The patient may need to rest for short periods during eating.	
___	___	___	15. **When the meal is completed or the patient is unable to eat any more, remove the tray from the room. Note the amount and types of food consumed.**	
___	___	___	16. Reposition the overbed table, remove the protective covering, offer hand hygiene as needed, and offer the bedpan. Assist the patient to a position of comfort and relaxation.	
___	___	___	17. Perform hand hygiene.	

Skill Checklists to Accompany Taylor's Clinical Nursing Skills:
A Nursing Process Approach, 2nd edition

Name _____ Date _____

Unit _____ Position _____

Instructor/Evaluator: _____ Position _____

Excellent	Satisfactory	Needs Practice	SKILL 11-2 **Inserting a Nasogastric Tube**	Comments
			Goal: The tube is passed into the patient's stomach without any complications.	
——	——	——	1. Check physician's order for insertion of NG tube and consider the risks associated with NG tube insertion.	
——	——	——	2. Identify the patient.	
——	——	——	3. Explain the procedure to the patient and provide the rationale as to why the tube is needed. Discuss the associated discomforts that may be experienced and possible interventions that may allay this discomfort. Answer any questions as needed.	
——	——	——	4. Gather equipment including selection of the appropriate NG polyurethane tube.	
——	——	——	5. Perform hand hygiene. Put on nonsterile gloves.	
——	——	——	6. Close the patient's bedside curtain or door. Raise the bed. Assist the patient to high Fowler's position and elevate the head of the bed 45 degrees. Drape chest with bath towel or disposable pad. Have emesis basin and tissues handy.	
——	——	——	7. **Measure the distance to insert tube by placing tip of tube at patient's nostril and extending to tip of ear lobe and then to tip of xiphoid process.** Mark tube with an indelible marker.	
——	——	——	8. Lubricate tip of tube (at least 2″–4″) with water-soluble lubricant. Apply topical anesthetic to nostril and oropharynx, as appropriate.	
——	——	——	9. After selecting the appropriate nostril, ask patient to slightly flex head back against the pillow. Gently insert the tube into the nostril while directing the tube upward and backward along the floor of the nose. Patient may gag when tube reaches pharynx. Provide tissues for tearing or watering of eyes. Offer comfort and reassurance to the patient.	

Excellent | Satisfactory | Needs Practice

10. **When pharynx is reached, instruct patient to touch chin to chest.** Encourage patient to sip water through a straw or swallow even if no fluids are permitted. Advance tube in downward and backward direction when patient swallows. Stop when patient breathes. **If gagging and coughing persist, stop advancing the tube and check placement of tube with tongue blade and flashlight.** If tube is curled, straighten the tube and attempt to advance again. Keep advancing tube until pen marking is reached. **Do not use force. Rotate tube if it meets resistance.**

11. **Discontinue procedure and remove tube if there are signs of distress, such as gasping, coughing, cyanosis, and inability to speak or hum.**

12. **While keeping one hand on tube or temporarily securing with tape, determine that tube is in patient's stomach:**

    a. Attach syringe to end of tube and aspirate a small amount of stomach **contents.**

    b. Measure the pH of aspirated fluid using pH paper or a meter. Place a drop of gastric secretions onto pH paper or place small amount in plastic cup and dip the pH paper into it. Within 30 seconds, compare the color on the paper with the chart supplied by the manufacturer.

    c. Visualize aspirated contents, checking for color and consistency.

    d. Obtain radiograph (x-ray) of placement of tube (as ordered by physician).

13. Apply tincture of benzoin or other skin adhesive to tip of nose and allow to dry. Secure tube with tape to patient's nose:

    a. Cut a 4″ piece of tape and split bottom 2″ or use packaged nose tape for NG tubes.

    b. Place unsplit end over bridge of patient's nose.

    c. Wrap split ends under tubing and up and over onto nose. **Be careful not to pull tube too tightly against nose.**

14. Clamp tube and cap or attach tube to suction according to the physician's orders.

Inserting a Nasogastric Tube *(Continued)*

Excellent	Satisfactory	Needs Practice		Comments
——	——	——	15. Secure tube to patient's gown by using rubber band or tape and safety pin. For additional support, tube can be taped onto patient's cheek using a piece of tape. **If double-lumen tube (eg, Salem sump) is used, secure vent above stomach level.** Attach at shoulder level.	
——	——	——	16. Assist with or provide oral hygiene at every 2- to 4-hour interval. Lubricate the lips generously and clean nares and lubricate as needed. Offer analgesic throat lozenges or anesthetic spray for throat irritation if needed.	
——	——	——	17. Remove all equipment, lower the bed, and make the patient comfortable. Remove nonsterile gloves and perform hand hygiene.	

Skill Checklists to Accompany Taylor's Clinical Nursing Skills:
A Nursing Process Approach, 2nd edition

Name _____ Date _____

Unit _____ Position _____

Instructor/Evaluator: _____ Position _____

SKILL 11-3
Administering a Tube Feeding

Excellent	Satisfactory	Needs Practice		Comments
			Goal: The patient will receive the tube feeding without complaints of nausea or episodes of vomiting.	
——	——	——	1. Identify the patient.	
——	——	——	2. Explain the procedure to the patient and why this intervention is needed. Raise the bed. Pull the patient's bedside curtain. Perform key abdominal assessments as described above.	
——	——	——	3. Assemble equipment. Check amount, concentration, type, and frequency of tube feeding on patient's chart. Check expiration date of formula.	
——	——	——	4. Perform hand hygiene. Put on nonsterile gloves.	
——	——	——	5. **Position patient with head of bed elevated at least 30 to 45 degrees or as near normal position for eating as possible.**	
——	——	——	6. Unpin tube from patient's gown. **Check to see that the NG tube is properly located in the stomach, by first instilling air, then aspirate for gastric contents.** At times, due to the tendency of small-bore tubes to collapse upon aspiration, several attempts may be necessary to aspirate gastric contents. After repeated instillations of 30 mL of air, accompanied by repositioning the patient, if unable to aspirate gastric contents, the tube placement should be checked by radiograph verified by physician's order. Check the pH as described in Skill 11-2.	
——	——	——	7. After multiple steps have been taken to ensure that the feeding tube is located in the stomach or small intestine, **aspirate all gastric contents with a syringe and measure to check for the residual amount of feeding in the stomach.** Flush tube with 30 mL of water for irrigation. Proceed with feeding if amount of residual does not exceed agency policy or physician's guideline. Disconnect syringe from tubing and cap end of tubing while preparing the formula feeding equipment. Remove gloves.	
——	——	——	8. Put on nonsterile gloves before preparing, assembling and handling any part of the feeding system.	
——	——	——	9. Administer feeding.	

Excellent	Satisfactory	Needs Practice		Comments

When Using a Feeding Bag (Open System)

a. Hang bag on IV pole and adjust to about 12″ above the stomach. Clamp tubing.

b. Check the expiration date of the formula. Cleanse top of feeding container with a disinfectant before opening it. **Pour formula into feeding bag and allow solution to run through tubing.** Close clamp.

c. Attach feeding setup to feeding tube, open clamp, and regulate drip according to physician's order, or allow feeding to run in over 30 minutes.

d. **Add 30 to 60 mL (1–2 oz) of water for irrigation to feeding bag when feeding is almost completed and allow it to run through the tube.**

e. Clamp tubing immediately after water has been instilled. Disconnect from feeding tube. Clamp tube and cover end with cap.

When Using a Large Syringe (Open System)

a. Remove plunger from 30- or 60-mL syringe.

b. Attach syringe to feeding tube, pour premeasured amount of tube feeding into syringe, open clamp, and allow food to enter tube. **Regulate rate, fast or slow, by height of the syringe. Do not push formula with syringe plunger.**

c. **Add 30 to 60 mL (1–2 oz) of water for irrigation to syringe when feeding is almost completed, and allow it to run through the tube.**

d. When syringe has emptied, hold syringe high and disconnect from tube. Clamp tube and cover end with cap.

When Using an Enteral Feeding Pump

a. Close flow-regulator clamp on tubing and fill feeding bag with prescribed formula. Amount used depends on agency policy. Place label on container with patient's name, date, and time the feeding was hung.

b. Hang feeding container on IV pole. **Allow solution to flow through tubing.**

Administering a Tube Feeding *(Continued)*

Excellent	Satisfactory	Needs Practice		Comments
——	——	——	c. Connect to feeding pump following manufacturer's directions. Set rate. Maintain the patient in the upright position throughout the feeding. If the patient needs to temporarily lie flat, the feeding should be paused. The feeding may be resumed after the patient's position has been changed back to 30 to 45 degrees.	
——	——	——	d. **Check residual every 4 to 8 hours.**	
——	——	——	10. Observe the patient's response during and after tube feeding and assess the abdomen at least once a shift.	
——	——	——	11. **Have patient remain in upright position for at least 1 hour after feeding.**	
——	——	——	12. Wash and clean equipment or replace according to agency policy. Remove gloves and perform hand hygiene.	

Skill Checklists to Accompany Taylor's Clinical Nursing Skills:
A Nursing Process Approach, 2nd edition

Name _____   Date _____

Unit _____   Position _____

Instructor/Evaluator: _____   Position _____

SKILL 11-4

Removing a Nasogastric Tube

Goal: The tube is removed with minimal discomfort to the patient, and the patient maintains an adequate nutritional intake.

Columns: Excellent | Satisfactory | Needs Practice | | Comments

1. Check physician's order for removal of NG tube.
2. Identify the patient.
3. Explain the procedure to the patient and why this intervention is warranted. Describe that it will entail a quick few moments of discomfort. Perform key abdominal assessments as described above.
4. Gather equipment.
5. Perform hand hygiene. Put on nonsterile disposable gloves.
6. Pull the patient's bedside curtain. Raise the bed to the appropriate height and place the patient in a 30- to 45-degree position. Place towel or disposable pad across patient's chest. Give tissues and emesis basin to patient.
7. Discontinue suction and separate tube from suction. Unpin tube from patient's gown and carefully remove adhesive tape from patient's nose.
8. Check placement and **attach syringe and flush with 10 mL of water or normal saline solution (optional) or clear with 30 to 50 cc of air.**
9. **Instruct patient to take a deep breath and hold it.**
10. **Clamp tube with fingers by doubling tube on itself. Quickly and carefully remove tube while patient holds breath. Coil the tube in a disposable towel as you remove from the patient.**
11. Dispose of tube per agency policy. Remove gloves and place in bag. Perform hand hygiene.
12. Offer mouth care to patient and facial tissue to blow nose. Lower the bed and assist the patient to a position of comfort as needed.
13. Put on gloves and measure the amount of nasogastric drainage in the collection device and record on output flow record, subtracting irrigant fluids if necessary. Add solidifying agent to nasogastric drainage according to hospital policy.
14. Remove gloves and perform hand hygiene.

Skill Checklists to Accompany Taylor's Clinical Nursing Skills:
A Nursing Process Approach, 2nd edition

Name _____ Date _____

Unit _____ Position _____

Instructor/Evaluator: _____ Position _____

SKILL 11-5

Irrigating a Nasogastric Tube Connected to Suction

Excellent   **Satisfactory**   **Needs Practice**

Goal: The tube will maintain patency with irrigation.   **Comments**

—— —— ——	1.	Check the physician's order
—— —— ——	2.	Identify the patient.
—— —— ——	3.	Explain the procedure to the patient and why this intervention is warranted. Perform key abdominal assessments as described above.
—— —— ——	4.	Gather necessary equipment. Check expiration dates on irrigating solution and irrigation set.
—— —— ——	5.	Perform hand hygiene. Put on gloves.
—— —— ——	6.	Pull the patient's bedside curtain. Raise the bed. Assist patient to 30- to 45-degree position, unless this is contraindicated.
—— —— ——	7.	**Check placement of NG tube.** (Refer to Skill 11-2.)
—— —— ——	8.	Pour irrigating solution into container. Draw up 30 mL of saline solution (or amount ordered by physician) into syringe.
—— —— ——	9.	Clamp suction tubing near connection site. If needed, disconnect tube from suction apparatus and lay on disposable pad or towel, or hold both tubes upright in nondominant hand.
—— —— ——	10.	Place tip of syringe in tube. **If Salem sump or double-lumen tube is used, make sure that syringe tip is placed in drainage port and not in blue air vent.** Hold syringe upright and gently insert the irrigant (or allow solution to flow in by gravity if agency policy or physician indicates). **Do not force solution into tube.**
—— —— ——	11.	**If unable to irrigate tube, reposition patient and attempt irrigation again. Inject 10 to 20 cc of air and aspirate again. Check with physician or follow agency policy, if repeated attempts to irrigate tube fail.**

Excellent	Satisfactory	Needs Practice	SKILL 11-5 **Irrigating a Nasogastric Tube Connected to Suction** *(Continued)*

				Comments
___	___	___	12. After irrigant has been instilled, observe for return flow of NG drainage into available container. Alternately, the nurse may reconnect the NG tube to suction and observe the return drainage as it drains into the suction container. **Inject air into blue air vent after irrigation is complete. Position the blue air vent above the patient's stomach.**	
___	___	___	13. Measure and record amount and description of irrigant and returned solution if measured at this time.	
___	___	___	14. Rinse equipment if it will be reused. Label with the date, patient's name, room number, and purpose (for NG tube/irrigation). Remove gloves and perform hand hygiene.	
___	___	___	15. Lower the bed. Assist the patient to a position of comfort. Perform hand hygiene.	

Skill Checklists to Accompany Taylor's Clinical Nursing Skills:
A Nursing Process Approach, 2nd edition

Name _____ Date _____

Unit _____ Position _____

Instructor/Evaluator: _____ Position _____

SKILL 11-6

Caring for a Gastrostomy Tube

Goal: The patient ingests an adequate diet and exhibits no signs and symptoms of irritation, excoriation, or infection at the tube insertion site.

Excellent	Satisfactory	Needs Practice		Comments
――	――	――	1. Check the physician's order.	
――	――	――	2. Identify the patient.	
――	――	――	3. Explain the procedure to the patient.	
――	――	――	4. Assess patient for presence of pain at the tube insertion site. If pain is present, offer patient analgesic medication per physician's order and wait for medication absorption before beginning insertion site care.	
――	――	――	5. Perform hand hygiene. Put on nonsterile gloves.	
――	――	――	6. Raise the bed to the appropriate height. Pull the patient's bedside curtain.	
――	――	――	7. If gastrostomy tube is new and still has sutures holding it in place, dip cotton-tipped applicator into sterile saline solution and gently clean around the insertion site, removing any crust or drainage. Avoid adjusting or lifting the external disk for the first few days after placement except to clean the area. If the gastric tube insertion site has healed and the sutures are removed, wet a washcloth and apply a small amount of soap onto washcloth. Gently cleanse around the insertion, removing any crust or drainage. **Rinse site, removing all soap.**	
――	――	――	8. Pat skin around insertion site dry.	
――	――	――	9. If the sutures have been removed, gently **rotate the guard or external bumper 90 degrees at least once a day. Assess that the guard or external bumper is not digging into the surrounding skin. Avoid placing any tension on the feeding tube.**	
――	――	――	10. Leave the stoma open to air unless there is drainage. If drainage is present, place one thickness of gauze pad under the external bumper and change as needed to keep the area dry. Use a skin protectant or substance such as zinc oxide to prevent skin breakdown.	
――	――	――	11. Remove gloves and perform hand hygiene.	
――	――	――	12. Lower the bed and assist the patient to a position of comfort as needed. Perform hand hygiene.	

Skill Checklists to Accompany Taylor's Clinical Nursing Skills:
A Nursing Process Approach, 2nd edition

Name _____ Date _____

Unit _____ Position _____

Instructor/Evaluator: _____ Position _____

Excellent	**Satisfactory**	**Needs Practice**	

SKILL 12-1
Assisting With the Use of a Bedpan

Goal: The patient is able to void with assistance.　　　　　**Comments**

Excellent	Satisfactory	Needs Practice		Comments
——	——	——	1. Identify the patient. Discuss procedure with patient and assess patient's ability to assist with the procedure, as well as personal hygiene preferences. Review chart for any limitations in physical activity.	
——	——	——	2. Bring bedpan and other necessary equipment to bedside. Perform hand hygiene. Put on disposable gloves.	
——	——	——	3. Warm bedpan, if it is made of metal, by rinsing it with warm water.	
——	——	——	4. Unless contraindicated, apply powder to the rim of the bedpan.	
——	——	——	5. Place bedpan and cover on chair next to bed. Close curtains around bed and close door to room if possible.	
——	——	——	6. If bed is adjustable, place it in high position. Place the patient in a supine position, with the head of the bed elevated about 30 degrees, unless contraindicated.	
——	——	——	7. Fold top linen back just enough to allow placement of bedpan. If there is no waterproof pad on the bed and time allows, consider placing a waterproof pad under patient's buttocks before placing bedpan.	
——	——	——	8. Ask the patient to bend the knees. Have the patient lift his or her hips upward. Assist patient, if necessary, by placing your hand that is closest to the patient palm up, under the lower back and assist with lifting. Slip the bedpan into place with other hand.	
——	——	——	9. **Ensure that bedpan is in proper position and patient's buttocks are resting on the rounded shelf of the regular bedpan or the shallow rim of the fracture bedpan.**	
——	——	——	10. Raise head of bed as near to sitting position as tolerated, unless contraindicated. Cover the patient with bed linens.	
——	——	——	11. **Place call device and toilet tissue within easy reach. Place the bed in the lowest position.** Leave patient if it is safe to do so. Use side rails appropriately.	
——	——	——	12. Remove gloves and perform hand hygiene.	

SKILL 12-1

Assisting With the Use of a Bedpan *(Continued)*

Excellent	Satisfactory	Needs Practice		Comments

Removing the Bedpan

___ ___ ___ 13. Perform hand hygiene and put on disposable gloves. Raise the bed to a comfortable working height. Have a receptacle, such as plastic trash bag, handy for discarding tissue.

___ ___ ___ 14. Lower the head of the bed, if necessary, to about 30 degrees. Remove bedpan in the same manner in which it was offered, being careful to hold it steady. Ask the patient to bend the knees and lift the buttocks up from the bedpan. Assist patient, if necessary, by placing your hand that is closest to the patient palm up, under the lower back and assist with lifting. Place the bedpan on the bedside chair and cover it.

___ ___ ___ 15. If patient needs assistance with hygiene, wrap tissue around the hand several times, and wipe patient clean, using one stroke from the pubic area toward the anal area. Discard tissue, and use more until patient is clean. Place patient on his or her side and spread buttocks to clean anal area.

___ ___ ___ 16. Do not place toilet tissue in the bedpan if a specimen is required or if output is being recorded. Place toilet tissue in appropriate receptacle.

___ ___ ___ 17. Return the patient to a comfortable position. Make sure the linens under the patient are dry. Replace or remove pad under the patient as necessary. Remove your gloves and ensure that the patient is covered.

___ ___ ___ 18. Raise side rail. Lower bed height and adjust head of bed to a comfortable position. Reattach call bell.

___ ___ ___ 19. Offer patient supplies to wash and dry his or her hands, assisting as necessary.

___ ___ ___ 20. Put on clean gloves. Empty and clean the bedpan, measuring urine in graduated container, as necessary. Discard trash receptacle with used toilet paper per facility policy. Perform hand hygiene.

Skill Checklists to Accompany Taylor's Clinical Nursing Skills:
A Nursing Process Approach, 2nd edition

Name _____ Date _____

Unit _____ Position _____

Instructor/Evaluator: _____ Position _____

Excellent	Satisfactory	Needs Practice	SKILL 12-2 **Assisting With the Use of a Urinal**	
			Goal: The patient is able to void with assistance.	**Comments**
___	___	___	1. Identify the patient. Discuss procedure with patient and assess patient's ability to assist with the procedure, as well as personal hygiene preferences. Review chart for any limitations in physical activity.	
___	___	___	2. Bring urinal and other necessary equipment to bedside. Perform hand hygiene. Put on disposable gloves.	
___	___	___	3. Close curtains around bed and close door to room if possible.	
___	___	___	4. Assist the patient to an appropriate position as necessary: standing at the bedside, lying on one side or back, sitting in bed with the head elevated, or sitting on the side of the bed.	
___	___	___	5. If the patient remains in the bed, fold the linens just enough to allow for proper placement of the urinal.	
___	___	___	6. If the patient is not standing, have him spread his legs slightly. **Hold the urinal close to the penis and position the penis completely within the urinal. Keep the bottom of the urinal lower than the penis. If necessary, assist the patient to hold the urinal in place.**	
___	___	___	7. Cover the patient with the bed linens.	
___	___	___	8. Place call device and toilet tissue within easy reach. Have a receptacle, such as plastic trash bag, handy for discarding tissue. Place the bed in the lowest position. Leave patient if it is safe to do so. Use side rails appropriately.	
___	___	___	9. Remove gloves and perform hand hygiene.	
			Removing the Urinal	
___	___	___	10. Perform hand hygiene and put on disposable gloves.	
___	___	___	11. Pull back the patient's bed linens just enough to remove the urinal. Cover the open end of the urinal. Place on the bedside chair. If patient needs assistance with hygiene, wrap tissue around the hand several times, and wipe patient clean. Place tissue in receptacle.	

SKILL 12-2

Assisting With the Use of a Urinal *(Continued)*

Excellent	Satisfactory	Needs Practice		Comments
——	——	——	12. Return the patient to a comfortable position. Make sure the linens under the patient are dry. Remove your gloves and ensure that the paitent is covered.	
——	——	——	13. Ensure patient call bell is in reach.	
——	——	——	14. Offer patient supplies to wash and dry his or her hands, assisting as necessary.	
——	——	——	15. Put on clean gloves. Empty and clean the urinal, measuring urine in graduated container, as necessary. Discard trash receptacle with used toilet paper per facility policy. Remove gloves and perform hand hygiene.	

Skill Checklists to Accompany Taylor's Clinical Nursing Skills:
A Nursing Process Approach, 2nd edition

Name _____   Date _____

Unit _____   Position _____

Instructor/Evaluator: _____   Position _____

Excellent	Satisfactory	Needs Practice	SKILL 12-3 **Assisting With the Use of a Bedside Commode**	
			Goal: The patient is able to void with assistance.	**Comments**
___	___	___	1. Identify the patient. Discuss procedure with patient and assess patient's ability to assist with the procedure, as well as personal hygiene preferences. Review chart for any limitations in physical activity.	
___	___	___	2. Bring the commode and other necessary equipment to bedside. Obtain assistance from another staff member, if necessary. Perform hand hygiene. Put on disposable gloves.	
___	___	___	3. Close curtains around bed and close door to room if possible.	
___	___	___	4. Place the commode close to and parallel with the bed. Raise or remove the seat cover.	
___	___	___	5. Assist the patient to a standing position and to pivot to the commode. **While bracing one commode leg with your foot, ask patient to place his or her hands one at a time on the arm rests. Assist the patient to slowly lower himself/herself onto the commode seat.**	
___	___	___	6. Cover the patient with a blanket. Place call device and toilet tissue within easy reach. Leave patient if it is safe to do so.	
___	___	___	7. Remove gloves and perform hand hygiene.	
			Assisting Patient Off Commode	
___	___	___	8. Perform hand hygiene and put on disposable gloves.	
___	___	___	9. Assist the patient to a standing position. If patient needs assistance with hygiene, wrap toilet tissue around your hand several times, and wipe patient clean, using one stroke from the pubic area toward the anal area. Discard tissue in an appropriate receptacle, according to facility policy, and continue with additional tissue until patient is clean.	
___	___	___	10. Do not place toilet tissue in the commode if a specimen is required or if output is being recorded. Replace or lower the seat cover.	

Excellent	Satisfactory	Needs Practice	SKILL 12-3 **Assisting With the Use of a** **Bedside Commode** *(Continued)*	
				Comments
——	——	——	11. Remove your gloves. Return the patient to the bed or chair. If the patient returns to the bed, raise side rails as appropriate. Ensure that the patient is covered and call device is readily within reach.	
——	——	——	12. Offer patient supplies to wash and dry his or her hands, assisting as necessary.	
——	——	——	13. Put on clean gloves. Empty and clean the commode, measuring urine in graduated container, as necessary. Remove gloves and perform hand hygiene.	

Skill Checklists to Accompany Taylor's Clinical Nursing Skills:
A Nursing Process Approach, 2nd edition

Name _____   Date _____

Unit _____   Position _____

Instructor/Evaluator: _____   Position _____

Excellent	Satisfactory	Needs Practice	SKILL 12-4 **Assessing Bladder Volume Using an Ultrasound Bladder Scanner**	Comments
			Goal: The volume of urine in the bladder will be accurately measured.	
____	____	____	1. Identify the patient. Discuss procedure with patient. Review chart for any limitations in physical activity.	
____	____	____	2. Bring the bladder scanner and other necessary equipment to bedside. Obtain assistance from another staff member, if necessary. Perform hand hygiene.	
____	____	____	3. Close curtains around bed and close door to room if possible.	
____	____	____	4. Raise the bed to a comfortable working height. Stand on the patient's right side if you are right handed, patient's left side if you are left handed.	
____	____	____	5. Assist patient to a supine position. Drape patient.	
____	____	____	6. Put on clean gloves.	
____	____	____	7. Press the "On" button. Wait until the device warms up. Press the "Scan" button to turn on the scanning screen.	
____	____	____	8. Press the appropriate gender button. The appropriate icon for male or female will appear on the screen.	
____	____	____	9. Clean the scanner head with the appropriate cleaner.	
____	____	____	10. **Gently palpate the patient's symphysis pubis. Place a generous amount of ultrasound gel or gel pad midline on the patient's abdomen, about 1″ to 1½″ above the symphysis pubis (anterior midline junction of pubic bones).**	
____	____	____	11. **Place the scanner head on the gel or gel pad, with the directional icon on the scanner head toward the patient's head. Aim the scanner head toward the bladder (point the scanner head slightly downward toward the coccyx). Press and release the "Scan" button.**	
____	____	____	12. Observe the image on the scanner screen. **Adjust the scanner head to center the bladder image on the crossbars.**	
____	____	____	13. Press and hold the "Done" button until it beeps. Read the volume measurement on the screen. Print the results if required by pressing "Print."	

Excellent	Satisfactory	Needs Practice	SKILL 12-4 **Assessing Bladder Volume Using an** **Ultrasound Bladder Scanner** *(Continued)*	
				Comments
——	——	——	14. Use a washcloth or paper towel to remove remaining gel from the patient's skin. Alternately, gently remove gel pad from patient's skin. Return the patient to a comfortable position. Remove your gloves and ensure that the patient is covered.	
——	——	——	15. Lower bed height and adjust head of bed to a comfortable position. Reattach call bell if necessary.	

Skill Checklists to Accompany Taylor's Clinical Nursing Skills:
A Nursing Process Approach, 2nd edition

Name _____   Date _____

Unit _____   Position _____

Instructor/Evaluator: _____   Position _____

Excellent	Satisfactory	Needs Practice	SKILL 12-5 **Catheterizing the Female Urinary Bladder** **Goal:** The patient's urinary elimination will be maintained, with a urine output of at least 30 mL/hour, and the patient's bladder will not be distended.	Comments
___	___	___	1. Identify the patient. Discuss procedure with patient and assess patient's ability to assist with the procedure. Discuss any allergies with patient, especially to iodine and latex. Review chart for any limitations in physical activity.	
___	___	___	2. Bring the catheter kit and other necessary equipment to bedside. Obtain assistance from another staff member, if necessary. Perform hand hygiene.	
___	___	___	3. Close curtains around bed and close door to room if possible.	
___	___	___	4. Provide for good light. Artificial light is recommended (use of a flashlight requires an assistant to hold and position it). Place a trash receptacle within easy reach.	
___	___	___	5. Raise the bed to a comfortable working height. Stand on the patient's right side if you are right handed, patient's left side if you are left handed.	
___	___	___	6. Assist patient to dorsal recumbent position with knees flexed, feet about 2 feet apart, with her legs abducted. Drape patient. Alternately, the Sims', or lateral, position can be used. Place the patient's buttocks near the edge of the bed with her shoulders at the opposite edge and her knees drawn toward her chest. Allow the patient to lie on either side, depending on which position is easiest for the nurse and best for the patient's comfort. Slide waterproof pad under patient.	
___	___	___	7. Put on clean gloves. Clean the perineal area with washcloth, skin cleanser, and warm water, using a different corner of the washcloth with each stroke. Wipe from above orifice downward toward sacrum (front to back). Rinse and dry. Remove gloves. Perform hand hygiene again.	
___	___	___	8. Prepare urine drainage setup if a separate urine collection system is to be used. Secure to bed frame according to manufacturer's directions.	
___	___	___	9. Open sterile catheterization tray on a clean overbed table using sterile technique.	

Excellent	Satisfactory	Needs Practice	SKILL 12-5 **Catheterizing the Female Urinary Bladder** *(Continued)*
			Comments
___	___	___	10. Put on sterile gloves. Grasp upper corners of drape and unfold drape without touching unsterile areas. Fold back a corner on each side to make a cuff over gloved hands. Ask patient to lift her buttocks and slide sterile drape under her with gloves protected by cuff.
___	___	___	11. Place a fenestrated sterile drape over the perineal area, exposing the labia.
___	___	___	12. Place sterile tray on drape between patient's thighs.
___	___	___	13. Open all the supplies. **Test the catheter balloon by removing protective cap on tip of syringe and attaching syringe prefilled with sterile water to injection port. Inject appropriate amount of fluid. If balloon inflates properly, withdraw fluid and leave syringe attached to port.**
___	___	___	14. Fluff cotton balls in tray before pouring antiseptic solution over them. Alternately, open package of antiseptic swabs. Open specimen container if specimen is to be obtained.
___	___	___	15. Lubricate 1″ to 2″ of catheter tip.
___	___	___	16. With thumb and one finger of nondominant hand, spread labia and identify meatus. **Be prepared to maintain separation of labia with one hand until catheter is inserted and urine is flowing well and continuously.** If the patient is in the sidelying position, lift the upper buttock and labia to expose the urinary meatus
___	___	___	17. Use your dominant hand to pick up a cotton ball. **Clean one labial fold, top to bottom (from above the meatus down toward the rectum), then discard the cotton ball. Using a new cotton ball for each stroke, continue to clean the other labial fold, then directly over the meatus.**
___	___	___	18. With your uncontaminated, dominant hand, place drainage end of catheter in receptacle. If the catheter is preattached to sterile tubing and drainage container (closed drainage system), position catheter and setup within easy reach on sterile field. Ensure that clamp on drainage bag is closed.
___	___	___	19. **Using your dominant hand, hold the catheter 2″ to 3″ from the tip and insert slowly into the urethra. Advance the catheter until there is a return of urine (approx. 2″–3″ [4.8–7.2 cm]). Once urine drains, advance catheter another 2″–3″ (4.8–7.2 cm). Do not force catheter through urethra into bladder.** Ask patient to breathe deeply, and rotate catheter gently if slight resistance is met as catheter reaches external sphincter.

Catheterizing the Female Urinary Bladder *(Continued)*

Excellent	Satisfactory	Needs Practice		Comments
——	——	——	20. Hold the catheter securely at the meatus with your nondominant hand. Use your dominant hand to inflate the catheter balloon. Inject entire volume supplied in prefilled syringe.	
——	——	——	21. Pull gently on catheter after balloon is inflated to feel resistance.	
——	——	——	22. Attach catheter to drainage system if not already preattached.	
——	——	——	23. Remove equipment and dispose of according to facility policy. Wash and dry the perineal area as needed.	
——	——	——	24. Remove gloves. **Secure catheter tubing to the patient's inner thigh with Velcro leg strap or tape.** Leave some slack in catheter for leg movement.	
——	——	——	25. Assist the patient to a comfortable position. Cover the patient with bed linens. Place the bed in the lowest position.	
——	——	——	26. Secure drainage bag below the level of the bladder. Check that drainage tubing is not kinked and that movement of side rails does not interfere with catheter or drainage bag.	
——	——	——	27. Put on clean gloves. Obtain urine specimen immediately, if needed, from drainage bag. Label specimen. Send urine specimen to the laboratory promptly or refrigerate it.	
——	——	——	28. Remove gloves. Perform hand hygiene.	

Skill Checklists to Accompany Taylor's Clinical Nursing Skills:
A Nursing Process Approach, 2nd edition

Name _____   Date _____

Unit _____   Position _____

Instructor/Evaluator: _____   Position _____

Excellent	Satisfactory	Needs Practice	SKILL 12-6 **Catheterizing the Male Urinary Bladder** **Goal:** The patient's urinary elimination will be maintained, with a urine output of at least 30 mL/hour, and the patient's bladder will not be distended.	Comments
——	——	——	1. Identify the patient. Discuss procedure with patient and assess patient's ability to assist with the procedure. Discuss any allergies with patient, especially to iodine and latex. Review chart for any limitations in physical activity.	
——	——	——	2. Bring the catheter kit and other necessary equipment to bedside. Obtain assistance from another staff member, if necessary. Perform hand hygiene. Put on disposable gloves.	
——	——	——	3. Close curtains around bed and close door to room if possible.	
——	——	——	4. Provide for good light. Artificial light is recommended. Place a trash receptacle within easy reach.	
——	——	——	5. Raise the bed to a comfortable working height. Stand on the patient's right side if you are right handed, patient's left side if you are left handed.	
——	——	——	6. Position patient on his back with thighs slightly apart. Drape patient so that only the area around the penis is exposed. Slide waterproof pad under patient.	
——	——	——	7. Put on clean gloves. Clean the genital area with washcloth, skin cleanser, and warm water. Clean the tip of the penis first, moving the washcloth in a circular motion from the meatus outward. Wash the shaft of the penis using downward strokes toward the pubic area. Rinse and dry. Remove gloves. Perform hand hygiene again.	
——	——	——	8. Prepare urine drainage setup if a separate urine collection system is to be used. Secure to bed frame according to manufacturer's directions.	
——	——	——	9. Open sterile catheterization tray on a clean overbed table, using sterile technique.	
——	——	——	10. Put on sterile gloves. Open sterile drape and place on patient's thighs. Place fenestrated drape with opening over penis.	
——	——	——	11. Place catheter set on or next to patient's legs on sterile drape.	

SKILL 12-6
Catheterizing the Male Urinary Bladder *(Continued)*

Excellent	Satisfactory	Needs Practice		Comments
——	——	——	12. Open all the supplies. **Test the catheter balloon by removing protective cap on tip of syringe and attaching syringe prefilled with sterile water to injection port. Inject appropriate amount of fluid. If balloon inflates properly, withdraw fluid and leave syringe attached to port.**	
——	——	——	13. Fluff cotton balls in tray before pouring antiseptic solution over them. Alternately, open package of antiseptic swabs. Open specimen container if specimen is to be obtained.	
——	——	——	14. With your uncontaminated, dominant hand, place drainage end of catheter in receptacle. If the catheter is preattached to sterile tubing and drainage container (closed drainage system), position catheter and setup within easy reach on sterile field. Ensure that clamp on drainage bag is closed.	
——	——	——	15. Remove cap from syringe prefilled with lubricant.	
——	——	——	16. Lift penis with nondominant hand. Retract foreskin in uncircumcised patient. **Be prepared to keep this hand in this position until catheter is inserted and urine is flowing well and continuously. Using your dominant hand and the forceps, pick up a cotton ball. Using a circular motion, clean the penis, moving from the meatus down the glans of the penis. Repeat this cleansing motion two more times, using a new cotton ball each time. Discard each cotton ball after one use.**	
——	——	——	17. Hold penis with slight upward tension and perpendicular to patient's body. Use your dominant hand to pick up the lubricant syringe. **Gently insert tip of syringe with lubricant into urethra and instill the 10 mL of lubricant.**	
——	——	——	18. Use your dominant hand to pick up the catheter and hold it an inch or two from the tip. Ask patient to bear down as if voiding. **Insert catheter tip into meatus. Ask the patient to take deep breaths as you advance the catheter to the bifurcation or "Y" level of the ports. Do not use force to introduce catheter.** If catheter resists entry, ask patient to breathe deeply and rotate catheter slightly.	
——	——	——	19. Hold the catheter securely at the meatus with your nondominant hand. Use your dominant hand to inflate the catheter balloon. **Inject entire volume supplied in prefilled syringe. Once balloon is inflated, catheter may be gently pulled back into place. Replace foreskin over catheter.** Lower penis.	

Catheterizing the Male Urinary Bladder *(Continued)*

Excellent	Satisfactory	Needs Practice		Comments
___	___	___	20. Pull gently on catheter after balloon is inflated to feel resistance.	
___	___	___	21. Attach catheter to drainage system if necessary.	
___	___	___	22. Remove equipment and dispose of according to facility policy. Wash and dry the perineal area as needed.	
___	___	___	23. Remove gloves. Secure catheter tubing to the patient's inner thigh or lower abdomen (with the penis directed toward the patient's chest) with Velcro leg strap or tape. Leave some slack in catheter for leg movement.	
___	___	___	24. Assist the patient to a comfortable position. Cover the patient with bed linens. Place the bed in the lowest position.	
___	___	___	25. Secure drainage bag below the level of the bladder. Check that drainage tubing is not kinked and that movement of side rails does not interfere with catheter or drainage bag.	
___	___	___	26. Put on clean gloves. Obtain urine specimen immediately, if needed, from drainage bag. Cover and label specimen. Send urine specimen to the laboratory promptly or refrigerate it.	
___	___	___	27. Remove gloves. Perform hand hygiene.	

Skill Checklists to Accompany Taylor's Clinical Nursing Skills:
A Nursing Process Approach, 2nd edition

Name _____   Date _____

Unit _____   Position _____

Instructor/Evaluator: _____   Position _____

SKILL 12-7
Removing an Indwelling Catheter

Goal: The catheter will be removed without difficulty and with minimal patient discomfort.

Excellent	Satisfactory	Needs Practice		Comments
——	——	——	1. Identify the patient. Discuss procedure with patient.	
——	——	——	2. Perform hand hygiene.	
——	——	——	3. Close curtains around bed and close door to room if possible.	
——	——	——	4. Raise the bed to a comfortable working height. Stand on the patient's right side if you are right handed, patient's left side if you are left handed.	
——	——	——	5. Position patient as for catheter insertion. Drape patient so that only the area around the catheter is exposed. Slide waterproof pad between the female patient's legs or over the male patient's thighs.	
——	——	——	6. Remove the tape used to secure the catheter to the patient's thigh or abdomen.	
——	——	——	7. **Insert the syringe into the balloon inflation port. Aspirate the entire amount of fluid used to inflate the balloon.**	
——	——	——	8. Ask the patient to take several slow deep breaths. **Slowly and gently remove the catheter.** Place it on the waterproof pad and wrap it in the pad.	
——	——	——	9. Wash and dry the perineal area as needed.	
——	——	——	10. Remove gloves. Assist the patient to a comfortable position. Cover the patient with bed linens. Place the bed in the lowest position.	
——	——	——	11. Put on clean gloves. Remove equipment and dispose of according to facility policy. Note characteristics and amount of urine in drainage bag.	
——	——	——	12. Remove gloves. Perform hand hygiene.	

Skill Checklists to Accompany Taylor's Clinical Nursing Skills:
A Nursing Process Approach, 2nd edition

Name _____ Date _____

Unit _____ Position _____

Instructor/Evaluator: _____ Position _____

Excellent	Satisfactory	Needs Practice	SKILL 12-8 **Performing Intermittent Closed Catheter Irrigation**	Comments
			Goal: The patient exhibits the free flow of urine through the catheter.	
____	____	____	1. Identify the patient. Discuss procedure with patient.	
____	____	____	2. Perform hand hygiene.	
____	____	____	3. Provide privacy by closing the curtains or door and draping patient with bath blanket.	
____	____	____	4. Raise the bed to a comfortable working height.	
____	____	____	5. Empty the catheter drainage bag and measure the amount of urine, noting the amount and characteristics of the urine.	
____	____	____	6. Assist patient to comfortable position and expose access port on catheter setup. Place waterproof pad under catheter and aspiration port. Remove tape anchoring catheter to the patient.	
____	____	____	7. Open supplies, using aseptic technique. Pour sterile solution into sterile basin. Aspirate the prescribed amount of irrigant (usually 30–60 mL) into sterile syringe and attach capped, sterile, blunt-ended needle, if necessary. Put on gloves.	
____	____	____	8. **Cleanse the access port with antimicrobial swab.**	
____	____	____	9. Clamp or fold catheter tubing below the access port.	
____	____	____	10. Remove cap and insert needle into port. Alternately, attach the syringe to the port using a twisting motion, if needleless system is in place. **Gently instill solution into catheter.**	
____	____	____	11. Remove syringe/needle from port. Apply needle guard, if needle used. **Unclamp or unfold tubing and allow irrigant and urine to flow into the drainage bag.** Repeat procedure as necessary.	
____	____	____	12. Remove gloves. Secure catheter tubing to the patient's inner thigh or lower abdomen (if a male patient) with Velcro leg strap or tape. Leave some slack in catheter for leg movement.	
____	____	____	13. Assist the patient to a comfortable position. Cover the patient with bed linens. Place the bed in the lowest position.	

Excellent	Satisfactory	Needs Practice	SKILL 12-8 **Performing Intermittent Closed** **Catheter Irrigation** *(Continued)*	
				Comments
___	___	___	14. Secure drainage bag below the level of the bladder. Check that drainage tubing is not kinked and that movement of side rails does not interfere with catheter or drainage bag.	
___	___	___	15. Remove equipment and discard needle and syringe in appropriate receptacle. Perform hand hygiene.	
___	___	___	16. Assess patient's response to procedure and quality and amount of drainage after the irrigation.	

Skill Checklists to Accompany Taylor's Clinical Nursing Skills: A Nursing Process Approach, 2nd edition

Name _____ Date _____

Unit _____ Position _____

Instructor/Evaluator: _____ Position _____

Excellent	Satisfactory	Needs Practice	SKILL 12-9 **Administering a Continuous Closed Bladder Irrigation**	Comments
			Goal: The patient exhibits free-flowing urine through the catheter.	
___	___	___	1. Assemble equipment and double-check physician's order. Identify the patient. Discuss procedure with patient.	
___	___	___	2. Calculate drip rate for prescibed infusion rate.	
___	___	___	3. Perform hand hygiene.	
___	___	___	4. Provide privacy by closing the curtains or door and draping patient with bath blanket.	
___	___	___	5. Raise the bed to a comfortable working height.	
___	___	___	6. Empty the catheter drainage bag and measure the amount of urine, noting the amount and characteristics of the urine.	
___	___	___	7. Assist patient to comfortable position and expose the irrigation port on the catheter setup. Place waterproof pad under catheter and aspiration port. Remove tape anchoring catheter to patient.	
___	___	___	8. Prepare sterile irrigation bag for use as directed by manufacturer. Clearly label the solution as "Bladder Irrigant". Include the date and time on the label. Secure tubing clamp and attach sterile tubing with drip chamber to container using aseptic technique. Hang bag on IV pole $2\frac{1}{2}'$ to $3'$ above level of patient's bladder. Release clamp and remove protective cover on end of tubing without contaminating it. Allow solution to flush tubing and remove air. Clamp tubing and replace end cover.	
___	___	___	9. Put on gloves. **Cleanse the irrigation port with an alcohol swab. Using aseptic technique, attach irrigation tubing to irrigation port of three-way indwelling catheter.**	
___	___	___	10. Check the drainage tubing to make sure clamp, if present, is open.	
___	___	___	11. **Release clamp on irrigation tubing and regulate flow at determined drip rate, according to physician's order.** At times, the physician may order the bladder irrigation to be done with a medicated solution. In these cases, use an IV pump to regulate the flow.	

SKILL 12-9

Administering a Continuous Closed Bladder Irrigation *(Continued)*

Excellent	Satisfactory	Needs Practice		Comments
——	——	——	12. Remove gloves. Assist the patient to a comfortable position. Cover the patient with bed linens. Place the bed in the lowest position.	
——	——	——	13. Perform hand hygiene.	
——	——	——	14. Assess patient's response to procedure, and quality and amount of drainage.	
——	——	——	15. As irrigation fluid container nears empty, clamp the administration tubing. Do not allow drip chamber to empty. Disconnect empty bag and attach a new full irrigation solution bag. Continue as ordered by physician.	
——	——	——	16. Record amount of irrigant used on intake/output record. Put on gloves and empty drainage collection bag as each new container is hung and recorded.	

Skill Checklists to Accompany Taylor's Clinical Nursing Skills:
A Nursing Process Approach, 2nd edition

Name _____   Date _____

Unit _____   Position _____

Instructor/Evaluator: _____   Position _____

Excellent	Satisfactory	Needs Practice	SKILL 12-10 **Applying an External Condom Catheter**	Comments
			Goal: The patient's urinary elimination will be maintained, with a urine output of at least 30 mL/hour, and the bladder will not be distended.	
____	____	____	1. Identify the patient. Discuss procedure with patient and assess patient's ability to assist with the procedure. Discuss any allergies with patient, especially to latex.	
____	____	____	2. Bring the necessary equipment to bedside. Obtain assistance from another staff member, if necessary. Perform hand hygiene. Put on disposable gloves.	
____	____	____	3. Close curtains around bed and close door to room if possible.	
____	____	____	4. Raise the bed to a comfortable working height. Stand on the patient's right side if you are right handed, patient's left side if you are left handed.	
____	____	____	5. Prepare urinary drainage setup or reusable leg bag for attachment to condom sheath.	
____	____	____	6. Position patient on his back with thighs slightly apart. Drape patient so that only the area around the penis is exposed. Slide waterproof pad under patient.	
____	____	____	7. Put on disposable gloves. Trim any long pubic hair that is in contact with penis.	
____	____	____	8. Clean the genital area with washcloth, skin cleanser, and warm water. If patient is uncircumcised, retract foreskin and clean glans of penis. Replace foreskin. Clean the tip of the penis first, moving the washcloth in a circular motion from the meatus outward. Wash the shaft of the penis using downward strokes toward the pubic area. Rinse and dry. Remove gloves. Perform hand hygiene again.	
____	____	____	9. Apply skin protectant to penis and allow to dry.	
____	____	____	10. Roll condom sheath outward onto itself. Grasp penis firmly with nondominant hand. **Apply condom sheath by rolling it onto penis with dominant hand. Leave 1″ to 2″ (2.5–5 cm) of space between tip of penis and end of condom sheath.**	
____	____	____	11. **Apply pressure to sheath at the base of penis for 10 to 15 seconds.**	

Applying an External Condom Catheter *(Continued)*

Excellent	Satisfactory	Needs Practice		Comments
——	——	——	12. Connect condom sheath to drainage setup. Avoid kinking or twisting drainage tubing.	
——	——	——	13. Remove gloves. Secure drainage tubing to the patient's inner thigh with Velcro leg strap or tape. Leave some slack in tubing for leg movement.	
——	——	——	14. Assist the patient to a comfortable position. Cover the patient with bed linens. Place the bed in the lowest position.	
——	——	——	15. Secure drainage bag below the level of the bladder. Check that drainage tubing is not kinked and that movement of side rails does not interfere with the drainage bag.	

Skill Checklists to Accompany Taylor's Clinical Nursing Skills:
A Nursing Process Approach, 2nd edition

Name _____ Date _____

Unit _____ Position _____

Instructor/Evaluator: _____ Position _____

Excellent	Satisfactory	Needs Practice	SKILL 12-11 **Changing a Stoma Appliance on an Ileal Conduit**	Comments
			Goal: The stoma appliance is applied correctly to the skin to allow urine to drain freely.	
____	____	____	1. Identify the patient. Explain procedure and encourage patient to observe or participate if possible.	
____	____	____	2. Perform hand hygiene.	
____	____	____	3. Close curtains around bed and close door to room if possible.	
____	____	____	4. Have patient sit or stand if able to assist with skill or assume supine position in bed. If in bed, raise the bed to a comfortable working height. Place waterproof pad under the patient at the stoma site.	
____	____	____	5. Place a disposable waterproof pad on the overbed table. Set up the wash basin with warm water and the rest of the supplies. Place a trash bag within reach.	
____	____	____	6. Put on nonsterile gloves. Empty pouch being worn into graduated container if it is not attached to straight drainage.	
____	____	____	7. **Gently remove pouch faceplate from skin by pushing skin from appliance rather than pulling appliance from skin. Start at the top of the appliance, while keeping the abdominal skin taut. If resistance is felt, use warm water or adhesive remover to aid in removal.**	
____	____	____	8. Place the used appliance in the trash bag, if disposable. If reusable, set aside to wash in lukewarm soap and water and allow to air dry after the new appliance is in place.	
____	____	____	9. Clean skin around stoma with mild soap and water or a cleansing agent and a washcloth. Remove all old adhesive from skin; use an adhesive remover if necessary.	
____	____	____	10. Gently pat area dry. **Make sure skin around stoma is thoroughly dry.** Assess stoma and condition of surrounding skin.	
____	____	____	11. Place one or two gauze squares over stoma opening.	
____	____	____	12. Apply skin protectant to a 2″ (5-cm) radius around the stoma, and allow it to dry completely, which takes about 30 seconds.	

Changing a Stoma Appliance on an Ileal Conduit *(Continued)*

Excellent	Satisfactory	Needs Practice		Comments
——	——	——	13. Lift the gauze squares for a moment and measure the stoma opening, using the measurement guide. Replace the gauze. Trace the same size opening on the back center of the appliance. Cut the opening 1/8″ larger than the stoma size.	
——	——	——	14. Remove the backing from the appliance. Quickly remove the gauze squares and discard appropriately; ease the appliance over the stoma. **Gently press onto the skin while smoothing over the surface. Apply gentle pressure to appliance for 5 minutes.**	
——	——	——	15. Secure optional belt to appliance and around patient.	
——	——	——	16. Remove gloves. Assist the patient to a comfortable position. Cover the patient with bed linens. Place the bed in the lowest position.	
——	——	——	17. Put on clean gloves. Remove or discard any remaining equipment and assess patient's response to procedure. Remove gloves and perform hand hygiene.	

Skill Checklists to Accompany Taylor's Clinical Nursing Skills:
A Nursing Process Approach, 2nd edition

Name _____ Date _____

Unit _____ Position _____

Instructor/Evaluator: _____ Position _____

SKILL 12-12

Caring for a Suprapubic Urinary Catheter

Goal: The patient's skin remains clean, dry and intact, without evidence of irritation or breakdown; and the patient verbalizes an understanding of the purpose for and care of the catheter, as appropriate.

Excellent	Satisfactory	Needs Practice		Comments
___	___	___	1. Identify the patient. Discuss procedure with patient. Encourage patient to observe or participate if possible.	
___	___	___	2. Assemble equipment.	
___	___	___	3. Perform hand hygiene.	
___	___	___	4. Provide privacy by closing the curtains or door and draping patient with bath blanket.	
___	___	___	5. Raise the bed to a comfortable working height.	
___	___	___	6. Put on clean gloves. Gently remove old dressing, if one is in place. Place dressing in trash bag. Remove gloves. Perform hand hygiene.	
___	___	___	7. Assess the insertion site and surrounding skin.	
___	___	___	8. Wet washcloth with warm water and apply skin cleanser. **Gently cleanse around suprapubic exit site.** Remove any encrustations. If this is a new suprapubic catheter, sterile cotton-tipped applicators and sterile saline should be used to clean the site until incision has healed. **Moisten the applicators with the saline and clean in circular motion from the insertion site outward.**	
___	___	___	9. Rinse area of all cleanser. Pat dry.	
___	___	___	10. If exit site has been draining, place small drain sponge around catheter to absorb any drainage. Be prepared to change this sponge throughout the day, depending on the amount of drainage. Do not cut a 4 × 4 to make a drain sponge.	
___	___	___	11. Remove gloves. Form a loop in tubing and anchor the tubing on the patient's abdomen.	
___	___	___	12. Assist the patient to a comfortable position. Cover the patient with bed linens. Place the bed in the lowest position.	
___	___	___	13. Put on clean gloves. Remove or discard equipment and assess patient's response to procedure. Remove gloves and perform hand hygiene.	

Skill Checklists to Accompany Taylor's Clinical Nursing Skills:
A Nursing Process Approach, 2nd edition

Name _____   Date _____

Unit _____   Position _____

Instructor/Evaluator: _____   Position _____

Excellent	Satisfactory	Needs Practice	SKILL 12-13 **Caring for a Peritoneal Dialysis Catheter** **Goal:** The peritoneal dialysis catheter dressing change is completed using aseptic technique without trauma to the site or patient; the site is clean, dry, and intact without evidence of inflammation or infection; and the patient exhibits fluid balance and participates in care as appropriate.	Comments
____	____	____	1. Identify the patient. Explain procedure and encourage patient to observe or participate if possible.	
____	____	____	2. Bring the necessary equipment to the bedside. Close curtains around bed and close door to room if possible.	
____	____	____	3. Perform hand hygiene and put on nonsterile gloves.	
____	____	____	4. Raise the bed to a comfortable working height.	
____	____	____	5. Assist patient to supine position. Expose abdomen, draping the patient's chest with the bath blanket, exposing only the catheter site.	
____	____	____	6. Put on one of the face masks; have patient put on the other mask.	
____	____	____	7. Gently remove old dressing, noting odor, amount and color of drainage, leakage, and condition of skin around catheter. Discard dressing in appropriate container.	
____	____	____	8. Remove nonsterile gloves and discard. Set up sterile field. Open packages. Using aseptic technique, place two sterile 4 × 4s in basin with antimicrobial agent. Leave two sterile 4 × 4s opened on sterile field. Alternately (based on facility's policy), place sterile antimicrobial swabs on the sterile field. Place sterile applicator on field. Squeeze a small amount of the topical antibiotic on one of the gauze squares on the sterile field.	
____	____	____	9. Put on sterile gloves.	
____	____	____	10. Pick up dialysis catheter with nondominant hand. **With the antimicrobial-soaked gauze or swab, cleanse the skin around the exit site using a circular motion, starting at the exit site and then slowly going outward 3″ to 4″. Gently remove crusted scabs if necessary.**	

Caring for a Peritoneal Dialysis Catheter *(Continued)*

Excellent	Satisfactory	Needs Practice		Comments

——	——	——	11. Continue to hold catheter with nondominant hand. After skin has dried, clean the catheter with an antimicrobial-soaked gauze, beginning at exit site, going around catheter, and then moving up to end of catheter. Gently remove crusted secretions on the tube if necessary.	
——	——	——	12. Using the sterile applicator, apply the topical antibiotic to the catheter exit site, if prescribed.	
——	——	——	13. Place sterile drain sponge around exit site. Then place a 4 × 4 over exit site. Remove your gloves and secure edges of gauze pad with tape. Some institutions recommend placing a transparent dressing over the gauze pads instead of tape. Remove masks.	
——	——	——	14. Coil the exposed length of tubing and secure to the dressing or patient's abdomen with tape.	
——	——	——	15. Assist the patient to a comfortable position. Cover the patient with bed linens. Place the bed in the lowest position.	
——	——	——	16. Put on clean gloves and dispose of equipment per facility policy. Remove gloves and perform hand hygiene.	

Skill Checklists to Accompany Taylor's Clinical Nursing Skills:
A Nursing Process Approach, 2nd edition

Name _____ Date _____

Unit _____ Position _____

Instructor/Evaluator: _____ Position _____

Excellent	Satisfactory	Needs Practice	SKILL 12-14 **Caring for a Hemodialysis Access (Arteriovenous Fistula or Graft)** **Goal:** The patient verbalizes appropriate care measures and observations to be made, demonstrates care measures, and the graft or fistula remains patent.	Comments
___	___	___	1. Identify the patient. Explain procedure and encourage patient to observe or participate if possible.	
___	___	___	2. Close curtains around bed and close door to room if possible.	
___	___	___	3. Perform hand hygiene.	
___	___	___	4. **Inspect area over access site for any redness, warmth, tenderness, or blemishes. Palpate over access site, feeling for a thrill or vibration. Palpate pulses distal to the site. Auscultate over access site with bell of stethoscope, listening for a bruit or vibration.**	
___	___	___	5. Ensure that a sign is placed over head of bed informing the healthcare team which arm is affected. **Do not perform a venipuncture or start an IV on the access arm.**	
___	___	___	6. Instruct patient not to sleep with the arm with the access site under head or body.	
___	___	___	7. Instruct patient not to lift heavy objects with or put pressure on the arm with the access site. Advise the patient not to carry heavy bags (including purses) on the shoulder of that arm.	
___	___	___	8. Remove gloves and perform hand hygiene.	
___	___	___	9. Document assessment findings and any patient education performed.	

Skill Checklists to Accompany Taylor's Clinical Nursing Skills:
A Nursing Process Approach, 2nd edition

Name _____ Date _____

Unit _____ Position _____

Instructor/Evaluator: _____ Position _____

Excellent	Satisfactory	Needs Practice	SKILL 13-1 **Inserting a Rectal Tube**	Comments
			Goal: The tube is inserted and removed without adverse effect and the patient expels flatus.	
——	——	——	1. Identify the patient. Discuss the procedure with the patient and assess the patient's ability to assist with the procedure.	
——	——	——	2. Bring rectal tube and other necessary equipment to bedside. Perform hand hygiene. Put on disposable clean gloves.	
——	——	——	3. Close curtains around bed and close door to room if possible.	
——	——	——	4. If bed is adjustable, place it in high position. Place the patient in a prone or knee–chest position, unless contraindicated. A right side-lying position is also acceptable.	
——	——	——	5. Fold top linen back just enough to allow access to the patient's rectal area. Place a waterproof pad under the patient's hip.	
——	——	——	6. Lubricate approximately 4″ (10 cm) of the rectal tube with water-soluble lubricant.	
——	——	——	7. Separate buttocks so that anus is visible. Have patient take a slow, deep breath, inhaling through nose and exhaling through mouth. Gently insert the rectal tube beyond the anal canal into the rectum, angling toward the umbilicus, approximately 3″ to 4″ (10 cm) for an adult.	
——	——	——	8. Place end of rectal tube into the bedpan or waterproof pad. Instruct the patient to maintain his/her position while the tube is in place.	
——	——	——	9. Leave rectal tube in place for no longer than 20 minutes. Tube may be taped in place.	
——	——	——	10. Cover the patient with the bed linens.	
——	——	——	11. Stay with the patient while the tube is in place. While tube is in place, monitor patient for any change in heart rate or complaints of dizziness, lightheadedness, diaphoresis, and clammy skin.	
			Removing the Tube	
——	——	——	12. Perform hand hygiene and replace gloves if they have been removed.	

SKILL 13-1

Inserting a Rectal Tube *(Continued)*

Excellent	Satisfactory	Needs Practice		Comments
——	——	——	13. Have patient take a slow, deep breath, inhaling through nose and exhaling through mouth. Gently remove the tube at the same angle it was inserted.	
——	——	——	14. Wrap contaminated end of rectal tube in paper towel and discard.	
——	——	——	15. Clean perineal area.	
——	——	——	16. Return the patient to a comfortable position. Make sure the linens under the patient are dry. Remove your gloves and ensure that the patient is covered.	
——	——	——	17. Raise side rail. Lower bed height and adjust head of bed to a comfortable position.	
——	——	——	18. Remove any remaining equipment. Perform hand hygiene.	

Skill Checklists to Accompany Taylor's Clinical Nursing Skills:
A Nursing Process Approach, 2nd edition

Name _____   Date _____

Unit _____   Position _____

Instructor/Evaluator: _____   Position _____

Excellent	Satisfactory	Needs Practice	SKILL 13-2 **Administering a Large-Volume Cleansing Enema**	
			Goal: The patient expels feces.	**Comments**
——	——	——	1. Verify the order for the enema. Identify the patient. Explain procedure to patient. Discuss where the patient will defecate. Have a bedpan, commode, or nearby bathroom ready for use.	
——	——	——	2. Warm solution in amount ordered, and check temperature with a bath thermometer if available. If bath thermometer is not available, warm to room temperature or slightly higher, and test on inner wrist. If tap water is used, adjust temperature as it flows from faucet.	
——	——	——	3. Perform hand hygiene.	
——	——	——	4. Add enema solution to container. Release clamp and allow fluid to progress through tube before reclamping.	
——	——	——	5. Pull the curtains around the bed and close the room door. If bed is adjustable, place it in high position.	
——	——	——	6. Position the patient on the left side (Sims' position), as dictated by patient comfort and condition. Fold top linen back just enough to allow access to the patient's rectal area. Place a waterproof pad under the patient's hip.	
——	——	——	7. Put on nonsterile gloves.	
——	——	——	8. Elevate solution so that it is no higher than 18″ (45 cm) above level of anus. Plan to give the solution slowly over a period of 5 to 10 minutes. The container may be hung on an IV pole or held in the nurse's hands at the proper height.	
——	——	——	9. Generously lubricate end of rectal tube 2″ to 3″ (5–7 cm). A disposable enema set may have a prelubricated rectal tube.	
——	——	——	10. Lift buttock to expose anus. Slowly and gently insert the enema tube 3″ to 4″ (7–10 cm) for an adult. Direct it at an angle pointing toward the umbilicus, not bladder. Ask patient to take several deep breaths.	
——	——	——	11. If resistance is met while inserting tube, permit a small amount of solution to enter, withdraw tube slightly, and then continue to insert it. Do not force entry of the tube. Ask patient to take several deep breaths.	

			SKILL 13-2 **Administering a Large-Volume** **Cleansing Enema** *(Continued)*	
Excellent	**Satisfactory**	**Needs Practice**		**Comments**
——	——	——	12. Introduce solution slowly over a period of 5 to 10 minutes. Hold tubing all the time that solution is being instilled.	
——	——	——	13. Clamp tubing or lower container if patient has desire to defecate or cramping occurs. Patient also may be instructed to take small, fast breaths or to pant.	
——	——	——	14. After solution has been given, clamp tubing and remove tube. Have paper towel ready to receive tube as it is withdrawn.	
——	——	——	15. Return the patient to a comfortable position. Encourage the patient to hold the solution until the urge to defecate is strong, usually in about 5 to 15 minutes. Make sure the linens under the patient are dry. Remove your gloves and ensure that the patient is covered.	
——	——	——	16. Raise side rail. Lower bed height and adjust head of bed to a comfortable position.	
——	——	——	17. Remove any remaining equipment. Perform hand hygiene.	
——	——	——	18. When patient has a strong urge to defecate, place him or her in a sitting position on a bedpan or assist to commode or bathroom. Stay with patient or have call light readily accessible.	
——	——	——	19. Remind patient not to flush commode before nurse inspects results of enema.	
——	——	——	20. Put on gloves and assist patient if necessary with cleaning of anal area. Offer washcloths, soap, and water for handwashing. Remove gloves.	
——	——	——	21. Leave the patient clean and comfortable. Care for equipment properly.	
——	——	——	22. Perform hand hygiene.	

Skill Checklists to Accompany Taylor's Clinical Nursing Skills:
A Nursing Process Approach, 2nd edition

Name _____ Date _____

Unit _____ Position _____

Instructor/Evaluator: _____ Position _____

SKILL 13-3
Administering a Small-Volume Cleansing Enema

Goal: The patient expels feces and reports a decrease in pain and discomfort.

Excellent	Satisfactory	Needs Practice		Comments
——	——	——	1. Verify the order for the enema. Identify the patient. Explain procedure to patient. Discuss where the patient will defecate. Have a bedpan, commode, or nearby bathroom ready for use.	
——	——	——	2. Perform hand hygiene.	
——	——	——	3. Pull the curtains around the bed and close the room door. If bed is adjustable, place it in high position.	
——	——	——	4. Position the patient on the left side (Sims' position), as dictated by patient comfort and condition. Fold top linen back just enough to allow access to the patient's rectal area. Place a waterproof pad under the patient's hip.	
——	——	——	5. Put on nonsterile gloves.	
——	——	——	6. Remove the cap and generously lubricate end of rectal tube 2″ to 3″ (5–7 cm).	
——	——	——	7. Lift buttock to expose anus. Slowly and gently insert the rectal tube 3″ to 4″ (7–10 cm) for an adult. Direct it at an angle pointing toward the umbilicus, not bladder. Ask patient to take several deep breaths.	
——	——	——	8. Do not force entry of the tube. Ask patient to take several deep breaths.	
——	——	——	9. Compress the container with your hands. Roll the end up on itself, toward the rectal tip. Administer all the solution in the container.	
——	——	——	10. After solution has been given, remove tube, keeping the container compressed. Have paper towel ready to receive tube as it is withdrawn. Encourage the patient to hold the solution until the urge to defecate is strong, usually in about 5 to 15 minutes.	
——	——	——	11. Remove gloves. Return the patient to a comfortable position. Make sure the linens under the patient are dry. Ensure that the patient is covered.	
——	——	——	12. Raise side rail. Lower bed height and adjust head of bed to a comfortable position.	

Excellent	Satisfactory	Needs Practice		Comments

Administering a Large-Volume Cleansing Enema *(Continued)*

⎯ ⎯ ⎯		13. Remove any remaining equipment. Perform hand hygiene.	
⎯ ⎯ ⎯		14. When patient has a strong urge to defecate, place him or her in a sitting position on a bedpan or assist to commode or bathroom. Stay with patient or have call light readily accessible.	
⎯ ⎯ ⎯		15. Remind patient not to flush commode before nurse inspects results of enema.	
⎯ ⎯ ⎯		16. Put on gloves and assist patient if necessary with cleaning of anal area. Offer washcloths, soap, and water for handwashing. Remove gloves.	
⎯ ⎯ ⎯		17. Leave the patient clean and comfortable. Care for equipment properly.	
⎯ ⎯ ⎯		18. Perform hand hygiene.	

Skill Checklists to Accompany Taylor's Clinical Nursing Skills:
A Nursing Process Approach, 2nd edition

Name _____ Date _____

Unit _____ Position _____

Instructor/Evaluator: _____ Position _____

Excellent	Satisfactory	Needs Practice	SKILL 13-4 **Administering a Retention Enema** **Goal:** The patient retains the solution for the prescribed, appropriate length of time and experiences the expected therapeutic effect of the solution.	Comments
——	——	——	1. Verify physician's orders. Identify the patient. Explain to patient procedure and rationale for enema, including where he or she will defecate, and have a bedpan, commode, or nearby bathroom ready for use. Gather equipment. Allow solution to warm to room temperature.	
——	——	——	2. Perform hand hygiene.	
——	——	——	3. Pull the curtains around the bed and close the room door. If bed is adjustable, place it in high position.	
——	——	——	4. Position the patient on the left side (Sims' position), as dictated by patient comfort and condition. Fold top linen back just enough to allow access to the patient's rectal area. Place a waterproof pad under the patient's hip.	
——	——	——	5. Put on nonsterile gloves.	
——	——	——	6. Remove cap of prepackaged enema solution and ensure that rectal tube is prelubricated. If not, apply a generous amount of lubricant to the tube.	
——	——	——	7. Lift buttock to expose anus. Slowly and gently insert rectal tube 3″ to 4″ (7–10 cm) for an adult. Direct it at an angle pointing toward the umbilicus. Ask patient to take several deep breaths.	
——	——	——	8. If resistance is met while inserting tube, permit a small amount of solution to enter, withdraw tube slightly, and then continue to insert it. **Do not force entry of tube.**	
——	——	——	9. Slowly squeeze enema container, emptying entire contents.	
——	——	——	10. **Remove container while keeping it compressed.** Have paper towel ready to receive tube as it is withdrawn.	
——	——	——	11. **Instruct patient to retain enema solution for at least 30 minutes or as indicated.**	
——	——	——	12. Return the patient to a comfortable position. Make sure the linens under the patient are dry. Remove your gloves and ensure that the patient is covered.	
——	——	——	13. Raise side rail. Lower bed height and adjust head of bed to a comfortable position.	

			SKILL 13-4 **Administering a Retention Enema** (*Continued*)	

Excellent	Satisfactory	Needs Practice		Comments
___	___	___	14. Remove any remaining equipment. Perform hand hygiene.	
___	___	___	15. When patient has a strong urge to defecate, place him or her in a sitting position on bedpan or assist to commode or bathroom. Stay with patient or have call light readily accessible.	
___	___	___	16. Remind patient not to flush commode before nurse inspects results of enema. Record character of stool and patient's reaction to enema.	
___	___	___	17. Assist patient if necessary with cleaning of anal area (putting on gloves if necessary). Offer washcloths, soap, and water for handwashing.	
___	___	___	18. Leave patient clean and comfortable. Care for equipment properly.	
___	___	___	19. Perform hand hygiene.	

*Skill Checklists to Accompany Taylor's Clinical Nursing Skills:
A Nursing Process Approach, 2nd edition*

Name _____   Date _____

Unit _____   Position _____

Instructor/Evaluator: _____   Position _____

Excellent	Satisfactory	Needs Practice	SKILL 13-5 **Digital Removal of Stool**	
			Goal: The patient will expel feces with assistance.	**Comments**
——	——	——	1. Verify physician's order. Identify the patient. Explain procedure to patient, discussing signs and symptoms of a slow heart rate. Instruct patient to alert you if any of these symptoms are felt during the procedure.	
——	——	——	2. Gather necessary equipment.	
——	——	——	3. Perform hand hygiene.	
——	——	——	4. Pull the curtains around the bed and close the room door. If bed is adjustable, place it in high position.	
——	——	——	5. Position the patient in a side-lying position, as dictated by patient comfort and condition. Fold top linen back just enough to allow access to the patient's rectal area. Place a waterproof pad under the patient's hip.	
——	——	——	6. Put on nonsterile gloves.	
——	——	——	7. Generously lubricate index finger with water-soluble lubricant and insert finger gently into anal canal, pointing toward the umbilicus.	
——	——	——	8. Gently work the finger around and into the hardened mass to break it up and then remove pieces of it. Instruct patient to bear down, if possible, while extracting feces to ease in removal. Place extracted stool in bedpan.	
——	——	——	9. Remove impaction at intervals if it is severe. Instruct patient to alert you if he or she begins to feel light-headed or nauseated. If patient reports either symptom, stop removal and assess patient.	
——	——	——	10. Put on clean gloves. Assist patient if necessary with cleaning of anal area. Offer washcloths, soap, and water for handwashing. If patient is able, offer sitz bath.	
——	——	——	11. Remove gloves. Return the patient to a comfortable position. Make sure the linens under the patient are dry. Ensure that the patient is covered.	
——	——	——	12. Raise side rail. Lower bed height and adjust head of bed to a comfortable position.	
——	——	——	13. Perform hand hygiene.	

Skill Checklists to Accompany Taylor's Clinical Nursing Skills:
A Nursing Process Approach, 2nd edition

Name _____   Date _____

Unit _____   Position _____

Instructor/Evaluator: _____   Position _____

Excellent	Satisfactory	Needs Practice	SKILL 13-6 **Applying a Fecal Incontinence Pouch**	Comments
			Goal: The patient expels feces into the pouch and maintains intact perianal skin.	
___	___	___	1. Gather necessary equipment. Identify the patient. Discuss reason for fecal incontinence bag with patient.	
___	___	___	2. Perform hand hygiene.	
___	___	___	3. Pull the curtains around the bed and close the room door. If bed is adjustable, place it in high position.	
___	___	___	4. Position the patient in a side-lying position, as dictated by patient comfort and condition. Fold top linen back just enough to allow access to the patient's rectal area. Place a waterproof pad under the patient's hip.	
___	___	___	5. Put on nonsterile gloves. Cleanse perianal area. Pat dry thoroughly.	
___	___	___	6. Trim perianal hair if needed.	
___	___	___	7. Apply the skin protectant or barrier and allow to dry.	
___	___	___	8. Remove paper backing from adhesive of pouch.	
___	___	___	9. With nondominant hand, separate buttocks. Apply fecal pouch to anal area with dominant hand, ensuring that opening of bag is over anus.	
___	___	___	10. Release buttocks. Attach connector of fecal incontinence pouch to urinary drainage bag. Hang drainage bag below patient.	
___	___	___	11. Remove gloves. Return the patient to a comfortable position. Make sure the linens under the patient are dry. Ensure that the patient is covered.	
___	___	___	12. Raise side rail. Lower bed height and adjust head of bed to a comfortable position.	
___	___	___	13. Perform hand hygiene.	

Name _____ Date _____

Unit _____ Position _____

Instructor/Evaluator: _____ Position _____

Excellent	Satisfactory	Needs Practice	SKILL 13-7 **Changing and Emptying an Ostomy Appliance**	Comments
			Goal: The stoma appliance is applied correctly to the skin to allow stool to drain freely.	
____	____	____	1. Gather necessary equipment. Identify the patient. Explain procedure and encourage patient to observe or participate if possible.	
____	____	____	2. Close curtains around bed and close door to room if possible.	
____	____	____	3. Perform hand hygiene.	
____	____	____	4. Assist patient to a comfortable sitting or lying position in bed or a standing or sitting position in the bathroom.	
			Emptying an Appliance	
____	____	____	5. Put on disposable gloves. Remove clamp and fold end of pouch upward like a cuff.	
____	____	____	6. Empty contents into bedpan, toilet, or measuring device. Rinse appliance or pouch with tepid water in a squeeze bottle.	
____	____	____	7. Wipe the lower 2″ of the appliance or pouch with toilet tissue.	
____	____	____	8. Uncuff edge of appliance or pouch and apply clip or clamp. Remove gloves. If appliance is not to be changed, perform hand hygiene. Assist patient to comfortable position.	
			Changing an Appliance	
____	____	____	9. Place a disposable pad on the work surface. Set up the wash basin with warm water and the rest of the supplies. Place a trash bag within reach.	
____	____	____	10. Put on clean gloves. Place waterproof pad under the patient at the stoma site. Empty the appliance as previously described.	
____	____	____	11. Gently remove pouch faceplate from skin by pushing skin from appliance rather than pulling appliance from skin. Start at the top of the appliance, while keeping the abdominal skin taut. Push the skin from the appliance rather than pulling the appliance from the skin.	

Excellent	Satisfactory	Needs Practice		Comments
			SKILL 13-7 ## Changing and Emptying an ## Ostomy Appliance *(Continued)*	
——	——	——	12. Place the appliance in the trash bag, if disposable. If reusable, set aside to wash in lukewarm soap and water and allow to air dry after the new appliance is in place.	
——	——	——	13. Use toilet tissue to remove any excess stool from stoma. Cover stoma with gauze pad. Clean skin around stoma with mild soap and water or a cleansing agent and a washcloth. Remove all old adhesive from skin; an adhesive remover may be used. Do not apply lotion to peristomal area.	
——	——	——	14. Gently pat area dry. Make sure skin around stoma is thoroughly dry. Assess stoma and condition of surrounding skin.	
——	——	——	15. Apply skin protectant to a 2″ (5-cm) radius around the stoma, and allow it to dry completely, which takes about 30 seconds.	
——	——	——	16. Lift the gauze squares for a moment and measure the stoma opening, using the measurement guide. Replace the gauze. Trace the same-size opening on the back center of the appliance. Cut the opening 1/8″ larger than the stoma size.	
——	——	——	17. Remove the backing from the appliance. Quickly remove the gauze squares and ease the appliance over the stoma. Gently press onto the skin while smoothing over the surface. Apply gentle pressure to appliance for 5 minutes.	
——	——	——	18. Close bottom of appliance or pouch by folding the end upward and using clamp or clip that comes with product.	
——	——	——	19. Remove gloves. Assist the patient to a comfortable position. Cover the patient with bed linens. Place the bed in the lowest position.	
——	——	——	20. Put on clean gloves. Remove or discard equipment and assess patient's response to procedure. Remove gloves and perform hand hygiene.	

Name _____ Date _____

Unit _____ Position _____

Instructor/Evaluator: _____ Position _____

SKILL 13-8

Irrigating a Colostomy

Excellent	Satisfactory	Needs Practice	**Goal:** The patient expels soft formed stool.	Comments
___	___	___	1. Assemble necessary equipment. Verify the order for the enema. Identify the patient. Explain procedure to patient. Plan where he or she will receive irrigation. Assist patient onto bedside commode or into nearby bathroom.	
___	___	___	2. Pull the curtains around the bed and close the room door. Drape the patient to keep him/her covered.	
___	___	___	3. Warm solution in amount ordered, and check temperature with a bath thermometer if available. If bath thermometer is not available, warm to room temperature or slightly higher, and test on inner wrist. If tap water is used, adjust temperature as it flows from faucet.	
___	___	___	4. Perform hand hygiene.	
___	___	___	5. Add irrigation solution to container. Release clamp and allow fluid to progress through tube before reclamping.	
___	___	___	6. Hang container so that bottom of bag will be at patient's shoulder level when seated.	
___	___	___	7. Put on nonsterile gloves.	
___	___	___	8. Remove ostomy appliance and attach irrigation sleeve. Place drainage end into toilet bowl or commode.	
___	___	___	9. Lubricate end of cone with water-soluble lubricant.	
___	___	___	10. Insert the cone into the stoma. Introduce solution slowly over a period of 5 to 6 minutes. Hold tubing (or if patient is able, allow patient to hold tubing) all the time that solution is being instilled. Control rate of flow by closing or opening the clamp.	
___	___	___	11. **Hold cone in place for an additional 10 seconds after fluid is infused.**	
___	___	___	12. Remove cone. Patient should remain seated on toilet or bedside commode.	
___	___	___	13. After majority of solution has returned, allow patient to clip (close) bottom of irrigating sleeve and continue with daily activities.	

Excellent

Satisfactory

Needs Practice

SKILL 13-8

Irrigating a Colostomy *(Continued)*

Comments

——— ——— ———   14. After solution has stopped flowing from stoma, put on clean gloves. Remove irrigating sleeve and cleanse skin around stoma opening with mild soap and water. Gently pat peristomal skin dry.

——— ——— ———   15. Attach new appliance to stoma or stoma cover (see Skill 13-7) as needed.

——— ——— ———   16. Remove gloves. Return the patient to a comfortable position. Make sure the linens under the patient are dry, if appropriate. Ensure that the patient is covered.

——— ——— ———   17. Raise side rail. Lower bed height and adjust head of bed to a comfortable position.

——— ——— ———   18. Perform hand hygiene.

Skill Checklists to Accompany Taylor's Clinical Nursing Skills:
A Nursing Process Approach, 2nd edition

Name _____   Date _____

Unit _____   Position _____

Instructor/Evaluator: _____   Position _____

Excellent	Satisfactory	Needs Practice	SKILL 14-1 **Using a Pulse Oximeter**	Comments
			Goal: The patient will exhibit arterial blood oxygen saturation within acceptable parameters, or greater than 95%.	
⎯	⎯	⎯	1. Identify the patient using at least two methods.	
⎯	⎯	⎯	2. Explain what you are going to do and why you are going to do it to the patient.	
⎯	⎯	⎯	3. Perform hand hygiene.	
⎯	⎯	⎯	4. Select an adequate site for application of the sensor.	
⎯	⎯	⎯	a. Use the patient's index, middle, or ring finger.	
⎯	⎯	⎯	b. Check the proximal pulse and capillary refill at the pulse closest to the site.	
⎯	⎯	⎯	c. If circulation at site is inadequate, consider using the earlobe or bridge of nose.	
⎯	⎯	⎯	d. Use a toe only if lower extremity circulation is not compromised.	
⎯	⎯	⎯	5. Select proper equipment:	
⎯	⎯	⎯	a. If one finger is too large for the probe, use a smaller one. A pediatric probe may be used for a small adult.	
⎯	⎯	⎯	b. Use probes appropriate for patient's age and size.	
⎯	⎯	⎯	c. Check if patient is allergic to adhesive. A nonadhesive finger clip or reflectance sensor is available.	
⎯	⎯	⎯	6. Prepare the monitoring site. Cleanse the selected area with the alcohol wipe or disposable cleansing cloth. Allow the area to dry. If necessary, remove nail polish and artificial nails after checking manufacturer's instructions.	
⎯	⎯	⎯	7. **Apply probe securely to skin. Make sure that the light-emitting sensor and the light-receiving sensor are aligned opposite each other (not necessary to check if placed on forehead or bridge of nose).**	
⎯	⎯	⎯	8. Connect the sensor probe to the pulse oximeter, turn the oximeter on, and check operation of the equipment (audible beep, fluctuation of bar of light or waveform on face of oximeter).	

Excellent	Satisfactory	Needs Practice		Comments
——	——	——	9. Set alarms on pulse oximeter. Check manufacturer's alarm limits for high and low pulse rate settings.	
——	——	——	10. **Check oxygen saturation at regular intervals, as ordered by physician and signaled by alarms. Monitor hemoglobin level.**	
——	——	——	11. Remove sensor on a regular basis and check for skin irritation or signs of pressure (every 2 hours for spring tension sensor or every 4 hours for adhesive finger or toe sensor).	
——	——	——	12. Clean nondisposable sensors according to the manufacturer's directions. Perform hand hygiene.	

Skill Checklists to Accompany Taylor's Clinical Nursing Skills:
A Nursing Process Approach, 2nd edition

Name _____   Date _____

Unit _____   Position _____

Instructor/Evaluator: _____   Position _____

SKILL 14-2

Teaching Patient to Use an Incentive Spirometer

Excellent	Satisfactory	Needs Practice	**Goal:** The patient accurately demonstrates the procedure for using the spirometer.	Comments
___	___	___	1. Identify the patient.	
___	___	___	2. Explain what you are going to do and the reason to the patient.	
___	___	___	3. Perform hand hygiene.	
___	___	___	4. Assist patient to an upright or semi-Fowler's position if possible. Remove dentures if they fit poorly. Administer pain medication as prescribed, if needed. Wait the appropriate amount of time for the medication to take effect. **If patient has recently undergone abdominal surgery, place a pillow or folded blanket over a chest or abdominal incision for splinting.**	
___	___	___	5. Demonstrate how to steady the device with one hand and hold mouthpiece with other hand. If patient cannot use hands, nurse may assist patient with the incentive spirometer.	
___	___	___	6. Instruct patient to exhale normally and then place lips securely around the mouthpiece.	
___	___	___	7. **Instruct patient to inhale slowly and as deeply as possible through the mouthpiece without using nose (if desired, a nose clip may be used).**	
___	___	___	8. When the patient cannot inhale anymore, **the patient should hold his breath and count to three.** Check position of gauge to determine progress and level attained. If patient begins to cough, splint an abdominal or chest incision.	
___	___	___	9. Instruct patient to remove lips from mouthpiece and exhale normally. **If patient becomes light-headed during the process, tell him or her to stop and take a few normal breaths before resuming incentive spirometry.**	
___	___	___	10. Encourage patient to perform incentive spirometry 5 to 10 times every 1 to 2 hours if possible.	
___	___	___	11. Clean the mouthpiece with water and shake to dry. Perform hand hygiene.	

Skill Checklists to Accompany Taylor's Clinical Nursing Skills:
A Nursing Process Approach, 2nd edition

Name _____   Date _____

Unit _____   Position _____

Instructor/Evaluator: _____   Position _____

Excellent	Satisfactory	Needs Practice	SKILL 14-3 **Suctioning the Nasopharyngeal and Oropharyngeal Airways** **Goal:** The patient will exhibit improved breath sounds and a clear, patent airway.	Comments
——	——	——	1. Identify the patient.	
——	——	——	2. Determine the need for suctioning. Verify the suction order in the patient's chart, if necessary. **For postoperative patient, administer pain medication before suctioning.**	
——	——	——	3. Explain what you are going to do and the reason to the patient, even if the patient does not appear to be alert. Reassure patient you will interrupt procedure if he or she indicates respiratory difficulty.	
——	——	——	4. Perform hand hygiene.	
——	——	——	5. Adjust bed to comfortable working position. Lower side rail closer to you. If patient is conscious, place him or her in a semi-Fowler's position. **If patient is unconscious, place him or her in the lateral position, facing you. Move the bed table close to your work area and raise to waist height.**	
——	——	——	6. Place towel or waterproof pad across patient's chest.	
——	——	——	7. **Adjust suction to appropriate pressure.** For a wall unit for an adult: 100–150 mm Hg; neonates: 60–80 mm Hg; infants: 80–100 mm Hg; children: 100–120 mm Hg For a portable unit for an adult: 10–15 cm Hg; neonates: 6–8 cm Hg; infants 8–10 cm Hg; children 10–12 cm Hg **Put on a disposable, clean glove and occlude the end of the connecting tubing to check suction pressure. Place the connecting tubing in a convenient location.**	
——	——	——	8. **Open sterile suction package using aseptic technique. The open wrapper or container becomes a sterile field to hold other supplies. Carefully remove the sterile container, touching only the outside surface. Set it up on the work surface and pour sterile saline into it.**	
——	——	——	9. Place a small amount of water-soluble lubricant on the sterile field, taking care to avoid touching the sterile field with the lubricant package.	
——	——	——	10. Increase the patient's supplemental oxygen level or apply supplemental oxygen per facility policy or physician order.	

Excellent	Satisfactory	Needs Practice	SKILL 14-3 **Suctioning the Nasopharyngeal and Oropharyngeal Airways** *(Continued)*	Comments
——	——	——	11. Put on face shield or goggles and mask. Put on sterile gloves. **The dominant hand will manipulate the catheter and must remain sterile. The nondominant hand is considered clean rather than sterile and will control the suction valve (Y port) on the catheter.**	
——	——	——	12. With dominant gloved hand, pick up sterile catheter. Pick up the connecting tubing with the nondominant hand and connect the tubing and suction catheter.	
——	——	——	13. Moisten the catheter by dipping it into the container of sterile saline. Occlude Y-tube to check suction.	
——	——	——	14. Encourage the patient to take several deep breaths.	
——	——	——	15. Apply lubricant to the first 2″–3″ of the catheter, using the lubricant that was placed on the sterile field.	
——	——	——	16. Remove the oxygen delivery device, if appropriate. Do not apply suction as the catheter is inserted. Hold the catheter between your thumb and forefinger.	
			For Nasopharyngeal Suctioning **Gently insert catheter through the naris and along the floor of the nostril toward trachea.** Roll the catheter between your fingers to help advance it. Advance the catheter approximately 5″–6″ to reach the pharynx.	
			For Oropharyngeal Suctioning Insert catheter through the mouth, along the side of the mouth toward trachea. Advance the catheter 3″–4″ to reach the pharynx.	
——	——	——	17. Apply suction by intermittently occluding the Y port on the catheter with the thumb of your nondominant hand and gently rotate the catheter as it is being withdrawn. **Do not suction for more than 10 to 15 seconds at a time.**	
——	——	——	18. Replace the oxygen-delivery device using your nondominant hand, if appropriate, and have the patient take several deep breaths.	
——	——	——	19. Flush catheter with saline. Assess effectiveness of suctioning and repeat as needed and according to patient's tolerance. Wrap the suction catheter around your dominant hand between attempts.	

Excellent	Satisfactory	Needs Practice	SKILL 14-3 **Suctioning the Nasopharyngeal and Oropharyngeal Airways** *(Continued)*	Comments
——	——	——	20. Allow at least a 30-second to 1-minute interval if additional suctioning is needed. No more than three suction passes should be made per suctioning episode. Alternate the nares, unless contraindicated, if repeated suctioning is required. Do not force catheter through the nares. Encourage patient to cough and deep breathe between suctioning. Suction the oropharynx after suctioning the nasopharynx.	
——	——	——	21. When suctioning is completed, remove gloves from dominant hand over the coiled catheter, pulling it off inside out. Remove glove from nondominant hand and dispose of gloves, catheter, and container with solution in the appropriate receptacle. Remove face shield or goggles and mask. Perform hand hygiene.	
——	——	——	22. Turn off suction. Remove supplemental oxygen placed for suctioning, if appropriate. Assist patient to a comfortable position. Raise bed rail.	
——	——	——	23. Offer oral hygiene after suctioning.	
——	——	——	24. Reassess patient's respiratory status, including respiratory rate, effort, oxygen saturation, and lung sounds.	

Skill Checklists to Accompany Taylor's Clinical Nursing Skills:
A Nursing Process Approach, 2nd edition

Name _____   Date _____

Unit _____   Position _____

Instructor/Evaluator: _____   Position _____

SKILL 14-4

Administering Oxygen by Nasal Cannula

Excellent	Satisfactory	Needs Practice	**Goal:** The patient will exhibit an oxygen saturation level within acceptable parameters.	Comments
____	____	____	1. Identify the patient using at least two methods.	
____	____	____	2. Explain what you are going to do and the reason to the patient. Review safety precautions necessary when oxygen is in use. Place "No Smoking" signs in appropriate areas.	
____	____	____	3. Perform hand hygiene.	
			4. **Connect nasal cannula to oxygen setup with humidification, if one is in use.** Adjust flow rate as ordered by physician. Check that oxygen is flowing out of prongs.	
____	____	____	5. Place prongs in patient's nostrils. Place tubing over and behind each ear with adjuster comfortably under chin or around the patient's head, with adjuster at the back of the head or neck. Place gauze pads at ear beneath the tubing as necessary.	
____	____	____	6. Adjust the fit of the cannula as necessary. Tubing should be snug but not tight against the skin.	
____	____	____	7. **Encourage patient to breathe through the nose, with mouth closed.**	
____	____	____	8. Reassess patient's respiratory status, including respiratory rate, effort, and lung sounds. Note any signs of respiratory distress, such as tachypnea, nasal flaring, use of accessory muscles, or dyspnea.	
____	____	____	9. Perform hand hygiene.	
____	____	____	10. Put on clean gloves. Remove and clean the cannula and assess nares at least every 8 hours, or according to agency recommendations. Check nares for evidence of irritation or bleeding.	

Skill Checklists to Accompany Taylor's Clinical Nursing Skills: A Nursing Process Approach, 2nd edition

Name _____   Date _____

Unit _____   Position _____

Instructor/Evaluator: _____   Position _____

Excellent	Satisfactory	Needs Practice	SKILL 14-5 **Administering Oxygen by Mask**	Comments
			Goal: The patient exhibits an oxygen saturation level within acceptable parameters.	
——	——	——	1. Identify the patient.	
——	——	——	2. Explain what you are going to do and the reason to the patient. Review safety precautions necessary when oxygen is in use. Place "No Smoking" signs in appropriate areas.	
——	——	——	3. Perform hand hygiene.	
——	——	——	4. Attach face mask to oxygen source (with humidification, if appropriate for the specific mask). Start the flow of oxygen at the specified rate. For a mask with a reservoir, be sure to allow oxygen to fill the bag before proceeding to the next step.	
——	——	——	5. Position face mask over patient's nose and mouth. Adjust the elastic strap so that the mask fits snugly but comfortably on the face. Adjust the flow rate to the prescribed rate.	
——	——	——	6. If the patient reports irritation or redness is noted, use gauze pads under the elastic strap at pressure points to reduce irritation to ears and scalp.	
——	——	——	7. Reassess patient's respiratory status, including respiratory rate, effort, and lung sounds. Note any signs of respiratory distress, such as tachypnea, nasal flaring, use of accessory muscles, or dyspnea.	
——	——	——	8. Perform hand hygiene.	
——	——	——	9. **Remove the mask and dry the skin every 2 to 3 hours if the oxygen is running continuously. Do not use powder around the mask.**	

Skill Checklists to Accompany Taylor's Clinical Nursing Skills: A Nursing Process Approach, 2nd edition

Name _____ Date _____

Unit _____ Position _____

Instructor/Evaluator: _____ Position _____

Excellent	Satisfactory	Needs Practice	SKILL 14-6 **Using an Oxygen Hood**	Comments
			Goal: The patient exhibits an oxygen saturation level within acceptable parameters.	
____	____	____	1. Identify the patient.	
____	____	____	2. Explain what you are going to do and the reason to the patient and parents/guardians. Review safety precautions necessary when oxygen is in use.	
____	____	____	3. Perform hand hygiene.	
____	____	____	4. Calibrate the oxygen analyzer according to manufacturer's directions.	
____	____	____	5. Place hood on crib. Connect humidifier to oxygen source in the wall. Connect the oxygen tubing to the hood. Adjust flow rate as ordered by physician. Check that oxygen is flowing into hood.	
____	____	____	6. Turn analyzer on. **Place oxygen analyzer probe in hood.**	
____	____	____	7. Adjust oxygen flow as necessary, based on sensor readings. Once oxygen levels reach the prescribed amount, place hood over patient's head. The hood should not rub against the infant's neck, chin, or shoulder.	
____	____	____	8. If using the soft vinyl hood, roll small blankets or towels and place around edges where hood meets crib (if needed) to keep oxygen concentration at desired level. **Do not block hole in top of hood if present. If using a vinyl hood, the vent hole covering may need to be removed.**	
____	____	____	9. Instruct family members not to raise edges of the hood.	
____	____	____	10. Reassess patient's respiratory status, including respiratory rate, effort, oxygen saturation, and lung sounds. Note any signs of respiratory distress, such as tachypnea, nasal flaring, grunting, retractions, or dyspnea.	
____	____	____	11. Perform hand hygiene.	
____	____	____	12. Frequently check bedding and patient's head for moisture.	
____	____	____	13. Monitor the patient's body temperature at regular intervals.	

Skill Checklists to Accompany Taylor's Clinical Nursing Skills:
A Nursing Process Approach, 2nd edition

Name _____   Date _____

Unit _____   Position _____

Instructor/Evaluator: _____   Position _____

Excellent	Satisfactory	Needs Practice	SKILL 14-7 **Using an Oxygen Tent**	Comments
			Goal: The patient exhibits an oxygen saturation level within acceptable parameters.	
——	——	——	1. Identify the patient.	
——	——	——	2. Explain what you are going to do and the reason to the patient and parents/guardians. Review safety precautions necessary when oxygen is in use.	
——	——	——	3. Perform hand hygiene.	
——	——	——	4. Calibrate the oxygen analyzer according to manufacturer's directions.	
——	——	——	5. Place tent over crib or bed. Connect the humidifier to the oxygen source in the wall and connect the tent tubing to the humidifier. Adjust flow rate as ordered by physician. Check that oxygen is flowing into tent.	
——	——	——	6. Turn analyzer on. Place oxygen analyzer probe in tent, out of patient's reach.	
——	——	——	7. Adjust oxygen as necessary, based on sensor readings. Once oxygen levels reach the prescribed amount, place patient in the tent.	
——	——	——	8. Roll small blankets like a jelly roll and tuck tent edges under blanket rolls, as necessary.	
——	——	——	9. **Encourage patient and family members to keep tent flap closed.**	
——	——	——	10. Reassess patient's respiratory status, including respiratory rate, effort, and lung sounds. Note any signs of respiratory distress, such as tachypnea, nasal flaring, use of accessory muscles, grunting, retractions, or dyspnea.	
——	——	——	11. Perform hand hygiene.	
——	——	——	12. Frequently check bedding and patient's pajamas for moisture.	

Skill Checklists to Accompany Taylor's Clinical Nursing Skills:
A Nursing Process Approach, 2nd edition

Name _____   Date _____

Unit _____   Position _____

Instructor/Evaluator: _____   Position _____

Excellent	Satisfactory	Needs Practice	SKILL 14-8 **Inserting an Oropharyngeal Airway**	Comments
			Goal: The patient will sustain a patent airway.	
____	____	____	1. Identify the patient.	
____	____	____	2. Explain to the patient what you are going to do and the reason, even though the patient does not appear to be alert.	
____	____	____	3. Perform hand hygiene.	
____	____	____	4. Put on disposable gloves.	
____	____	____	5. Measure the oropharyngeal airway for correct size. The oropharyngeal airway is measured by holding the airway on the side of the patient's face. The airway should reach from the opening of the mouth to the back angle of the jaw.	
____	____	____	6. **Check mouth for any loose teeth, dentures, or other foreign material. Remove dentures or material if present.**	
____	____	____	7. Position patient in semi-Fowler's position.	
____	____	____	8. Suction patient if necessary.	
____	____	____	9. Open patient's mouth by using your thumb and index finger to gently pry teeth apart. **Insert the airway with the curved tip pointing up toward the roof of the mouth.**	
____	____	____	10. Slide the airway across the tongue to the back of the mouth. Rotate the airway 180 degrees as it passes the uvula. The tip should point down and the curvature should follow the contour of the roof of the mouth. A flashlight can be used to confirm the position of the airway with the curve fitting over the tongue.	
____	____	____	11. Ensure accurate placement and adequate ventilation by auscultating breath sounds.	
____	____	____	12. Position patient on his or her side when airway is in place.	
____	____	____	13. Remove gloves and perform hand hygiene.	
____	____	____	14. Remove the airway for a brief period every 4 hours, or according to facility policy. Assess mouth, provide mouth care, and clean the airway according to facility policy before reinserting it.	

Skill Checklists to Accompany Taylor's Clinical Nursing Skills:
A Nursing Process Approach, 2nd edition

Name _____   Date _____

Unit _____   Position _____

Instructor/Evaluator: _____   Position _____

Excellent	Satisfactory	Needs Practice	SKILL 14-9 **Inserting a Nasopharyngeal Airway**	
			Goal: The patient will sustain and maintain a patent airway.	**Comments**
___	___	___	1. Identify the patient.	
___	___	___	2. Explain what you are going to do and the reason to the patient, even if the patient does not appear to be alert.	
___	___	___	3. Perform hand hygiene.	
___	___	___	4. Put on disposable gloves. If patient is coughing or has copious secretions, a mask and goggles should also be worn.	
___	___	___	5. **Measure the nasopharyngeal airway for correct size.** The nasopharyngeal airway length is measured by holding the airway on the side of the patient's face. The airway should reach from the tragus of the ear to the nostril plus 1″. The diameter should be slightly smaller than the diameter of the nostril.	
___	___	___	6. Adjust bed to a comfortable working level. Lower side rail closer to you. If patient is awake and alert, position patient supine in semi-Fowler's position. If patient is not conscious or alert, position patient in a side-lying position.	
___	___	___	7. Suction patient if necessary.	
___	___	___	8. Lubricate the nasopharyngeal airway generously with the water-soluble lubricant, covering the airway from the tip to the guard rim.	
___	___	___	9. Gently insert the airway into the naris, narrow end first, until the rim is touching the naris. If resistance is met, stop and try other naris.	
___	___	___	10. Check placement by closing the patient's mouth and place your fingers in front of the tube opening to check for air movement. Assess the pharynx to visualize the tip of the airway behind the uvula. Assess the nose for blanching or stretching of the skin.	
___	___	___	11. Remove gloves and other personal protective equipment. Raise bed rail. Perform hand hygiene.	
___	___	___	12. **Remove the airway, clean in warm soapy water, and place in other naris at least every 8 hours, or according to facility policy.**	

Skill Checklists to Accompany Taylor's Clinical Nursing Skills:
A Nursing Process Approach, 2nd edition

Name _____   Date _____

Unit _____   Position _____

Instructor/Evaluator: _____   Position _____

Excellent	Satisfactory	Needs Practice	SKILL 14-10 **Suctioning an Endotracheal Tube: Open System** **Goal:** The patient will exhibit improved breath sounds and a clear, patent airway.	Comments
___	___	___	1. Identify the patient.	
___	___	___	2. Determine the need for suctioning. Verify the suction order in the patient's chart. **For postoperative patient, administer pain medication as prescribed before suctioning.**	
___	___	___	3. Explain what you are going to do and the reason to the patient, even if the patient does not appear to be alert. Reassure patient you will interrupt procedure if he or she indicates respiratory difficulty.	
___	___	___	4. Perform hand hygiene.	
___	___	___	5. Adjust bed to comfortable working position. Lower side rail closer to you. If patient is conscious, place him or her in a semi-Fowler's position. **If patient is unconscious, place him or her in the lateral position, facing you. Move the overbed table close to your work area and raise to waist height.**	
___	___	___	6. Place towel or waterproof pad across patient's chest.	
___	___	___	7. **Turn suction to appropriate pressure.** For a wall unit for an adult: 100–150 mm Hg; neonates: 60–80 mm Hg; infants: 80–100 mm Hg; children: 100–120 mm Hg For a portable unit for an adult: 10–15 cm Hg; neonates: 6–8 cm Hg; infants: 8–10 cm Hg; children: 1–12 cm Hg	
___	___	___	8. **Put on a disposable, clean glove and occlude the end of the connecting tubing to check suction pressure. Place the connecting tubing in a convenient location. Place the resuscitation bag connected to oxygen within convenient reach, if using.**	
___	___	___	9. Open sterile suction package using aseptic technique. The open wrapper becomes a sterile field to hold other supplies. Carefully remove the sterile container, touching only the outside surface. Set it up on the work surface and pour sterile saline into it.	

SKILL 14-10
Suctioning an Endotracheal Tube: Open System *(Continued)*

Excellent	Satisfactory	Needs Practice		Comments
——	——	——	10. Put on face shield or goggles and mask. Put on sterile gloves. **The dominant hand will manipulate the catheter and must remain sterile. The nondominant hand is considered clean rather than sterile and will control the suction valve (Y port) on the catheter.**	
——	——	——	11. With dominant gloved hand, pick up sterile catheter. Pick up the connecting tubing with the nondominant hand and connect the tubing and suction catheter.	
——	——	——	12. Moisten the catheter by dipping it into the container of sterile saline, unless it is a silicone catheter. Occlude Y-tube to check suction.	
——	——	——	13. Hyperventilate the patient using your nondominant hand and a manual resuscitation bag and delivering 3 to 6 breaths or use the sigh mechanism on a mechanical ventilator.	
——	——	——	14. Open the adapter on the mechanical ventilator tubing or remove the manual resuscitation bag with your nondominant hand.	
——	——	——	15. Using your dominant hand, gently and quickly insert catheter into trachea. **Advance the catheter to the predetermined length. Do not occlude Y-port when inserting catheter.**	
——	——	——	16. Apply suction by intermittently occluding the Y port on the catheter with the thumb of your nondominant hand, and gently rotate the catheter as it is being withdrawn. **Do not suction for more than 10 to 15 seconds at a time.**	
——	——	——	17. Hyperventilate the patient using your nondominant hand and a manual resuscitation bag and delivering 3 to 6 breaths. Replace the oxygen delivery device, if applicable, using your nondominant hand and have the patient take several deep breaths. If the patient is mechanically ventilated, close the adapter on the mechanical ventilator tubing or replace ventilator tubing and use the sigh mechanism on a mechanical ventilator.	
——	——	——	18. Flush catheter with saline. Assess effectiveness of suctioning and repeat as needed and according to patient's tolerance. Wrap the suction catheter around your dominant hand between attempts.	

SKILL 14-10
Suctioning an Endotracheal Tube:
Open System *(Continued)*

Excellent	Satisfactory	Needs Practice		Comments
____	____	____	19. Allow at least a 30-second to 1-minute interval if additional suctioning is needed. No more than three suction passes should be made per suctioning episode. Suction the oropharynx after suctioning the trachea. Do not reinsert in the endotracheal tube after suctioning the mouth.	
____	____	____	20. When suctioning is completed, remove glove from dominant hand over the coiled catheter, pulling it off inside out. Remove glove from nondominant hand and dispose of gloves, catheter, and container with solution in the appropriate receptacle. Remove face shield or goggles and mask. Perform hand hygiene.	
____	____	____	21. Turn off suction. Assist patient to a comfortable position. Raise bed rail. Offer oral hygiene after suctioning.	
____	____	____	22. Reassess patient's respiratory status, including respiratory rate, effort, oxygen saturation, and lung sounds.	

Name _____   Date _____

Unit _____   Position _____

Instructor/Evaluator: _____   Position _____

Excellent	Satisfactory	Needs Practice	SKILL 14-11 **Suctioning an Endotracheal Tube: Closed System** **Goal:** The patient will exhibit improved breath sounds and a clear, patent airway.	Comments
___	___	___	1. Identify the patient.	
___	___	___	2. Determine the need for suctioning. Verify the suction order in the patient's chart. **For postoperative patient, administer pain medication as prescribed before suctioning.**	
___	___	___	3. Explain what you are going to do and the reason to the patient, even if the patient does not appear to be alert. Reassure patient you will interrupt procedure if he or she indicates respiratory difficulty.	
___	___	___	4. Perform hand hygiene.	
___	___	___	5. Adjust bed to comfortable working position. Lower side rail closer to you. If patient is conscious, place him or her in a semi-Fowler's position. **If patient is unconscious, place him or her in the lateral position, facing you. Move the overbed table close to your work area and raise to waist height.**	
___	___	___	6. **Turn suction to appropriate pressure:** For a wall unit for an adult: 100–150 mm Hg; neonates: 60–80 mm Hg; infants: 80–100 mm Hg; children: 100–120 mm Hg For a portable unit for an adult: 10–15 cm Hg; neonates: 6–8 cm Hg; infants: 8–10 cm Hg; children: 10–12 cm Hg **Put on a disposable, clean glove and occlude the end of the connecting tubing to check suction pressure. Place the connecting tubing in a convenient location.**	
___	___	___	7. Open the package of closed suction device using aseptic technique. **Make sure that the device remains sterile.**	
___	___	___	8. Put on sterile gloves.	
___	___	___	9. Using nondominant hand, disconnect ventilator from endotracheal tube. Place ventilator tubing in a convenient location so that the inside of the tubing remains sterile or continue to hold the tubing in your nondominant hand.	
___	___	___	10. **Using dominant hand and keeping device sterile, connect the closed suctioning device so that the suctioning catheter is in line with the endotracheal tube.**	

SKILL 14-11
Suctioning an Endotracheal Tube:
Closed System *(Continued)*

Excellent	Satisfactory	Needs Practice		Comments

—— —— —— **11. Keeping the inside of the ventilator tubing sterile, attach ventilator tubing to port perpendicular to the endotracheal tube.** Attach suction tubing to suction catheter.

—— —— —— 12. Pop top off sterile normal saline dosette. Open plug to port by suction catheter and insert saline dosette or syringe.

—— —— —— **13. Hyperoxygenate or hyperventilate the patient by using the sigh button on the ventilator before suctioning.** Turn safety cap on suction button of catheter so that button is easily depressed.

—— —— —— 14. Grasp suction catheter through protective sheath, about 6″ (15 cm) from the endotracheal tube. Gently insert the catheter into the endotracheal tube. Release the catheter while holding onto the protective sheath. Move hand further back on catheter. **Grasp catheter through sheath and repeat movement, advancing the catheter to the predetermined length. Do not occlude Y-port when inserting catheter.**

—— —— —— **15. Apply intermittent suction by depressing the suction button with thumb of nondominant hand. Gently rotate catheter with thumb and index finger of dominant hand as catheter is being withdrawn. Do not suction for more than 10 to 15 seconds at a time. Hyperoxygenate or hyperventilate with sigh button on ventilator as ordered.**

—— —— —— 16. Once catheter is withdrawn back into sheath, depress the suction button while gently squeezing the normal saline dosette until catheter is clean. **Allow at least a 30-second to 1-minute interval if additional suctioning is needed. No more than three suction passes should be made per suctioning episode.**

—— —— —— **17. When procedure is completed, ensure that catheter is withdrawn into sheath, and turn safety button. Remove normal saline dosette and apply cap to port.**

—— —— —— 18. Suction the oral cavity with a separate single-use, disposable catheter and perform oral hygiene.

—— —— —— 19. Remove gloves and perform hand hygiene.

—— —— —— 20. Adjust the patient's position and raise the side rail. Reassess patient's respiratory status, including respiratory rate, effort, oxygen saturation, and lung sounds.

Skill Checklists to Accompany Taylor's Clinical Nursing Skills:
A Nursing Process Approach, 2nd edition

Name _____ Date _____

Unit _____ Position _____

Instructor/Evaluator: _____ Position _____

Excellent	Satisfactory	Needs Practice	SKILL 14-12 **Securing an Endotracheal Tube**	Comments
			Goal: The tube remains in place and the patient maintains bilaterally equal and clear lung sounds.	
——	——	——	1. Identify the patient.	
——	——	——	2. Assess the need for endotracheal tube retaping. **Administer pain medication or sedation as prescribed before attempting to retape endotracheal tube.** Explain the procedure to the patient.	
——	——	——	3. Obtain the assistance of a second individual to hold the endotracheal tube in place while the old tape is removed and the new tape is placed.	
——	——	——	4. Perform hand hygiene.	
——	——	——	5. Adjust bed to comfortable working position. Lower side rail closer to you. If patient is conscious, place him or her in a semi-Fowler's position. **If patient is unconscious, place him or her in the lateral position, facing you. Move the overbed table close to your work area. Place a trash receptacle within easy reach of work area.** Put on face shield or goggles and mask. Suction patient as described in Skill 14-10 or 14-11. Remove face shield or goggles and mask after suctioning.	
——	——	——	6. Measure a piece of tape for the length needed to reach around the patient's neck to the mouth plus 8″. Cut tape. Lay it adhesive side up on the table.	
——	——	——	7. Cut another piece of tape long enough to reach from one jaw around the back of the neck to the other jaw. Lay this piece on the center of the longer piece on the table, matching the tapes' adhesive sides together.	
——	——	——	8. Take one 3-mL syringe or tongue blade and wrap the sticky tape around the syringe until the nonsticky area is reached. Do this for the other side as well.	
——	——	——	9. Take one of the 3-mL syringes or tongue blades and pass it under the patient's neck so that there is a 3-mL syringe on either side of the patient's head.	
——	——	——	10. Put on disposable gloves. Have the assistant put on gloves as well.	
——	——	——	11. **Provide oral care, including suctioning the oral cavity.**	

Excellent	Satisfactory	Needs Practice		Comments

SKILL 14-12
Securing an Endotracheal Tube *(Continued)*

___	___	___	12. Take note of the "cm" position markings on the tube. Begin to unwrap old tape from around the endotracheal tube. After one side is unwrapped, have assistant hold the endotracheal tube as close to the lips or nares as possible to offer stabilization.	
___	___	___	13. Carefully remove the remaining tape from the endotracheal tube. **After tape is removed, have assistant gently and slowly move endotracheal tube (if orally intubated) to the other side of the mouth. Assess mouth for any skin breakdown. Before applying new tape, make sure that markings on endotracheal tube are at same spot as when re-taping began.**	
___	___	___	14. Remove old tape from cheeks and side of face. Use adhesive remover to remove excess adhesive from tape. Clean the face and neck with washcloth and cleanser. If patient has facial hair, consider shaving cheeks. Pat cheeks dry with the towel.	
___	___	___	15. Apply the skin barrier to the patient's face (under his nose, cheeks, under lower lip) where the tape will sit. Unroll one side of the tape. Ensure that nonsticky part of tape remains behind patient's neck while pulling firmly on the tape. **Place adhesive portion of tape snugly against patient's cheek.** Split the tape in half from the end to the corner of the mouth.	
___	___	___	16. Place the top-half piece of tape under the patient's nose. Wrap the lower half around the tube in one direction, such as over and around the tube. Fold over tab on end of tape.	
___	___	___	17. Unwrap second side of tape. Split to corner of the mouth. Place the bottom-half piece of tape along the patient's lower lip. Wrap the top half around the tube in the opposite direction, such as below and around the tube. Fold over tab on end of tape.	
___	___	___	18. **Auscultate lung sounds. Assess for cyanosis, oxygen saturation, chest symmetry, and stability of endotracheal tube. Again check to ensure that the tube is at the correct depth.**	
___	___	___	19. **If endotracheal tube is cuffed, check pressure of balloon by attaching a hand-held pressure gauge to the pilot balloon of the endotracheal tube.**	
___	___	___	20. Remove face shield or goggles and mask. Remove gloves and perform hand hygiene. Assist patient to a comfortable position. Raise bed rail.	

Skill Checklists to Accompany Taylor's Clinical Nursing Skills: A Nursing Process Approach, 2nd edition

Name _____ Date _____

Unit _____ Position _____

Instructor/Evaluator: _____ Position _____

Excellent	Satisfactory	Needs Practice	SKILL 14-13 **Suctioning the Tracheostomy: Open System**	Comments
			Goal: The patient will exhibit improved breath sounds and a clear, patent airway.	
____	____	____	1. Identify the patient.	
____	____	____	2. Determine the need for suctioning. Verify the suction order in the patient's chart. **For postoperative patient, administer pain medication as prescribed before suctioning.**	
____	____	____	3. Explain to the patient what you are going to do and the reason, even if the patient does not appear to be alert. Reassure patient you will interrupt procedure if he or she indicates respiratory difficulty.	
____	____	____	4. Perform hand hygiene.	
____	____	____	5. Adjust bed to comfortable working position. Lower side rail closer to you. If patient is conscious, place him or her in a semi-Fowler's position. **If patient is unconscious, place him or her in the lateral position, facing you. Move the overbed table close to your work area and raise to waist height.**	
____	____	____	6. Place towel or waterproof pad across patient's chest.	
____	____	____	7. **Turn suction to appropriate pressure:** For a wall unit for an adult: 100–150 mm Hg; neonates: 60–80 mm Hg; infants: 80–100 mm Hg; children: 100–120 mm Hg For a portable unit for an adult: 10–15 cm Hg; neonates: 6–8 cm Hg; infants: 8–10 cm Hg; children: 10–12 cm Hg **Put on a disposable, clean glove and occlude the end of the connecting tubing to check suction pressure. Place the connecting tubing in a convenient location. If using it, place resuscitation bag connected to oxygen within convenient reach.**	
____	____	____	8. Open sterile suction package using aseptic technique. The open wrapper or container becomes a sterile field to hold other supplies. Carefully remove the sterile container, touching only the outside surface. Set it up on the work surface and pour sterile saline into it.	

Excellent	Satisfactory	Needs Practice	SKILL 14-13 **Suctioning the Tracheostomy: Open System** *(Continued)*	
				Comments
⎯	⎯	⎯	9. Put on face shield or goggles and mask. Put on sterile gloves. **The dominant hand will manipulate the catheter and must remain sterile. The nondominant hand is considered clean rather than sterile and will control the suction valve (Y port) on the catheter.**	
⎯	⎯	⎯	10. With dominant gloved hand, pick up sterile catheter. Pick up the connecting tubing with the nondominant hand and connect the tubing and suction catheter.	
⎯	⎯	⎯	11. Moisten the catheter by dipping it into the container of sterile saline, unless it is a silicone catheter. Occlude Y-tube to check suction.	
⎯	⎯	⎯	12. Using your nondominant hand and a manual resuscitation bag, hyperventilate the patient delivering 3 to 6 breaths or use the sigh mechanism on a mechanical ventilator.	
⎯	⎯	⎯	13. Open the adapter on the mechanical ventilator tubing or remove oxygen delivery setup with your nondominant hand.	
⎯	⎯	⎯	14. Using your dominant hand, gently and quickly insert catheter into trachea. **Advance the catheter to the predetermined length. Do not occlude Y-port when inserting catheter.**	
⎯	⎯	⎯	15. Apply suction by intermittently occluding the Y port on the catheter with the thumb of your nondominant hand, and gently rotate the catheter as it is being withdrawn. **Do not suction for more than 10 to 15 seconds at a time.**	
⎯	⎯	⎯	16. Hyperventilate the patient using your nondominant hand and a manual resuscitation bag, delivering 3 to 6 breaths. Replace the oxygen delivery device, if applicable, using your nondominant hand and have the patient take several deep breaths. If the patient is mechanically ventilated, close the adapter on the mechanical ventilator tubing and use the sigh mechanism on a mechanical ventilator.	
⎯	⎯	⎯	17. Flush catheter with saline. Assess effectiveness of suctioning and repeat as needed and according to patient's tolerance. Wrap the suction catheter around your dominant hand between attempts.	
⎯	⎯	⎯	18. **Allow at least a 30-second to 1-minute interval if additional suctioning is needed. No more than three suction passes should be made per suctioning episode. Encourage patient to cough and deep breathe between suctionings.** Suction the oropharynx after suctioning the trachea. Do not reinsert in the tracheostomy after suctioning the mouth.	

Excellent	Satisfactory	Needs Practice		Comments
——	——	——	19. When suctioning is completed, remove glove from dominant hand over the coiled catheter, pulling it off inside out. Remove glove from nondominant hand and dispose of gloves, catheter, and container with solution in the appropriate receptacle. Remove face shield or goggles and mask. Perform hand hygiene.	
——	——	——	20. Turn off suction. Assist patient to a comfortable position. Raise bed rail. Offer oral hygiene after suctioning.	
——	——	——	21. Reassess patient's respiratory status, including respiratory rate, effort, oxygen saturation, and lung sounds.	

Skill Checklists to Accompany Taylor's Clinical Nursing Skills:
A Nursing Process Approach, 2nd edition

Name _____ Date _____

Unit _____ Position _____

Instructor/Evaluator: _____ Position _____

Excellent	Satisfactory	Needs Practice	SKILL 14-14 **Providing Tracheostomy Care** **Goal:** The patient will exhibit a tracheostomy tube and site free from drainage, secretions, and skin irritation or breakdown.	Comments
____	____	____	1. Identify the patient.	
____	____	____	2. Determine the need for tracheostomy care. **Assess patient's pain and administer pain medication, if indicated.**	
____	____	____	3. Explain what you are going to do and the reason to the patient, even if the patient does not appear to be alert. Reassure patient you will interrupt procedure if he or she indicates respiratory difficulty.	
____	____	____	4. Perform hand hygiene.	
____	____	____	5. Adjust bed to comfortable working position. Lower side rail closer to you. If patient is conscious, place him or her in a semi-Fowler's position. **If patient is unconscious, place him or her in the lateral position, facing you. Move the overbed table close to your work area and raise to waist height. Place a trash receptacle within easy reach of work area.**	
____	____	____	6. Put on face shield or goggles and mask. Suction tracheostomy if necessary. If tracheostomy has just been suctioned, remove soiled site dressing and discard before removal of gloves used to perform suctioning.	
			Cleaning the Tracheostomy: Nondisposable Inner Cannula	
____	____	____	7. Prepare supplies	
____	____	____	a. Open tracheostomy care kit and separate basins, touching only the edges. If kit is not available, open three sterile basins.	
____	____	____	b. Fill one basin 0.5″ deep with hydrogen peroxide or half hydrogen peroxide and half saline, based on facility policy.	
____	____	____	c. Fill other two basins 0.5″ deep with saline.	
____	____	____	d. Open sterile brush or pipe cleaners if they are not already available in cleaning kit. Open additional sterile gauze pad.	
____	____	____	8. Put on disposable gloves.	

Excellent	Satisfactory	Needs Practice		Comments

SKILL 14-14
Providing Tracheostomy Care *(Continued)*

——— ——— ———   9. Remove the oxygen source if one is present. If not already removed, remove site dressing and dispose of in the trash. Stabilize the outer cannula and faceplate of the tracheostomy with one hand. Rotate the lock on the inner cannula in a counterclockwise motion with your other hand to release it.

——— ——— ———   10. Continue to hold the faceplate. Gently remove the inner cannula and carefully drop it in the basin with hydrogen peroxide. Replace the oxygen source over the outer cannula. Remove gloves and discard.

——— ——— ———   11. Clean the inner cannula as follows:

——— ——— ———   a. Put on sterile gloves.

——— ——— ———   b. Remove inner cannula from soaking solution. Moisten brush or pipe cleaners in saline and insert into tube, using back-and-forth motion.

——— ——— ———   c. Agitate cannula in saline solution. Remove and tap against inner surface of basin.

——— ——— ———   d. Place on sterile gauze pad.

——— ——— ———   12. **Suction outer cannula using sterile technique if necessary.**

——— ——— ———   13. Stabilize the outer cannula and faceplate with one hand. Replace inner cannula into outer cannula. Turn lock clockwise and check that inner cannula is secure. Reapply oxygen source if needed.

Applying Clean Dressing and Ties/Tape

——— ——— ———   14. Remove oxygen source. Dip cotton-tipped applicator or gauze sponge in second basin with sterile saline and clean stoma under faceplate. **Use each applicator or sponge only once, moving from stoma site outward.**

——— ——— ———   15. Pat skin gently with dry 4″ × 4″ gauze sponge.

——— ——— ———   16. Slide commercially prepared tracheostomy dressing or prefolded non–cotton-filled 4″ × 4″ dressing under faceplate.

——— ——— ———   17. Change the tracheostomy tape:

——— ——— ———   a. **Leave soiled tape in place until new one is applied.**

——— ——— ———   b. Cut piece of tape the length of twice the neck circumference plus 4″. Trim ends of tape on the diagonal.

SKILL 14-14
Providing Tracheostomy Care *(Continued)*

Excellent	Satisfactory	Needs Practice		Comments
——	——	——	c. Insert one end of tape through faceplate opening alongside old tape. Pull through until both ends are even length.	
——	——	——	d. Slide both ends of the tape under patient's neck and insert one end through remaining opening on other side of faceplate. Pull snugly and tie ends in double square knot. You should be able to fit one finger between the neck and the ties. Check to make sure that the patient can flex neck comfortably.	
——	——	——	e. Carefully remove old tape. Reapply oxygen source if necessary.	
——	——	——	18. Remove face shield or mask and goggles. Remove gloves and discard. Perform hand hygiene. Reassess patient's respiratory status, including respiratory rate, effort, oxygen saturation, and lung sounds.	

Skill Checklists to Accompany Taylor's Clinical Nursing Skills:
A Nursing Process Approach, 2nd edition

Name _____   Date _____

Unit _____   Position _____

Instructor/Evaluator: _____   Position _____

SKILL 14-15
Providing Care of a Chest Drainage System

Goal: The patient will not experience any complications related to the chest drainage system or respiratory distress.

Excellent	Satisfactory	Needs Practice		Comments
___	___	___	1. Identify the patient.	
___	___	___	2. Explain what you are going to do and the reason to the patient.	
___	___	___	3. Perform hand hygiene.	
___	___	___	4. Put on clean gloves.	
			Assessing the Drainage System	
___	___	___	5. Move the patient's gown to expose chest tube insertion site. Keep the patient covered as much as possible, using a bath blanket to drape the patient if necessary. **Observe the dressing around the chest tube insertion site and ensure that it is dry, intact, and occlusive.**	
___	___	___	6. Check that all connections are securely taped. Gently palpate around the insertion site, feeling for subcutaneous emphysema, a collection of air or gas under the skin. This may feel crunchy or spongy, or like "popping" under your fingers.	
___	___	___	7. Check drainage tubing to ensure that there are no dependent loops or kinks. The drainage collection device must be positioned below the tube insertion site.	
___	___	___	8. If the chest tube is ordered to be to suctioned, note the fluid level in the suction chamber and check it with the amount of ordered suction. **Look for bubbling in the suction chamber.** Temporarily disconnect the suction to check the level of water in the chamber. Add sterile water or saline if necessary to maintain correct amount of suction.	
___	___	___	9. Observe the water-seal chamber for fluctuations of the water level with the patient's inspiration and expiration (tidaling). If suction is used, temporarily disconnect the suction to observe for fluctuation. Assess for the presence of bubbling in the water-seal chamber. Add water if necessary to maintain the level at the 2-cm mark, or the mark recommended by the manufacturer.	

Excellent	Satisfactory	Needs Practice	

SKILL 14-15
Providing Care of a Chest
Drainage System *(Continued)*

Comments

____ ____ ____ 10. Assess the amount and type of fluid drainage. Measure drainage output at the end of each shift by marking the level on the container or placing a small piece of tape at the drainage level to indicate date and time. The amount should be a running total, because the drainage system is never emptied. If the drainage system fills, it is removed and replaced.

____ ____ ____ 11. Remove gloves. Perform hand hygiene.

Changing the Drainage System

____ ____ ____ 12. Obtain two padded Kelly clamps, a new drainage system, and bottle of sterile water. Add water to the water-seal chamber until it reaches the 2-cm mark or the mark recommended by the manufacturer. Follow manufacturer's directions to add water to suction system if suction is ordered.

____ ____ ____ 13. Put on clean gloves.

____ ____ ____ 14. **Apply Kelly clamps 1.5″ to 2.5″ from insertion site and 1″ apart, going opposite directions.**

____ ____ ____ 15. Remove the suction from the current drainage system. Unroll the band or use scissors to carefully cut away any foam tape on connection of chest tube and drainage system. Using a slight twisting motion, remove the drainage system. **Do not pull on the chest tube.**

____ ____ ____ 16. **Keeping the end of the chest tube sterile, insert the end of the new drainage system into the chest tube.** Remove Kelly clamps. Reconnect suction if ordered. Apply plastic bands or foam tape to chest tube/drainage system connection site.

____ ____ ____ 17. Assess the patient and the drainage system as outlined in Steps 5–10.

____ ____ ____ 18. Remove gloves. Perform hand hygiene.

Skill Checklists to Accompany Taylor's Clinical Nursing Skills:
A Nursing Process Approach, 2nd edition

Name _____   Date _____

Unit _____   Position _____

Instructor/Evaluator: _____   Position _____

SKILL 14-16

Assisting With Removal of a Chest Tube

Excellent	Satisfactory	Needs Practice	**Goal:** The patient will remain free of respiratory distress.	**Comments**
____	____	____	1. Identify the patient.	
____	____	____	2. Explain what you are going to do and the reason to the patient.	
____	____	____	3. Perform hand hygiene.	
____	____	____	4. Administer pain medication as prescribed. **Premedicate patient 10 to 15 minutes before chest tube removal.**	
____	____	____	5. Put on clean gloves.	
____	____	____	6. Provide reassurance to patient while physician removes dressing.	
____	____	____	7. **After physician has removed chest tube and secured occlusive dressing, assess patient's lung sounds, respiratory rate, oxygen saturation, and pain level.**	
____	____	____	8. Anticipate the physician ordering a chest x-ray.	
____	____	____	9. Dispose of equipment appropriately. Remove and dispose of gloves. Perform hand hygiene.	

Name _____ Date _____

Unit _____ Position _____

Instructor/Evaluator: _____ Position _____

Excellent	Satisfactory	Needs Practice	SKILL 14-17 **Using a Bag and Mask (Handheld Resuscitation Bag)**	Comments

Goal: The patient will exhibit signs and symptoms of adequate oxygen saturation.

Excellent	Satisfactory	Needs Practice		Comments
____	____	____	1. If not an emergency, identify the patient.	
____	____	____	2. Explain what you are going to do and the reason to the patient, even if the patient does not appear to be alert.	
____	____	____	3. Perform hand hygiene, if not crisis situation. Put on disposable gloves. Put on face shield or goggles and mask.	
____	____	____	4. **Ensure that the mask is connected to the bag device, the oxygen tubing is connected to the oxygen source, and the oxygen is turned on, at a flow rate of 10–15 liters/minute.** This may be done through visualization or by listening to the open end of the reservoir or tail: if air is heard flowing, the oxygen is attached and on.	
____	____	____	5. If possible, get behind head of bed and remove headboard. **Slightly hyperextend patient's neck (unless contraindicated). If unable to hyperextend, use jaw thrust maneuver to open airway.**	
____	____	____	6. Place mask over patient's face with opening over oral cavity. If mask is teardrop-shaped, the narrow portion should be placed over the bridge of the nose.	
____	____	____	7. **With dominant hand, place three fingers on mandible, keeping head slightly hyperextended. Place thumb and one finger in C position around the mask, pressing hard enough to form a seal around patient's face.**	
____	____	____	8. **Using nondominant hand, gently and slowly (over 2–3 seconds) squeeze the bag, watching chest for symmetric rise.** If two people are available, one person should maintain a seal on the mask with two hands while the other squeezes the bag to deliver the ventilation and oxygenation.	
____	____	____	9. Deliver the breaths with the patient's own inspiratory effort, if present. Avoid delivering breaths when the patient exhales. Deliver one breath every 5 seconds, if patient's own respiratory drive is absent. Continue delivering breaths until patient's drive returns or until patient is intubated and attached to mechanical ventilation.	
____	____	____	10. Remove face shield or goggles and mask. Remove gloves and perform hand hygiene.	

Skill Checklists to Accompany Taylor's Clinical Nursing Skills:
A Nursing Process Approach, 2nd edition

Name _____   Date _____

Unit _____   Position _____

Instructor/Evaluator: _____   Position _____

Excellent	Satisfactory	Needs Practice		Comments
			SKILL 15-1 **Starting an Intravenous Infusion**	
			Goal: The IV catheter is inserted using sterile technique on the first attempt. Also, the patient experiences minimal trauma and the IV solution flows freely.	
——	——	——	1. Verify IV order against the physician order. Clarify any inconsistencies. Check the patient's chart for allergies. Check for color, clarity, expiration date, etc.	
——	——	——	2. Know techniques for IV insertion, precautions, purpose of the IV administration, and medications if ordered.	
——	——	——	3. Gather all equipment and bring to bedside.	
——	——	——	4. Identify the patient. Ask the patient if allergic to any medication, iodine, or tape, as appropriate. If considering using an anesthetic (numbing) cream or 1% lidocaine injection, check for allergies for these substances as well.	
——	——	——	5. Explain the need for the IV and procedure to patient.	
——	——	——	6. Perform hand hygiene. If using an anesthetic cream, apply the anesthetic cream to a few potential insertion sites.	
——	——	——	7. Prepare IV solution and tubing:	
——	——	——	a. **Maintain strict aseptic technique when opening sterile packages and IV solution.** Remove administration set from package.	
——	——	——	b. Clamp IV tubing, uncap spike on administration set, and insert into entry site on IV bag or bottle as manufacturer directs.	
——	——	——	c. Squeeze drip chamber and allow it to fill at least halfway.	
——	——	——	d. Remove cap at end of the IV tubing and while maintaining its sterility, open the IV tubing clamp, and allow fluid to move through tubing. **Allow fluid to flow until all air bubbles have disappeared** and the entire length of the tubing is primed (filled) with IV solution. Close clamp and recap end of tubing, maintaining sterility of the setup.	
——	——	——	e. If an electronic device is to be used, follow manufacturer's instructions for inserting tubing and setting infusion rate.	

SKILL 15-1

Starting an Intravenous Infusion *(Continued)*

Excellent	Satisfactory	Needs Practice		Comments
____	____	____	f. Apply label if medication was added to container (pharmacy may have added medication and applied label). Label tubing with date and time that tubing was hung.	
____	____	____	g. Place time-tape on container and hang IV on pole.	
____	____	____	8. Place patient in low Fowler's position in bed. Place protective towel or pad under patient's arm. Close the door to the room or pull the bedside curtain.	
____	____	____	9. Provide emotional support as needed.	
____	____	____	10. **Select and palpate for an appropriate vein. Avoid an arm that has been compromised such as with presence of arteriovenous fistula.**	
____	____	____	11. If the site is hairy and agency policy permits, clip a 2″ area around the intended site of entry.	
____	____	____	12. Apply a tourniquet 3″ to 4″ above the venipuncture site to obstruct venous blood flow and distend the vein. Direct the ends of the tourniquet away from the site of entry. Make sure the radial pulse is still present.	
____	____	____	13. Instruct the patient to hold the arm lower than the heart.	
____	____	____	14. Ask patient to open and close fist. Observe and palpate for a suitable vein. Try the following techniques if a vein cannot be felt:	
____	____	____	a. Massage the patient's arm from proximal to distal end and gently tap over intended vein.	
____	____	____	b. Remove tourniquet and place warm, moist compresses over intended vein for 10 to 15 minutes.	
____	____	____	15. Put on clean gloves.	
____	____	____	16. If using intradermal lidocaine, cleanse insertion site with alcohol using a circular motion. Inject a small amount (0.2–0.3 mL) of lidocaine into the area. If numbing cream was used, wipe cream off insertion site. **Cleanse site with an antiseptic solution such as chlorhexidine or according to agency policy. Use a circular motion to move from the center outward for several inches.**	
____	____	____	17. Use the nondominant hand, placed about 1″ or 2″ below entry site, to hold the skin taut against the vein. **Avoid touching the prepared site.** Ask the patient to remain still while performing the venipuncture.	

Excellent	Satisfactory	Needs Practice	SKILL 15-1 **Starting an Intravenous Infusion** *(Continued)*	Comments
——	——	——	18. Enter the skin gently, holding the catheter by the hub in your dominant hand, bevel side up, at a 10- to 15-degree angle. Catheter may be inserted from directly over the vein or the side of the vein. While following the course of the vein, advance the needle or catheter into the vein. A sensation of "give" can be felt when the needle enters the vein.	
——	——	——	19. When blood returns through the lumen of the needle or the flashback chamber of the catheter, advance either device 1/8″ to 1/4″ farther into the vein. A catheter needs to be advanced until the hub is at the venipuncture site, but the exact technique depends on the type of device used.	
——	——	——	20. Release the tourniquet as soon as possible. Quickly remove the protective cap from the IV tubing and attach the tubing to the catheter or needle. Stabilize the catheter or needle with your nondominant hand.	
——	——	——	21. Start the flow of solution promptly by releasing the clamp on the tubing. Examine the tissue around the entry site for signs of infiltration.	
——	——	——	22. Secure the catheter with narrow nonallergenic tape (1/2″), placed sticky side up under the hub and crossed over the top of the hub.	
——	——	——	23. **Place sterile dressing over venipuncture site.** Agency policy may direct nurse to use gauze dressing or transparent dressing. Apply tape to dressing if necessary. Loop the tubing near the site of entry, and anchor to dressing.	
——	——	——	24. Label the IV dressing with the date, time, site, and type and size of catheter used for the infusion on the tape anchoring the tubing.	
——	——	——	25. Remove all equipment and dispose of properly. Remove gloves and perform hand hygiene.	
——	——	——	26. Anchor arm to an armboard for support if necessary, or apply a site protector or tube-shaped mesh netting over the insertion site. Explain to patient the purpose of the armboard and the importance of safeguarding the site when using the extremity.	
——	——	——	27. Adjust the rate of solution flow according to the amount prescribed, or follow manufacturer's directions for adjusting flow rate on infusion pump.	

Excellent	Satisfactory	Needs Practice	SKILL 15-1 **Starting an Intravenous Infusion** *(Continued)*	Comments
——	——	——	28. Document procedure and patient's response. Chart time, site, device used, and solution.	
——	——	——	29. Return to check flow rate and observe IV site for infiltration 30 minutes after starting infusion. Ask the patient if experiencing any pain or discomfort related to the IV infusion.	

Skill Checklists to Accompany Taylor's Clinical Nursing Skills:
A Nursing Process Approach, 2nd edition

Name _____   Date _____

Unit _____   Position _____

Instructor/Evaluator: _____   Position _____

Excellent	Satisfactory	Needs Practice	SKILL 15-2 **Changing IV Solution Container and Tubing**	Comments
			Goal: The patient experiences minimal to no trauma when solution and tubing are changed.	
____	____	____	1. Identify the patient. Ask the patient if allergic to any medication, iodine, or tape, as appropriate.	
____	____	____	2. Gather all equipment and bring to bedside. Check IV solution and medication additives against physician's order. Label IV if medication is added. Include the date, time, and your name or initials.	
____	____	____	3. Explain procedure and reason for change to patient.	
____	____	____	4. Perform hand hygiene.	
			To Change IV Solution Container	
____	____	____	5. Carefully remove protective cover from new IV solution container and expose bag entry site.	
____	____	____	6. **Close clamp on IV tubing. If using an electronic device, turn device to "hold" position.**	
____	____	____	7. Lift container off IV pole and invert it. **Quickly remove the spike from the old IV container, being careful not to contaminate it.**	
____	____	____	8. Steady new container and insert spike. Hang on IV pole.	
____	____	____	9. Reopen clamp, check the drip chamber of the administration set on tubing, and adjust flow. Readjust electronic device by turning the device "ON" and verify the programmed flow rate. Inspect for air bubbles in the tubing. If using an electronic device, check that the device is operating correctly.	
____	____	____	10. Label container according to agency policy. Record on intake and output record and document on chart according to agency policy. Discard used equipment properly. Perform hand hygiene.	
			To Change IV Solution Container and Tubing	
____	____	____	11. Prepare IV solution and tubing, checking IV order with the physician's order, and labeling the IV with date, time, and name or initials.	

Changing IV Solution Container and Tubing *(Continued)*

Excellent	Satisfactory	Needs Practice		Comments
___	___	___	a. **Maintain strict aseptic technique when opening sterile packages and IV solution.**	
___	___	___	b. Clamp IV tubing, uncap spike on administration set, and insert into entry site on IV bag or bottle as manufacturer directs.	
___	___	___	c. Squeeze drip chamber and allow it to fill at least halfway.	
___	___	___	d. Remove cap at end of the IV tubing and while maintaining its sterility, open the IV tubing clamp, and allow fluid to move through tubing. **Allow fluid to flow until all air bubbles have disappeared** and the entire length of the tubing is primed (filled) with IV solution. Close clamp and recap end of tubing, maintaining sterility of the setup.	
___	___	___	e. If an electronic device is to be used, follow manufacturer's instructions for inserting tubing and setting infusion rate.	
___	___	___	f. Label tubing with date and time that tubing was hung.	
___	___	___	g. Place time-tape on container and hang IV on pole.	
___	___	___	12. Close the clamp on the existing IV tubing. Also, close the clamp on the short extension tubing connected to the IV catheter in the patient's arm.	
___	___	___	13. Remove the current infusion tubing from the resealable cap on the short extension IV tubing. Using an antimicrobial wipe, swab the resealable cap and insert the new IV tubing into the cap.	
___	___	___	14. Open the clamp on the IV tubing and on the short extension tubing. Check the IV flow. Readjust electronic device as needed.	
___	___	___	15. **Regulate IV flow according to physician's order.**	
___	___	___	16. **Label IV tubing with date, time, and your initials. Label IV solution container and record procedure according to agency policy.** Discard used equipment properly and perform hand hygiene.	
___	___	___	17. Record patient's response to IV infusion.	

Skill Checklists to Accompany Taylor's Clinical Nursing Skills:
A Nursing Process Approach, 2nd edition

Name _____ Date _____

Unit _____ Position _____

Instructor/Evaluator: _____ Position _____

Excellent	Satisfactory	Needs Practice	SKILL 15-3 **Monitoring an IV Site and Infusion**	
			Goal: The patient remains free from complications and demonstrates signs and symptoms of fluid balance.	**Comments**
——	——	——	1. Identify the patient.	
——	——	——	2. **Monitor IV infusion every hour or per agency policy. More frequent checks may be necessary if medication is being infused.**	
——	——	——	a. Check physician's order for IV solution.	
——	——	——	b. Check drip chamber and time drops, if IV is not regulated by an infusion-control device.	
——	——	——	c. Check tubing for anything that might interfere with flow. Be sure that clamp is in the open position. **Observe dressing for leakage of IV solution.**	
——	——	——	d. Check settings, alarm, and indicator lights on infusion control device if one is being used. Educate patient related to alarm features on electronic infusion device.	
——	——	——	3. **Inspect site for swelling, leakage at the site, coolness, or pallor, which may indicate infiltration. Ask if patient is experiencing any pain or discomfort. This necessitates removing IV and restarting at another site. Check agency policy for treating infiltration.**	
——	——	——	4. **Inspect site for redness, swelling and heat. Palpate for induration. Ask if patient is experiencing pain. These findings may indicate phlebitis. IV will need to be discontinued and restarted at another site. Notify physician if you suspect phlebitis. Check agency policy for treatment of phlebitis.**	
——	——	——	5. **Check for local manifestations (redness, pus, warmth, induration, and pain) that may indicate an infection is present at the site, or systemic manifestations (chills, fever, tachycardia, hypotension) that may accompany local infection at the site. IV should be discontinued and physician notified. Be careful not to disconnect IV tubing when putting on patient's hospital gown.**	
——	——	——	6. Be alert for additional complications of IV therapy.	

Excellent	Satisfactory	Needs Practice	SKILL 15-3 **Monitoring an IV Site and Infusion** *(Continued)*	
				Comments
——	——	——	a. Fluid overload can result in signs of cardiac and/or respiratory failure. Monitor intake and output and vital signs. Assess for edema and auscultate lung sounds. Ask if patient is experiencing any shortness of breath.	
——	——	——	b. Bleeding at the site is most likely to occur when the IV is discontinued.	
——	——	——	7. If possible, instruct patient to call for assistance if any discomfort is noted at site, solution container is nearly empty, flow has changed in any way, or if the electronic pump alarm sounds.	

Skill Checklists to Accompany Taylor's Clinical Nursing Skills:
A Nursing Process Approach, 2nd edition

Name _____ Date _____

Unit _____ Position _____

Instructor/Evaluator: _____ Position _____

SKILL 15-4
Changing a Peripheral IV Dressing

Goal: The patient will exhibit an IV site that is clean, dry, and without evidence of any signs and symptoms of infection infiltration, or phlebitis.

Excellent	Satisfactory	Needs Practice		Comments
			1. Identify the patient. Ask the patient if allergic to any medication, iodine, or tape, as appropriate	
			2. Explain the need for the IV and procedure to patient.	
			3. **Perform hand hygiene. Put on clean gloves.**	
			4. Place towel or disposable pad under the arm with the IV site. **Carefully remove old dressing, but leave tape that anchors the IV needle or catheter in place.** Discard properly.	
			5. **Inspect IV site for presence of phlebitis (inflammation), infection, or infiltration. Discontinue and relocate IV if noted.**	
			6. Loosen and gently remove tape, being careful to steady catheter with one hand. Use adhesive remover if necessary.	
			7. **Cleanse the entry site with a chlorhexidine solution, using a circular motion and moving from the center outward. Allow to dry.**	
			8. Reapply tape strip to needle or catheter at entry site.	
			9. Apply transparent polyurethane dressing over entry site. Remove gloves and perform hand hygiene.	
			10. **Secure IV tubing with additional tape if necessary. Label dressing with date, time of change, and initials. Check that IV flow is accurate and system is patent.**	
			11. Discard equipment properly and perform hand hygiene.	
			12. Record patient's response to dressing change and observation of site.	

Skill Checklists to Accompany Taylor's Clinical Nursing Skills:
A Nursing Process Approach, 2nd edition

Name _____   Date _____

Unit _____   Position _____

Instructor/Evaluator: _____   Position _____

Excellent	Satisfactory	Needs Practice	SKILL 15-5 **Capping a Primary Line for Intermittent Use**	Comments
			Goal: The patient will remain free of injury and any signs and symptoms of IV complications.	
____	____	____	1. Gather equipment and verify physician's order. Fill syringe with normal saline or heparin flush according to agency policy. Recap syringe for use in Step 10.	
____	____	____	2. Identify the patient.	
____	____	____	3. Explain procedure to patient.	
____	____	____	4. Perform hand hygiene.	
____	____	____	5. Assess the IV site.	
____	____	____	6. **Clamp off primary IV tubing.**	
____	____	____	7. Put on clean gloves according to hospital policy. Clamp the extension tubing if a clamp is present. Remove the primary IV tubing from the extension set or adapter device. Cleanse adapter device with an antimicrobial swab.	
____	____	____	8. Unclamp the extension set and insert a saline or heparin flush syringe into the cap. Instill the solution over 1 minute or flush the line according to agency policy. Reclamp the extension tubing and remove the syringe.	
____	____	____	9. Remove gloves and dispose of them appropriately.	
____	____	____	10. Tape adapter device (and extension tubing if used).	
____	____	____	11. Perform hand hygiene and ensure the patient is comfortable.	
____	____	____	12. Chart on IV administration record, MAR, or CMAR per institutional policy.	

Skill Checklists to Accompany Taylor's Clinical Nursing Skills:
A Nursing Process Approach, 2nd edition

Name _____ Date _____

Unit _____ Position _____

Instructor/Evaluator: _____ Position _____

Excellent	Satisfactory	Needs Practice		Comments
			SKILL 15-6 **Administering a Blood Transfusion** **Goal:** The patient receives the blood transfusion without any evidence of a transfusion reaction or complication.	
— — —	— — —	— — —	1. Identify the patient. Ask if the patient is allergic to any medication, iodine, tape, or if the patient has had a transfusion or transfusion reaction in the past.	
— — —	— — —	— — —	2. Determine whether patient knows reason for the blood transfusion. Explain to patient what will happen. Check for signed consent for transfusion if required by agency. Advise patient to report any chills, itching, rash, or unusual symptoms. If the physician has ordered any premedication, administer it now.	
— — —	— — —	— — —	3. Perform hand hygiene and put on clean gloves.	
— — —	— — —	— — —	4. **Hang container of 0.9% normal saline with blood administration set to initiate IV infusion and follow administration of blood.**	
— — —	— — —	— — —	5. Start IV with 18- or 19-gauge catheter if not already present (see Skill 15-1). Keep IV open by starting flow of normal saline.	
— — —	— — —	— — —	6. Obtain blood product from blood bank according to agency policy. Scan for bar codes on blood products if required.	
— — —	— — —	— — —	7. **Complete identification and checks as required by agency:**	
— — —	— — —	— — —	• **Identification number**	
— — —	— — —	— — —	• **Blood group and type**	
— — —	— — —	— — —	• **Expiration date**	
— — —	— — —	— — —	• **Patient's name**	
— — —	— — —	— — —	• **Inspect blood for clots.**	
— — —	— — —	— — —	8. **Take baseline set of vital signs before beginning transfusion.**	
— — —	— — —	— — —	9. Start infusion of the blood product:	
— — —	— — —	— — —	a. Prime in-line filter with blood.	
— — —	— — —	— — —	b. **Start administration slowly (no more than 25–50 mL for the first 15 minutes). Stay with the patient for the first 5 to 15 minutes of transfusion.**	

Excellent	Satisfactory	Needs Practice	SKILL 15-6 **Administering a Blood Transfusion** *(Continued)*	Comments
——	——	——	c. Assess vital signs at least every 15 minutes for the first half hour. Follow institution's recommendations for taking vital signs during the remainder of the transfusion.	
——	——	——	d. Observe patient for flushing, dyspnea, itching, hives or rash, or any unusual comments.	
——	——	——	e. Never warm blood in a microwave. Use a blood-warming device, if indicated or ordered, especially with rapid transfusions through a CVP catheter.	
——	——	——	10. Maintain the prescribed flow rate as ordered or as deemed appropriate based on the patient's overall condition, keeping in mind the outer limits for safe administration. Ongoing monitoring is crucial throughout the entire duration of the blood transfusion for early identification of any adverse reactions. **Assess frequently for transfusion reaction. Stop blood transfusion if you suspect a reaction. Quickly replace the blood tubing with new tubing and 0.9% sodium chloride. Notify physician and blood bank.**	
——	——	——	11. When transfusion is complete, clamp off blood and begin to infuse 0.9% normal saline.	
——	——	——	12. Record administration of blood and patient's reaction as ordered by agency. Return blood-transfusion bag to blood bank according to agency policy.	

Skill Checklists to Accompany Taylor's Clinical Nursing Skills:
A Nursing Process Approach, 2nd edition

Name _____   Date _____

Unit _____   Position _____

Instructor/Evaluator: _____   Position _____

Excellent	Satisfactory	Needs Practice	SKILL 15-7 **Changing the Dressing and Flushing Central Venous Access Devices**	
			Goal: The patient will remain free of any signs and symptoms of infection.	**Comments**
——	——	——	1. Gather equipment and verify physician's order (often this will be a standing protocol).	
——	——	——	2. Identify the patient.	
——	——	——	3. Explain procedure to patient.	
——	——	——	4. Perform hand hygiene.	
——	——	——	5. Position the patient with the arm extended from body below heart level.	
——	——	——	6. **Apply a mask and have patient also put on a mask.** Put on clean gloves. Set up sterile field on area to be used. Have patient place the arm in the middle of the sterile field. Open dressing kit using sterile technique and place on sterile towel.	
——	——	——	7. Assess CVAD insertion site (for inflammation, redness, etc.) through old dressing. Remove old dressing by lifting it distally and then working proximally, making sure to stabilize the catheter with thumb. Remove and dispose of gloves properly. Put on sterile gloves.	
——	——	——	8. Starting at insertion site and continuing in a circle, wipe off any old blood or drainage with a sterile antimicrobial wipe. **Cleanse according to agency policy. Move in a circular fashion, cleansing thoroughly from the insertion site outward (2″–3″ area).** Allow to dry.	
——	——	——	9. **Reapply sterile dressing or securement device according to agency policy.** Secure tubing or lumens to prevent tugging on insertion site.	
——	——	——	10. **Clamp all lines of the CVAD and remove injection caps. Cleanse the catheter ends with antimicrobial swab and then apply new injection caps. Tape the distal ends down securely.**	

Excellent	Satisfactory	Needs Practice	SKILL 15-7 **Changing the Dressing and Flushing Central Venous Access Devices** *(Continued)*	Comments
____	____	____	11. Some agency policies incorporate the flushing of the different lumens or injection port after the dressing change. Flush with 3 to 5 mL of NSS using a 10-mL syringe and 3 mL of heparin (100U/mL) after each use or as agency policy directs.	
____	____	____	12. Note date, time of dressing change, size of catheter, and initials on tape or dressing.	
____	____	____	13. Discard equipment properly and perform hand hygiene.	
____	____	____	14. Record patient's response to dressing change and observation of site.	

Skill Checklists to Accompany Taylor's Clinical Nursing Skills:
A Nursing Process Approach, 2nd edition

Name _____   Date _____

Unit _____   Position _____

Instructor/Evaluator: _____   Position _____

Excellent	Satisfactory	Needs Practice	SKILL 15-8 **Accessing an Implanted Port**	Comments
			Goal: The port is accessed with minimal to no discomfort to the patient.	
——	——	——	1. Gather equipment and verify physician's order (many times this will be a standing protocol).	
——	——	——	2. Identify the patient.	
——	——	——	3. Explain procedure to patient.	
——	——	——	4. Perform hand hygiene.	
——	——	——	5. Raise bed to comfortable working height.	
——	——	——	6. Attach the blunt needles to the 10-mL syringes. Withdraw 10 mL of .9% sodium chloride (NSS) from the vial.	
——	——	——	7. Connect the intermittent injection cap to the extension tubing on the noncoring needle. Attach the 10-mL syringe to the intermittent injection cap and flush the needle with sodium chloride. Clamp the tubing. Remove the syringe from the injection cap.	
——	——	——	8. If transparent dressing is in place, put on clean gloves and gently pull it back, beginning with edges and proceeding around the edge of the dressing. Once dressing is removed, gently pull straight back on needle. Discard in appropriate receptacle and remove gloves.	
——	——	——	9. **Open the kit using sterile technique. Put on the mask and sterile gloves. Set up your sterile field.** If port is not accessed, proceed to Step 10.	
——	——	——	10. **Cleanse according to agency policy. For example, using an antimicrobial swab, cleanse in a circular fashion from the insertion site outward (2″–3″ area). Use each swab once and discard. Allow site to dry.**	
——	——	——	11. **Locate the port septum by palpation.** With your nondominant hand, hold the port stable, keeping the skin taut but without touching the port side.	
——	——	——	12. Visualize the center of the port. **Push the Huber needle (noncoring 90-degree) through the skin into the portal septum until it hits the back of the port septum.**	
——	——	——	13. Cleanse the injection cap with an antimicrobial swab and insert the syringe with normal saline.	

SKILL 15-8
Accessing an Implanted Port *(Continued)*

Excellent	Satisfactory	Needs Practice		Comments
――	――	――	14. **Open the clamp and push down on the syringe plunger, flushing the device with 3 to 5 mL of saline, while observing for fluid leak or infiltration. It should flush easily, without resistance.**	
――	――	――	15. Pull back on the syringe plunger to aspirate for blood return. Aspirate only a few milliliters of blood; do not allow blood to enter syringe.	
――	――	――	16. Flush with the remainder of saline in syringe.	
――	――	――	17. Clamp the tubing, remove the syringe, and attach the heparin-filled syringe (if appropriate for the institution). Clamp the tubing while maintaining positive pressure on the syringe barrel at the end of the flush.	
――	――	――	18. Remove the syringe. **If space exists between the skin and the needle, place a sterile folded 2 ×2 gauze in the space to support the needle.** If using a "Gripper" needle, remove the gripper portion from the needle by squeezing the sides together and lifting off the needle while holding the needle securely to the port with the other hand.	
――	――	――	19. Apply tape or Steri-Strips in a starlike pattern over the needle to secure it.	
――	――	――	20. Cover the entire needle and port with the transparent dressing, leaving the ports of the extension tubing uncovered for easy access.	
――	――	――	21. Remove gloves and discard. Perform hand hygiene.	
――	――	――	22. Label the dressing with the date, time, size needle used, and your initials, according to agency policy.	
――	――	――	23. Document procedure, including time, date, type and location of port, condition of skin at site, size needle used, presence of blood return, and any difficulties encountered.	

Skill Checklists to Accompany Taylor's Clinical Nursing Skills:
A Nursing Process Approach, 2nd edition

Name _____   Date _____

Unit _____   Position _____

Instructor/Evaluator: _____   Position _____

Excellent	Satisfactory	Needs Practice	SKILL 15-9 **Deaccessing an Implanted Port**	Comments
			Goal: The needle is removed with minimal to no discomfort to the patient.	
——	——	——	1. Gather equipment and verify physician's order (many times this will be a standing protocol).	
——	——	——	2. Identify the patient.	
——	——	——	3. Explain procedure to patient.	
——	——	——	4. Perform hand hygiene.	
——	——	——	5. Raise bed to comfortable working height.	
——	——	——	6. Put on clean gloves.	
——	——	——	7. Gently pull back transparent dressing, beginning with edges and proceeding around the edge of the dressing. Carefully remove all the tape that is securing the needle in place.	
——	——	——	8. Clean the injection cap and insert the saline-filled syringe. **Unclamp the catheter's extension tubing and begin to flush with a minimum of 10-mL normal saline.**	
——	——	——	9. **Remove the syringe and insert the heparin-filled syringe, flushing with 5-mL heparin (100 U/mL or agency's policy). Clamp the extension tubing while maintaining positive pressure on the barrel of the syringe. Remove the syringe.**	
——	——	——	10. Secure the port on either side with the fingers of your nondominant hand. Grasp the needle/wings with the fingers of your dominant hand. Firmly and smoothly, pull the needle straight up at a 90-degree angle from the skin to remove it from the septum.	
——	——	——	11. Apply gentle pressure with the gauze to the insertion site. A Band-Aid may be applied over the port if any oozing occurs.	
——	——	——	12. Remove gloves and place bed in the lowest position. Make sure that the patient is comfortable before you leave the room.	
——	——	——	13. Perform hand hygiene.	

Skill Checklists to Accompany Taylor's Clinical Nursing Skills:
A Nursing Process Approach, 2nd edition

Name _____   Date _____

Unit _____   Position _____

Instructor/Evaluator: _____   Position _____

SKILL 16-1

Obtaining an Electrocardiogram (ECG/EKG)

Goal: A cardiac electrical tracing is obtained without any complications.

Excellent	Satisfactory	Needs Practice		Comments
___	___	___	1. Place the ECG machine close to the patient's bed, and plug the power cord into the wall outlet.	
___	___	___	2. Perform hand hygiene.	
___	___	___	3. Check the patient's identification. Close curtains around bed and close door to room if possible.	
___	___	___	4. As you set up the machine to record a 12-lead ECG, explain the procedure to the patient. Tell the patient that the test records the heart's electrical activity, and it may be repeated at certain intervals. Emphasize that no electrical current will enter his or her body. Tell the patient the test typically takes about 5 minutes.	
___	___	___	5. If bed is adjustable, raise it to a comfortable working height.	
___	___	___	6. Have the patient lie supine in the center of the bed with the arms at the sides. Raise the head of the bed if necessary to promote comfort. Expose the patient's arms and legs, and drape appropriately. Encourage the patient to relax the arms and legs. If the bed is too narrow, place the patient's hands under the buttocks to prevent muscle tension. Also use this technique if the patient is shivering or trembling. Make sure the feet do not touch the bed's footboard.	
___	___	___	7. Select flat, fleshy areas on which to place the electrodes. Avoid muscular and bony areas. If the patient has an amputated limb, choose a site on the stump.	
___	___	___	8. If an area is excessively hairy, clip the hair. Do not shave hair. Clean excess oil or other substances from the skin with soap and water and dry it completely.	

Excellent	Satisfactory	Needs Practice		Comments

Excellent	Satisfactory	Needs Practice		Comments
——	——	——	9. Apply the limb lead electrodes. The tip of each lead wire is lettered and color-coded for easy identification. The white or RA lead goes to the right arm; the green or RL lead to the right leg; the red or LL lead to the left leg; the black or LA lead to the left arm. Peel the contact paper off the self-sticking disposable electrode and apply directly to the prepared site, as recommended by the manufacturer. **Position disposable electrodes on the legs with the lead connection pointing superiorly.**	
——	——	——	10. Connect the limb lead wires to the electrodes. Make sure the metal parts of the electrodes are clean and bright.	
——	——	——	11. Expose the patient's chest. Apply the precordial lead electrodes. The tip of each lead wire is lettered and color-coded for easy identification. The brown or V_1 to V_6 leads are applied to the chest. Peel the contact paper off the self-sticking disposable electrode and apply directly to the prepared site, as recommended by the manufacturer. Position chest electrodes as follows:	
——	——	——	• V_1: Fourth intercostal space at right sternal border	
——	——	——	• V_2: Fourth intercostal space at left sternal border	
——	——	——	• V_3: Halfway between V_2 and V_4	
——	——	——	• V_4: Fifth intercostal space at the left midclavicular line	
——	——	——	• V_5: Fifth intercostal space at anterior axillary line (halfway between V_4 and V_6)	
			• V_6: Fifth intercostal space at midaxillary line, level with V_4	
——	——	——	12. Connect the precordial lead wires to the electrodes. Make sure the metal parts of the electrodes are clean and bright.	
——	——	——	13. After the application of all the leads, make sure the paper-speed selector is set to the standard 25 m/second and that the machine is set to full voltage.	
——	——	——	14. If necessary, enter the appropriate patient identification data.	
——	——	——	15. Ask the patient to relax and breathe normally. **Tell him or her to lie still and not to talk while you record the ECG.**	

Obtaining an Electrocardiogram (ECG/EKG) *(Continued)*

Excellent	Satisfactory	Needs Practice		Comments

16. Press the AUTO button. Observe the tracing quality. The machine will record all 12 leads automatically, recording three consecutive leads simultaneously. Some machines have a display screen so you can preview waveforms before the machine records them on paper. Adjust waveform if necessary. If any part of the waveform extends beyond the paper when you record the ECG, adjust the normal standardization to half-standardization and repeat. Note this adjustment on the ECG strip, because this will need to be considered in interpreting the results.

17. When the machine finishes recording the 12-lead ECG, remove the electrodes and clean the patient's skin, if necessary, with adhesive remover for sticky residue.

18. After disconnecting the lead wires from the electrodes, dispose of the electrodes.

19. Return the patient to a comfortable position. Lower bed height and adjust head of bed to a comfortable position.

20. Remove any remaining equipment. Perform hand hygiene.

Skill Checklists to Accompany Taylor's Clinical Nursing Skills:
A Nursing Process Approach, 2nd edition

Name _____ Date _____

Unit _____ Position _____

Instructor/Evaluator: _____ Position _____

Excellent	Satisfactory	Needs Practice	SKILL 16-2 **Applying a Cardiac Monitor**	
			Goal: A clear waveform, free from artifact, is displayed on the cardiac monitor.	**Comments**
——	——	——	1. Gather all equipment and bring it to the bedside.	
——	——	——	2. Perform hand hygiene.	
——	——	——	3. Check the patient's identification. Explain the procedure to the patient. Close curtains around bed and close door to room if possible.	
——	——	——	4. Plug the cardiac monitor into an electrical outlet and turn it on to warm up the unit while preparing the equipment and the patient. For telemetry monitoring, insert a new battery into the transmitter. Match the poles on the battery with the polar markings on the transmitter case. Press the button at the top of the unit, test the battery's charge, and test the unit to ensure that the battery is operational.	
——	——	——	5. Insert the cable into the appropriate socket in the monitor.	
——	——	——	6. Connect the lead wires to the cable. In some systems, the lead wires are permanently secured to the cable. For telemetry, if the lead wires are not permanently affixed to the telemetry unit, attach them securely. If they must be attached individually, connect each one to the correct outlet.	
——	——	——	7. Connect an electrode to each of the lead wires, carefully checking that each lead wire is in its correct outlet.	
——	——	——	8. Expose the patient's chest and determine electrode positions, based on which system and leads are being used. If necessary, clip the hair from an area about 10 cm in diameter around each electrode site. Clean the area with soap and water and dry it completely to remove skin secretions that may interfere with electrode function.	
——	——	——	9. Remove the backing from the pregelled electrode. Check the gel for moisture. If the gel is dry, discard it and replace it with a fresh electrode. **Apply the electrode to the site and press firmly to ensure a tight seal.** Repeat with the remaining electrodes to complete the three-lead or five-lead system.	

SKILL 16-2

Applying a Cardiac Monitor *(Continued)*

Excellent	Satisfactory	Needs Practice		Comments
___	___	___	10. When all the electrodes are in place, connect the appropriate lead wire to each electrode. Check waveform for clarity, position, and size. **To verify that the monitor is detecting each beat, compare the digital heart rate display with an auscultated count of the patient's heart rate.** If necessary, use the gain control to adjust the size of the rhythm tracing, and use the position control to adjust the waveform position on the monitor.	
___	___	___	11. Set the upper and lower limits of the heart rate alarm, based on the patient's condition or unit policy.	
___	___	___	12. For telemetry, place the transmitter in the pouch in the hospital gown. If not available in gown, use a portable pouch. Place transmitter in pouch. Tie the pouch strings around the patient's neck and waist, making sure that the pouch fits snugly without causing discomfort. If no pouch is available, place the transmitter in the patient's bathrobe pocket.	
___	___	___	13. To obtain a rhythm strip, press the RECORD key either at the bedside for monitoring or at the central station for telemetry. Label the strip with the patient's name and room number, date, time, and rhythm identification. Place the rhythm strip in the appropriate location in the patient's chart. Analyze strip as appropriate.	
___	___	___	14. Return the patient to a comfortable position.	
___	___	___	15. Remove any remaining equipment. Perform hand hygiene.	

Name _____   Date _____

Unit _____   Position _____

Instructor/Evaluator: _____   Position _____

Excellent	Satisfactory	Needs Practice	SKILL 16-3 **Obtaining an Arterial Blood Sample From an Arterial Line–Stopcock System**	Comments
			Goal: A specimen is obtained without compromise to the patency of the arterial line.	
―	―	―	1. Gather all equipment and bring it to the bedside.	
―	―	―	2. Perform hand hygiene.	
―	―	―	3. Check the patient's identification. Compare the specimen label with the patient's identification. Explain the procedure to the patient. Close curtains around bed and close door to room if possible.	
―	―	―	4. If bed is adjustable, raise it to a comfortable working height.	
―	―	―	5. Perform hand hygiene and put on gloves and goggles.	
―	―	―	6. Turn off or temporarily silence the arterial pressure alarms, depending on your facility's policy (some facilities require that alarms be left on).	
―	―	―	7. Locate the stopcock nearest the arterial line insertion site. Use the alcohol swab or chlorhexidine to scrub the sampling port on the stopcock. Allow to air dry.	
―	―	―	8. Attach a 5-mL syringe into the sampling port on the stopcock to obtain the discard volume. Turn the stopcock off to the flush solution. Aspirate slowly until blood enters the syringe. Stop aspirating. Note the volume in the syringe, which is the dead-space volume. Continue to aspirate until the dead-space volume has been withdrawn a total of 3 times. For example, if the dead-space volume is 0.8 mL, aspirate 2.4 mL of blood.	
―	―	―	9. Turn the stopcock to the halfway position between the flush solution and the sampling port to close the system in all directions.	
―	―	―	10. Remove the discard syringe and dispose of appropriately.	
―	―	―	11. Place the syringe for the laboratory sample or the Vacutainer in the sampling port of the stopcock. Turn the stopcock off to the flush solution, and slowly withdraw the required amount of blood. For each additional sample required, repeat this procedure. If the physician has ordered coagulation tests, obtain blood for this sample from the final syringe.	

Excellent	Satisfactory	Needs Practice		Comments

___	___	___	12. Turn the stopcock to the halfway position between the flush solution and the sampling port to close the system in all directions. Remove the syringe or Vacutainer. Apply the rubber cap to the ABG syringe hub, if necessary.	
___	___	___	13. Insert a 5-mL syringe into the sampling port of the stopcock. Turn the stopcock off to the patient. Activate the in-line flushing device. Flush through the sampling port into the syringe to clear the stopcock and sampling port of any residual blood.	
___	___	___	14. Turn off the stopcock to the sampling port; remove the syringe. Remove sampling port cap and replace with new sterile one. Intermittently flush the arterial catheter with the in-line flushing device until the tubing is clear of blood.	
___	___	___	15. Reactivate the monitor alarms. Attach needles to the filled syringes and transfer the blood samples to the appropriate containers, if necessary. Record date and time the samples were obtained on the labels, as well as the required information to identify the person obtaining the samples. If ABG was collected, record oxygen flow rate (or room air) on label. Apply labels to the specimens, according to facility policy. Place in biohazard bags; place ABG sample in bag with ice.	
___	___	___	16. Check the monitor for return of the arterial waveform and pressure reading.	
___	___	___	17. Return the patient to a comfortable position. Lower bed height and adjust head of bed to a comfortable position.	
___	___	___	18. Remove any remaining equipment. Perform hand hygiene. Send specimens to the lab immediately.	

Skill Checklists to Accompany Taylor's Clinical Nursing Skills:
A Nursing Process Approach, 2nd edition

Name _____ Date _____

Unit _____ Position _____

Instructor/Evaluator: _____ Position _____

Excellent	Satisfactory	Needs Practice	SKILL 16-4 **Removing Arterial and Femoral Lines**
			Goal: The line is removed intact and without injury to the patient. **Comments**

Excellent	Satisfactory	Needs Practice	
___	___	___	1. Gather all equipment and bring it to the bedside.
___	___	___	2. Perform hand hygiene.
___	___	___	3. Check the patient's identification. Explain the procedure to the patient. Close curtains around bed and close door to room if possible.
___	___	___	4. Ask patient to empty bladder. Maintain an IV infusion of normal saline during procedure, as per medical orders or facility guidelines.
___	___	___	5. Put on clean gloves, goggles, and gown.
___	___	___	6. Use Doppler ultrasound to locate femoral artery, if line being removed is in a femoral site, 1″ to 2″ above entrance site of femoral line. Mark with "X" using special marker for skin.
___	___	___	7. Turn off the monitor alarms and then turn off the flow clamp to the flush solution. Carefully remove the dressing over the insertion site. Put on sterile gloves. Remove any sutures using the suture removal kit; make sure all sutures have been removed.
___	___	___	8. **Withdraw the catheter using a gentle, steady motion. Keep the catheter parallel to the blood vessel during withdrawal. Watch for hematoma formation during catheter removal by gently palpating surrounding tissue. If hematoma starts to form, reposition hands until optimal pressure is obtained to prevent further leakage of blood.**
___	___	___	9. **Immediately after withdrawing the catheter, apply pressure 1″ or 2″ above the site at the previously marked spot with a sterile 4 × 4 gauze pad. Maintain pressure for at least 10 minutes, or per facility policy (longer if bleeding or oozing persists). Apply additional pressure to a femoral site or if the patient has coagulopathy or is receiving anticoagulants.**
___	___	___	10. Assess distal pulses every 3 to 5 minutes while pressure is being applied. Note: dorsalis pedis and posterior tibial pulses should be markedly weaker from baseline if enough pressure is applied to femoral artery.

Excellent	Satisfactory	Needs Practice	SKILL 16-4 **Removing Arterial and Femoral Lines** *(Continued)*	
				Comments
——	——	——	11. Cover the site with an appropriate dressing and secure the dressing with tape. If stipulated by facility policy, make a pressure dressing for a femoral site by folding four sterile 4 × 4 gauze pads in half, and apply the dressing. Cover the dressing with a tight adhesive bandage, per policy, and then cover the femoral bandage with a sandbag. Maintain the patient on bed rest, with the head of the bed <30°, for 6 hours with the sandbag in place.	
——	——	——	12. Remind the patient not to lift his/her head while on bed rest. Use log roll to assist patient in using bedpan, if needed.	
——	——	——	13. Remove and properly dispose of gloves and personal protective equipment. Perform hand hygiene.	
——	——	——	14. Observe the site for bleeding. Assess circulation in the extremity distal to the site by evaluating color, pulses, and sensation. Repeat this assessment every 15 minutes for the first 1 hour, every 30 minutes for the next 2 hours, hourly for the next 2 hours, then every 4 hours, or according to facility policy.	

Skill Checklists to Accompany Taylor's Clinical Nursing Skills:
A Nursing Process Approach, 2nd edition

Name _____   Date _____

Unit _____   Position _____

Instructor/Evaluator: _____   Position _____

Excellent	Satisfactory	Needs Practice	SKILL 16-5 **Performing Cardiopulmonary Resuscitation (CPR)**	Comments
			Goal: CPR is performed effectively without adverse effect to the patient.	
⎯	⎯	⎯	1. Assess responsiveness. If the patient is not responsive, call for help, pull call bell, and call the facility emergency response number. Call for the automated external defibrillator (AED).	
⎯	⎯	⎯	2. Put on gloves, if available. Position the patient supine on his or her back on a firm, flat surface, with arms alongside the body. If the patient is in bed, place a backboard or other rigid surface under the patient (often the footboard of the patient's bed).	
⎯	⎯	⎯	3. Use the head tilt–chin lift maneuver to open the airway. Place one hand on the victim's forehead and apply firm, backward pressure with the palm to tilt the head back. Place the fingers of the other hand under the bony part of the lower jaw near the chin and lift the jaw upward to bring the chin forward and the teeth almost to occlusion. If trauma to the head or neck is present or suspected, use the jaw-thrust maneuver to open the airway. Place one hand on each side of the patient's head. Rest elbows on the flat surface under the patient, grasp the angle of the patient's lower jaw and lift with both hands.	
⎯	⎯	⎯	4. Look, listen, and feel for air exchange.	
⎯	⎯	⎯	5. If the patient resumes breathing or adequate respirations and signs of circulation are noted, place the patient in the recovery position.	
⎯	⎯	⎯	6. If no spontaneous breathing is noted, seal the patient's mouth and nose with the face shield, one-way valve mask, or Ambu-bag (resuscitation bag), if available. If not available, seal mouth with your mouth.	
⎯	⎯	⎯	7. Instill two breaths, each lasting 1 second, making the chest rise.	

Excellent	Satisfactory	Needs Practice		Comments

SKILL 16-5
Performing Cardiopulmonary Resuscitation (CPR) *(Continued)*

——— ——— ——— 8. If you are unable to ventilate or the chest does not rise during ventilation, reposition the patient's head and reattempt to ventilate. If still unable to ventilate, inspect oral airway. Remove any foreign matter or vomitus that is visible in the mouth. Use suction to remove material, if available. Perform five abdominal thrusts to remove the obstruction. If patient is obese or pregnant, perform five chest thrusts. Chest thrusts are delivered with the hands in the same position, using the same technique, as that for chest compressions during CPR. Attempt to ventilate. Repeat this cycle as necessary.

——— ——— ——— 9. Check the carotid pulse, simultaneously evaluating for breathing, coughing, or movement. This assessment should take no more than 10 seconds.
Place the patient in the recovery position if breathing resumes.

——— ——— ——— 10. If patient has a pulse, but remains without spontaneous breathing, continue rescue breathing at a rate of one breath every 5–6 seconds, for a rate of 10–12 breaths per minute.

——— ——— ——— 11. If the patient is without signs of circulation, position the heel of one hand in the center of the chest between the nipples, directly over the lower half of the sternum. Place the other hand directly on top of the first hand. Extend or interlace fingers to keep fingers above the chest.

——— ——— ——— 12. Perform 30 chest compressions at a rate of 100 per minute, counting "one, two, etc." up to 30, keeping elbows locked, arms straight, and shoulders directly over the hands. Chest compressions should depress the sternum approximately $1/3$ to $1/2$ the depth of the chest. Allow full chest recoil after each compression.

——— ——— ——— 13. Give two rescue breaths after each set of 30 compressions. Do five complete cycles of 30 compressions and two ventilations.

——— ——— ——— 14. Reassess breathing and circulation after each set of five compression/breathing cycles. Take no more than 10 seconds to do this.

——— ——— ——— 15. Defibrillation should be provided at the earliest possible moment, as soon as AED available.

——— ——— ——— 16. Continue CPR until the patient resumes spontaneous breathing and circulation, medical help arrives, you are too exhausted to continue, or a physician discontinues CPR.

Skill Checklists to Accompany Taylor's Clinical Nursing Skills:
A Nursing Process Approach, 2nd edition

Name _____   Date _____

Unit _____   Position _____

Instructor/Evaluator: _____   Position _____

Excellent	Satisfactory	Needs Practice	SKILL 16-6 **Performing Emergency Automated External Defibrillation**	Comments
			Goal: It is performed correctly without adverse effect to the patient and the patient regains signs of circulation, with organized electrical rhythm and pulse.	
——	——	——	1. Assess responsiveness. If the patient is not responsive, call for help and pull call bell, and call the facility emergency response number. Call for the AED. Perform cardiopulmonary resuscitation (CPR) until the defibrillator and other emergency equipment arrive.	
——	——	——	2. Prepare the AED. Power on the AED. Push the power button. Some devices will turn on automatically when the lid or case is opened.	
——	——	——	3. Attach AED connecting cables to the AED (may be preconnected). Attach AED cables to the adhesive electrode pads (may be preconnected).	
——	——	——	4. Stop chest compressions. Peel away the covering from the electrode pads to expose the adhesive surface. Attach the electrode pads to the patient's chest. Place one pad on the upper right sternal border, directly below the clavicle. Place the second pad lateral to the left nipple, with the top margin of the pad a few inches below the axilla.	
——	——	——	5. Once the pads are in place and the device is turned on, follow the prompts given by the device. Clear the patient and analyze the rhythm. Ensure no one is touching the patient. Loudly state a "Clear the patient" message. Press "Analyze" button to initiate analysis, if necessary. Some devices automatically begin analysis when the pads are attached. Avoid all movement affecting the patient during analysis.	
——	——	——	6. If ventricular tachycardia or ventricular fibrillation is present, the device will announce that a shock is indicated and begin charging. Once the AED is charged, a message will be delivered to shock the patient.	
——	——	——	7. Before pressing the "Shock" button, loudly state a "Clear the patient" message. Visually check that no one is in contact with the patient. Press the "Shock" button. If the AED is fully automatic, a shock will be delivered automatically.	

Excellent	Satisfactory	Needs Practice	

SKILL 16-6
Performing Emergency Automated External Defibrillation *(Continued)*

Comments

___ ___ ___   8. After the first shock, check the patient for signs of circulation, including a pulse. If the patient is without signs of circulation, resume CPR for 2 minutes. Rhythm checks should be performed every 2 minutes.

___ ___ ___   9. After any "no shock indicated" message, or 2 minutes, check the patient for signs of circulation, including a pulse. If no signs of circulation are present, press "Analyze" on the AED. Defibrillate if indicated by the AED. Continue with CPR and AED interpretation until the AED gives a "no shock indicated" message, the patient exhibits signs of circulation, or until ACLS is available. If signs of circulation do not return after an additional shock, resume CPR for 2 minutes.

___ ___ ___ 10. Continue with CPR and AED interpretation until the AED gives a "no shock indicated" message, the patient exhibits signs of circulation, or until ACLS is available.

___ ___ ___ 11. When "no shock indicated" message is received, check for signs of circulation. If signs of circulation are present, check breathing. If breathing is inadequate, assist breathing. Start rescue breathing (1 breath every 5 seconds). If breathing is adequate, place the patient in the recovery position, with the AED attached. Continue to assess the patient.

___ ___ ___ 12. Continue CPR until the patient resumes spontaneous breathing and circulation, medical help arrives, you are too exhausted to continue, or a physician discontinues CPR.

Skill Checklists to Accompany Taylor's Clinical Nursing Skills:
A Nursing Process Approach, 2nd edition

Name _____ Date _____

Unit _____ Position _____

Instructor/Evaluator: _____ Position _____

Excellent	Satisfactory	Needs Practice	SKILL 16-7 **Performing Emergency Manual External Defibrillation (Asynchronous)** **Goal:** It is performed correctly without adverse effect to the patient and the patient regains signs of circulation.	Comments
——	——	——	1. Assess responsiveness. If the patient is not responsive, call for help and pull call bell, and call the facility emergency response number. Call for the AED. Perform cardiopulmonary resuscitation (CPR) until the defibrillator and other emergency equipment arrive.	
——	——	——	2. Turn on the defibrillator.	
——	——	——	3. If the defibrillator has "quick-look" capability, place the paddles on the patient's chest. Otherwise, connect the monitoring leads of the defibrillator to the patient and assess the cardiac rhythm.	
——	——	——	4. Expose the patient's chest, and apply conductive pads at the paddle placement positions. For anterolateral placement, place one paddle to the right of the upper sternum, just below the right clavicle, and the other over the fifth or sixth intercostal space at the left anterior axillary line. "Hands-free" defibrillator pads can be used with the same placement positions, if available. For anteroposterior placement, place the anterior paddle directly over the heart at the precordium, to the left of the lower sternal border. Place the flat posterior paddle under the patient's body beneath the heart and immediately below the scapulae (but not on the vertebral column).	
——	——	——	5. Set the energy level for 360 joules for an adult patient when using monophasic defibrillator. Use clinically appropriate energy levels for biphasic defibrillators, beginning with 150 to 200 J.	
——	——	——	6. Charge the paddles by pressing the charge buttons, which are located either on the machine or on the paddles themselves.	
——	——	——	7. Place the paddles over the conductive pads and press firmly against the patient's chest, using 25 lb (11 kg) of pressure.	
——	——	——	8. Reassess the cardiac rhythm.	
——	——	——	9. If the patient remains in VF or pulseless VT, instruct all personnel to stand clear of the patient and the bed, including the operator.	

Excellent	Satisfactory	Needs Practice	SKILL 16-7 **Performing Emergency Manual External Defibrillation (Asynchronous)** *(Continued)*	Comments
___	___	___	10. Discharge the current by pressing both paddle charge buttons simultaneously.	
___	___	___	11. After the first shock, check the patient for signs of circulation, including a pulse. If the patient is without signs of circulation, resume CPR for 2 minutes. Rhythm checks should be performed every 2 minutes.	
___	___	___	12. If necessary, prepare to defibrillate a second time. Energy level on the defibrillator should remain at 360 J for subsequent shocks.	
___	___	___	13. Announce that you are preparing to defibrillate and follow the procedure described above.	
___	___	___	14. Reassess the patient.	
___	___	___	15. Reassess the patient for signs of circulation, including a pulse. If no signs of circulation are present, reassess heart rhythm. Defibrillate if indicated. Continue with CPR and rhythm interpretation until the patient exhibits adequate cardiac rhythm, signs of circulation, or until ACLS is available. If signs of circulation do not return after an additional shock, resume CPR for 2 minutes.	
			16. If defibrillation restores a normal rhythm:	
___	___	___	a. Check for signs of circulation; check the central and peripheral pulses, and obtain a blood pressure reading, heart rate, and respiratory rate.	
___	___	___	b. If signs of circulation are present, check breathing. If breathing is inadequate, assist breathing. Start rescue breathing (1 breath every 5 seconds).	
___	___	___	c. If breathing is adequate, place the patient in the recovery position. Continue to assess the patient.	
___	___	___	d. Assess the patient's level of consciousness, cardiac rhythm, breath sounds, and skin color and temperature.	
___	___	___	e. Obtain baseline ABG levels and a 12-lead ECG, if ordered.	
___	___	___	f. Provide supplemental oxygen, ventilation, and medications as needed.	
___	___	___	17. Check the chest for electrical burns and treat them, as ordered, with corticosteroid or lanolin-based creams. If using 'hands-free' pads, keep pads on in case of recurrent ventricular tachycardia or ventricular fibrillation.	
___	___	___	18. Prepare the defibrillator for immediate reuse.	

Skill Checklists to Accompany Taylor's Clinical Nursing Skills:
A Nursing Process Approach, 2nd edition

Name _____ Date _____

Unit _____ Position _____

Instructor/Evaluator: _____ Position _____

Excellent	Satisfactory	Needs Practice	SKILL 16-8 **Using an External (Transcutaneous) Pacemaker**	Comments
			Goal: It is applied correctly without adverse effect to the patient and the patient regains signs of circulation, including the capture of at least the minimal set heart rate.	
⎯	⎯	⎯	1. If patient is responsive, explain the procedure to the patient. Explain that it involves some discomfort and that you'll administer medication to keep him comfortable and help him relax. Perform hand hygiene. Check the patient's identification, if not an emergency situation.	
⎯	⎯	⎯	2. Close curtains around bed and close door to room if possible.	
⎯	⎯	⎯	3. If necessary, clip the hair over the areas of electrode placement. **However, do not shave the area.**	
⎯	⎯	⎯	4. Attach cardiac monitoring electrodes to the patient in the lead I, II, and III positions. Do this even if the patient is already on telemetry monitoring. If you select the lead II position, adjust the LL (left leg) electrode placement to accommodate the anterior pacing electrode and the patient's anatomy.	
⎯	⎯	⎯	5. Attach the patient monitoring electrodes to the ECG cable and into the ECG input connection on the front of the pacing generator. Set the selector switch to the MONITOR ON position.	
⎯	⎯	⎯	6. Note the ECG waveform on the monitor. Adjust the R-wave beeper volume to a suitable level and activate the alarm by pressing the ALARM ON button. Set the alarm for 10 to 20 beats lower and 20 to 30 beats higher than the intrinsic rate.	
⎯	⎯	⎯	7. Press the START/STOP button for a printout of the waveform.	
⎯	⎯	⎯	8. Apply the two pacing electrodes. Make sure the patient's skin is clean and dry to ensure good skin contact. Briskly rubbing the skin with your hand before placing the electrodes may improve monitor signal quality. Pull the protective strip from the posterior electrode (marked BACK) and apply the electrode on the left side of the thoracic spinal column, just below the scapula.	

Excellent	Satisfactory	Needs Practice		Comments

SKILL 16-8
Using an External (Transcutaneous) Pacemaker *(Continued)*

9. Apply the anterior pacing electrode (marked FRONT), which has two protective strips: one covering the gelled area and one covering the outer rim. Expose the gelled area and apply it to the skin in the anterior position, to the left side of the sternum in the usual V_2 to V_5 position, centered close to the point of maximal cardiac impulse. Move this electrode around to get the best waveform. Then expose the electrode's outer rim and firmly press it to the skin.

10. Prepare to pace the heart. After making sure the energy output in milliamperes (mA) is on 0, connect the electrode cable to the monitor output cable.

11. Check the waveform, looking for a tall QRS complex in lead II.

12. Check the selector switch to PACER ON. Select synchronous (demand) or asynchronous (fixed-rate or nondemand) mode, per medical orders. **Tell the patient he or she may feel a thumping or twitching sensation. Reassure the patient you will provide medication if the discomfort is intolerable.**

13. Set the pacing rate dial to 10 to 20 beats higher than the intrinsic rhythm. Look for pacer artifact or spikes, which will appear as you increase the rate. If the patient does not have an intrinsic rhythm, set the rate at 80 beats/minute.

14. Set the pacing current output (in milliamperes [mA]). For patients with bradycardia, start with the minimal setting and **slowly increase the amount of energy delivered to the heart by adjusting the OUTPUT mA dial. Do this until electrical capture is achieved: you will see a pacer spike followed by a widened QRS complex and a tall broad T wave that resembles a premature ventricular contraction.**

15. Increase output by 2 mA or 10%. **Do not go higher because of the increased risk of discomfort to the patient.**

16. Assess for mechanical capture: Presence of a pulse and signs of improved cardiac output (increased blood pressure, improved level of consciousness, improved body temperature).

17. For patients with asystole, start with the full output. If capture occurs, slowly decrease the output until capture is lost, then add 2 mA or 10% more.

18. Secure the pacing leads and cable to the patient's body.

Excellent	Satisfactory	Needs Practice		Comments

SKILL 16-8
Using an External (Transcutaneous) Pacemaker *(Continued)*

Excellent	Satisfactory	Needs Practice		Comments
——	——	——	19. Monitor the patient's heart rate and rhythm to assess ventricular response to pacing. Assess the patient's vital signs, skin color, level of consciousness, and peripheral pulses. Take blood pressure in both arms.	
——	——	——	20. Assess the patient's pain and administer analgesia/sedation as ordered to ease the discomfort of chest wall muscle contractions.	
——	——	——	21. Perform a 12-lead ECG and perform additional ECGs daily or with clinical changes.	
——	——	——	22. Continually monitor the ECG readings, noting capture, sensing, rate, intrinsic beats, and competition of paced and intrinsic rhythms. If the pacemaker is sensing correctly, the sense indicator on the pulse generator should flash with each beat.	
——	——	——	23. Perform hand hygiene.	

Skill Checklists to Accompany Taylor's Clinical Nursing Skills:
A Nursing Process Approach, 2nd edition

Name _____   Date _____

Unit _____   Position _____

Instructor/Evaluator: _____   Position _____

Excellent	Satisfactory	Needs Practice	SKILL 17-1 **Logrolling a Patient** **Goal:** The patient's spine remains in proper alignment, thereby reducing the risk for injury.	Comments
____	____	____	1. Review the medical record and nursing plan of care for conditions that may influence the patient's ability to move or to be positioned. Assess for tubes, IV lines, incisions, or equipment that may alter the positioning procedure. Identify any movement limitations.	
____	____	____	2. Identify the patient. Explain the procedure to the patient.	
____	____	____	3. Perform hand hygiene and put on gloves, if necessary.	
____	____	____	4. Close the door to the room or draw the bedside curtains.	
____	____	____	5. Adjust the bed to a comfortable working height.	
____	____	____	6. Stand on one side of the bed and have two assistants stand on the opposite side of the bed. Lower the side rails. Place the bed in flat position. Place a small pillow between the patient's knees.	
____	____	____	7. If a drawsheet or friction-reducing sheet is not in place under the patient, take the time to place one, to facilitate future movement of the patient.	
____	____	____	8. If the patient can move the arms, ask the patient to cross the arms on the chest. Roll or fanfold the drawsheet or friction-reducing sheet close to the patient's sides and grasp it. In unison, gently slide the patient to the side of the bed opposite to that which the patient will be turned.	
____	____	____	9. Make sure the drawsheet and sheet under the patient are straightened and wrinkle free. Reroll the drawsheet on the side from which the patient is being turned, if necessary, after straightening the sheets.	
____	____	____	10. If necessary, reposition personnel to ensure two nurses stand on the side of the bed to which the patient is turning. The third helper stands on the other side. **Grasp the drawsheet at hip and shoulder level; have assistants on the opposite side grasp the drawsheet above and below your area.**	

Excellent	Satisfactory	Needs Practice		Comments
—	—	—	11. Have everyone face the patient. On a predetermined signal, move the patient by holding the rolled drawsheet taut to support the body. Turn the patient as a unit in one smooth motion toward the side of the bed with the two nurses. The patient's head, shoulders, spine, hips, and knees should turn simultaneously.	
—	—	—	12. **Once the patient has been turned, use pillows to support the patient's back, buttocks, and legs in straight alignment in a side-lying position. Raise the side rails, if necessary.**	
—	—	—	13. **Stand at the foot of the bed and assess the spinal column. It should be straight, without any twisting or bending.** Ensure that the call bell and telephone are within reach. Replace covers. Lower bed height. Raise side rails as appropriate	
—	—	—	14. Reassess the patient's neurologic status and comfort level.	
—	—	—	15. Place the bed in lowest position. Make sure the call bell is in reach. Remove gloves, if worn, and perform hand hygiene.	

Name _____   Date _____

Unit _____   Position _____

Instructor/Evaluator: _____   Position _____

Excellent	Satisfactory	Needs Practice	SKILL 17-2 **Applying a Two-Piece Cervical Collar**	Comments
			Goal: The patient's cervical spine is immobilized, preventing further injury to the spinal cord.	
____	____	____	1. Review the medical record and nursing plan of care to determine need for placement of a cervical collar. Identify any movement limitations.	
____	____	____	2. Identify the patient. Explain the procedure to the patient.	
____	____	____	3. Assess patient for any changes in neurologic status.	
____	____	____	4. Perform hand hygiene and put on gloves, if necessary.	
____	____	____	5. Close the door to the room or draw the bedside curtains.	
____	____	____	6. Adjust the bed to a comfortable working height. Lower the side rails if necessary	
____	____	____	7. Gently clean the face and neck with a mild soap and water. If the patient has experienced trauma, inspect the area for broken glass or other material that could cut the patient or the nurse. Pat the area dry.	
____	____	____	8. With a second person stabilizing the cervical spine, measure from the bottom of the chin to the top of the sternum, and measure around the neck. Match these height and circumference measurements to the manufacturer's recommended size chart.	
____	____	____	9. Slide the flattened back portion of the collar under the patient's head. **The center of the collar should line up with the center of the patient's neck. Do not allow the patient's head to move when passing the collar under the head.**	
____	____	____	10. Place the front of the collar centered over the chin, while ensuring that the chin area fits snugly in the recess. Be sure that the front half of the collar overlaps the back half. Secure Velcro straps on both sides. Check to see that at least one finger can be inserted between collar and patient's neck.	
____	____	____	11. Place the bed in lowest position. Make sure the call bell is in reach. Raise the side rails. Remove gloves and perform hand hygiene.	

Excellent	Satisfactory	Needs Practice	SKILL 17-2 **Applying a Two-Piece Cervical Collar** *(Continued)*	
				Comments
——	——	——	12. Check the skin under the cervical collar at least every 4 hours for any signs of skin breakdown. Remove the top half of the collar daily and cleanse the skin under the collar. When the collar is removed, have a second person immobilize the cervical spine.	

Skill Checklists to Accompany Taylor's Clinical Nursing Skills:
A Nursing Process Approach, 2nd edition

Name _____ Date _____

Unit _____ Position _____

Instructor/Evaluator: _____ Position _____

Excellent	Satisfactory	Needs Practice	SKILL 17-3 **Caring for a Patient in Halo Traction**	Comments
			Goal: The patient maintains cervical alignment.	
____	____	____	1. Review the medical record and the nursing plan of care to determine the type of device being used and prescribed care.	
____	____	____	2. Identify the patient. Explain the procedure to the patient.	
____	____	____	3. Perform hand hygiene.	
____	____	____	4. Close the room door or curtains. Place the bed at a comfortable working height or have the patient sit up if appropriate.	
____	____	____	5. Monitor vital signs and perform a neurologic assessment, including level of consciousness, motor function, and sensation, per facility policy. This is usually at least every 2 hours for 24 hours, or possibly every hour for 48 hours.	
____	____	____	6. Examine the halo vest unit every 8 hours for stability, secure connections, and positioning. Make sure the patient's head is centered in the halo without neck flexion or extension. Check each bolt for loosening.	
____	____	____	7. Check the fit of the vest. With the patient in a supine position, you should be able to insert one or two fingers under the jacket at the shoulder and chest.	
____	____	____	8. Put on unsterile gloves, if appropriate. Wash the patient's chest and back daily. Place the patient on his or her back or sitting up if appropriate. Loosen the bottom Velcro straps.	
____	____	____	9. Wring out a bath towel soaked in warm water. Pull the towel back and forth in a drying motion beneath the front. Do not use soap or lotion under the vest.	
____	____	____	10. Thoroughly dry the skin in the same manner with a dry towel. Inspect the skin for tender, reddened areas or pressure spots. Lightly dust the skin with a prescribed medicated powder or cornstarch.	
____	____	____	11. Turn the patient on his or her side, less than 45 degrees if lying supine, and repeat the process on the back. Close the Velcro straps. Assist the patient with changing the shirt.	

SKILL 17-3

Caring for a Patient in Halo Traction *(Continued)*

Excellent	Satisfactory	Needs Practice		Comments
——	——	——	12. Perform a respiratory assessment. Check for respiratory impairment, such as absence of breath sounds, the presence of adventitious sounds, reduced inspiratory effort, or shortness of breath.	
——	——	——	13. Assess the pin sites for redness, tenting of the skin, prolonged or purulent drainage, swelling, and bowing, bending, or loosening of the pins. Monitor body temperature.	
——	——	——	14. Perform pin-site care. (See Skills 9-18 and 9-19.)	
——	——	——	15. Depending on physician order and facility policy, apply the antimicrobial ointment to pin sites and apply a dressing.	
——	——	——	16. Remove gloves and dispose of them appropriately. Place the bed in the lowest position.	
——	——	——	17. Perform hand hygiene.	

Skill Checklists to Accompany Taylor's Clinical Nursing Skills:
A Nursing Process Approach, 2nd edition

Name _____   Date _____

Unit _____   Position _____

Instructor/Evaluator: _____   Position _____

SKILL 17-4

Caring for an External Ventriculostomy (Intraventricular Catheter–Closed Fluid-Filled System)

Goal: The patient maintains intracranial pressure at less than 10 to 15 mm Hg and cerebral perfusion pressure at 60 to 90 mm Hg

Excellent	Satisfactory	Needs Practice		Comments
____	____	____	1. Identify the patient. Explain procedure to patient. Review physician's order for specific information about parameters.	
____	____	____	2. Perform hand hygiene; apply gloves if indicated.	
____	____	____	3. Assess patient for any changes in neurologic status.	
____	____	____	4. **Assess the height of the ventriculostomy system to ensure that the stopcock is at the level of midpoint between the outer canthus of the patient's eye and the tragus of the patient's ear or external auditory canal, using carpenter level, bubble-line level, or laser level, according to facility policy. Adjust the height of the system if needed. Move the drip chamber to the ordered height.** Assess the amount of CSF in the drip chamber if the ventriculostomy is draining.	
____	____	____	5. **Zero the transducer.** Turn stopcock off to the patient. Remove the cap from the transducer, being careful not to touch the end of the cap. Press and hold the calibration button on the monitor until the monitor beeps. Return the cap to the transducer. **Turn the stopcock off to the drip chamber to obtain an ICP reading. After obtaining the reading, turn the stopcock off to the transducer.**	
____	____	____	6. **Move the ventriculostomy to prevent too much drainage, too little drainage, or inaccurate ICP readings.**	
____	____	____	7. Care for the insertion site according to the institution's policy. Assess the site for any signs of infection, such as purulent drainage, redness, or warmth. Ensure the catheter is secured at site per facility policy.	
____	____	____	8. Calculate the CCP, if necessary. Calculate the difference between the systemic mean arterial pressure and the ICP.	
____	____	____	9. Remove gloves, if worn. Perform hand hygiene.	

Skill Checklists to Accompany Taylor's Clinical Nursing Skills:
A Nursing Process Approach, 2nd edition

Name _____ Date _____

Unit _____ Position _____

Instructor/Evaluator: _____ Position _____

SKILL 17-5
Caring for a Fiberoptic Intracranial Catheter

Excellent	Satisfactory	Needs Practice	**Goal:** The patient maintains intracranial pressure less than 10 to 15 mm Hg and cerebral perfusion pressure 60 to 90 mm Hg	Comments
___	___	___	1. Identify the patient. Explain procedure to patient. Review physician's order.	
___	___	___	2. Perform hand hygiene.	
___	___	___	3. Assess patient for any changes in neurologic status.	
___	___	___	4. **Assess ICP, MAP, and CPP at least hourly. Note ICP waveforms as shown on the monitor. Notify the physician if A or B waves are present.**	
___	___	___	5. Care for the insertion site according to the institution's policy. Assess the site for any signs of infection, such as drainage, redness, or warmth. Ensure the catheter is secured at site per facility policy.	
___	___	___	6. Calculate the CCP, if necessary. Calculate the difference between the systemic mean arterial pressure and the ICP.	
___	___	___	7. Perform hand hygiene.	

Skill Checklists to Accompany Taylor's Clinical Nursing Skills:
A Nursing Process Approach, 2nd edition

Name _____   Date _____

Unit _____   Position _____

Instructor/Evaluator: _____   Position _____

Excellent	Satisfactory	Needs Practice	SKILL 18-1 **Testing Stool for Occult Blood** **Goal:** An uncontaminated stool sample is obtained following collection guidelines and transported to the laboratory within the recommended time frame, without adverse effect.	Comments
____	____	____	1. Identify the patient. Discuss with patient the need for a stool sample. Explain to patient the process by which the stool will be collected, either from a bedpan, commode, or plastic receptacle in toilet.	
____	____	____	2. Close curtains around bed or close door to room if possible.	
____	____	____	3. Perform hand hygiene.	
____	____	____	4. Place the plastic collection receptacle in the toilet, if applicable. Assist the patient to the bathroom or onto the bedside commode, or assist the patient onto the bedpan. Instruct patient not to urinate or discard toilet paper with the stool, which may contaminate the specimen.	
____	____	____	5. After the patient defecates, assist the patient out of the bathroom, off the commode, or remove the bedpan. Perform hand hygiene and put on disposable gloves.	
____	____	____	6. **With wooden applicator, apply a small amount of stool from the center of the bowel movement onto one window of Hemoccult testing card. With opposite end of wooden applicator, obtain another sample of stool from another area and apply a small amount of stool onto second window of Hemoccult card.**	
____	____	____	7. Close flap over stool samples.	
____	____	____	8. If sending to laboratory, check specimen label with patient identification bracelet. Label should include patient's name and identification number, time specimen was collected, route of collection, identification for person obtaining sample, and any other information required by agency policy. Label the specimen card per facility policy. Place in sealable plastic biohazard bag and send to laboratory immediately.	
____	____	____	9. If testing at bedside, open flap on opposite side of card and **place two drops of developer over each window and wait the time stated in the manufacturer's instructions.**	

Excellent	Satisfactory	Needs Practice		Comments
			SKILL 18-1 **Testing Stool for Occult Blood** (Continued)	
——	——	——	10. Observe card for any blue areas.	
——	——	——	11. Discard Hemoccult testing slide appropriately, according to facility policy. Remove gloves and perform hand hygiene.	

Skill Checklists to Accompany Taylor's Clinical Nursing Skills:
A Nursing Process Approach, 2nd edition

Name _____   Date _____

Unit _____   Position _____

Instructor/Evaluator: _____   Position _____

Excellent	Satisfactory	Needs Practice	SKILL 18-2 **Collecting a Stool Specimen for Culture**	Comments
			Goal: An uncontaminated specimen is obtained and sent to the laboratory promptly.	
____	____	____	1. Gather necessary equipment. Identify the patient. Place disposable collection container (hat) in toilet or bedside commode to catch stool without urine. Instruct patient to void first and not to discard toilet paper with stool. Tell patient to call you as soon as bowel movement is completed.	
____	____	____	2. Perform hand hygiene and put on gloves.	
____	____	____	3. After patient has passed a stool, use the tongue blades to obtain a sample, free of blood or urine, and place it in a dry, clean container.	
____	____	____	4. Collect as much of the stool as possible to send to the laboratory.	
____	____	____	5. Place lid on container. Remove gloves and perform hand hygiene.	
____	____	____	6. Check specimen label with patient identification bracelet. Label should include patient's name and identification number, time specimen was collected, route of collection, identification for person obtaining sample, and any other information required by agency policy. Place label on the container per facility policy. Place container in plastic sealable biohazard bag.	
____	____	____	7. **Transport specimen to laboratory while stool is still warm. If immediate transport is impossible, check with laboratory personnel or policy manual as to whether refrigeration is contraindicated.**	

Skill Checklists to Accompany Taylor's Clinical Nursing Skills:
A Nursing Process Approach, 2nd edition

Name _____ Date _____

Unit _____ Position _____

Instructor/Evaluator: _____ Position _____

Excellent	Satisfactory	Needs Practice	SKILL 18-3 **Obtaining a Capillary Blood Sample** **for Glucose Testing**	
			Goal: The blood glucose level is measured accurately without adverse effect.	**Comments**
——	——	——	1. Check the patient's medical record or nursing plan of care for monitoring schedule. You may decide that additional testing is indicated based on nursing judgment and the patient's condition.	
——	——	——	2. Gather equipment.	
——	——	——	3. Close curtains around bed and close door to room if possible.	
——	——	——	4. Identify the patient. Explain procedure to patient and instruct patient about the need for monitoring blood glucose.	
——	——	——	5. Perform hand hygiene. Put on nonsterile gloves.	
——	——	——	6. Turn the monitor on.	
——	——	——	7. Enter the patient's identification number, if required, according to facility policy.	
——	——	——	8. Prepare lancet using aseptic technique.	
——	——	——	9. Remove test strip from the vial. **Recap container immediately.** Test strips also come individually wrapped. Turn monitor on. **Check that code number for the strip matches code number on monitor screen.**	
——	——	——	10. Insert strip into the meter according to directions for that specific device.	
——	——	——	11. For adult, massage side of finger toward puncture site.	
——	——	——	12. **Have patient wash hands with soap and warm water and dry thoroughly. Alternately, the skin may be cleansed with an alcohol swab. Allow skin to dry completely.**	
——	——	——	13. Hold lancet perpendicular to skin and pierce site with lancet.	
——	——	——	14. **Wipe away first drop of blood with gauze square or cotton ball if recommended by manufacturer of monitor.**	

SKILL 18-3

Obtaining a Capillary Blood Sample
for Glucose Testing *(Continued)*

Excellent	Satisfactory	Needs Practice		Comments
——	——	——	15. Encourage bleeding by lowering hand, making use of gravity. Lightly stroke the finger, if necessary, until sufficient amount of blood has formed to cover the sample area on the strip, based on monitor requirements (check instructions for monitor). Take care not to squeeze the finger, not to squeeze at puncture site, or not to touch puncture site or blood.	
——	——	——	16. **Gently touch drop of blood to pad on test strip without smearing it.**	
——	——	——	17. Press time button if directed by manufacturer.	
——	——	——	18. Apply pressure to puncture site with a cotton ball. **Do not use alcohol wipe.**	
——	——	——	19. Read blood glucose results and document appropriately at bedside. Inform patient of test result.	
——	——	——	20. Turn meter off, remove test strip and dispose of supplies appropriately. Place lancet in sharps container.	
——	——	——	21. Remove gloves and perform hand hygiene.	

Skill Checklists to Accompany Taylor's Clinical Nursing Skills:
A Nursing Process Approach, 2nd edition

Name _____ Date _____

Unit _____ Position _____

Instructor/Evaluator: _____ Position _____

SKILL 18-4
Collecting a Sputum Specimen for Culture

Excellent **Satisfactory** **Needs Practice**

Goal: The patient produces an adequate sample from the lungs. **Comments**

1. Identify the patient. Explain procedure to patient. If patient may have pain with coughing, administer pain medication if ordered. If patient can perform task without assistance after instruction, leave container at bedside with instructions to call nurse as soon as specimen is produced.
2. Assemble equipment.
3. Close curtains around bed and close door to room if possible.
4. Perform hand hygiene. Put on disposable gloves and goggles.
5. Adjust bed to comfortable working position. Lower side rail closer to you. Place patient in semi-Fowler's position. **Have patient clear nose and throat and rinse mouth with water before beginning procedure.**
6. **Instruct patient to inhale deeply and cough.** If patient has had abdominal surgery, assist patient to splint abdomen.
7. If patient produces sputum, open the lid to the container and have patient expectorate specimen into container.
8. If patient believes he or she can produce more specimen, have patient repeat the procedure.
9. Close lid to container. Offer oral hygiene to patient.
10. Remove goggles and gloves. Perform hand hygiene.
11. Check specimen label with patient identification bracelet. Label should include patient's name and identification number, time specimen was collected, route of collection, identification for person obtaining sample, and any other information required by agency policy. Place label on the container per facility policy. Place container in plastic sealable biohazard bag. Immediately transport to laboratory.

Skill Checklists to Accompany Taylor's Clinical Nursing Skills:
A Nursing Process Approach, 2nd edition

Name _____ Date _____

Unit _____ Position _____

Instructor/Evaluator: _____ Position _____

Excellent	Satisfactory	Needs Practice	SKILL 18-5 **Collecting a Urine Specimen (Clean Catch, Midstream)** **for Urinalysis and Culture**	
			Goal: An adequate amount of urine is obtained from the patient without contamination.	**Comments**
____	____	____	1. Identify the patient. Explain procedure to patient.	
____	____	____	2. Perform hand hygiene and put on nonsterile gloves. Have patient perform hand hygiene, if performing self collection.	
____	____	____	3. Close curtains around bed and close door to room if possible.	
____	____	____	4. Assist the patient to the bathroom, onto the bedside commode or bedpan. Instruct patient not to defecate or discard toilet paper into the urine, which may contaminate the specimen.	
____	____	____	5. Instruct the female patient to separate the labia for cleaning of the area and during collection of urine. Female patients should use the towelettes or wet washcloth to clean each side of the urinary meatus, then the center over the meatus, from front to back, using a new wipe for each stroke. Male patients should use a towlette to clean the tip of the penis, wiping in a circular motion away from the urethra. Instruct male patient who is not circumcised to retract foreskin before cleaning and during collection.	
____	____	____	6. **Have patient void about 25 mL into toilet, bedpan, or commode. The patient should then stop urinating briefly, then void into collection container. Collect specimen (10–20 mL is enough), and then finish voiding. Do not touch the inside of the container or the lid.**	
____	____	____	7. Place lid on container. If necessary, transfer specimen to appropriate containers for ordered test, according to facility policy.	
____	____	____	8. Assist the patient from the bathroom, off the commode, or off the bedpan. Provide perineal care if necessary.	
____	____	____	9. Remove gloves. Perform hand hygiene.	

Collecting a Urine Specimen (Clean Catch, Midstream) for Urinalysis and Culture *(Continued)*

Excellent	Satisfactory	Needs Practice		Comments
——	——	——	10. Check specimen label with patient identification bracelet. Label should include patient's name and identification number, time specimen was collected, route of collection, identification for person obtaining sample, and any other information required by agency policy. Place label on the container per facility policy. Place container in plastic sealable biohazard bag.	
——	——	——	11. Transport specimen to laboratory as soon as possible. If unable to take specimen to laboratory immediately, refrigerate it.	

Name _____ Date _____

Unit _____ Position _____

Instructor/Evaluator: _____ Position _____

SKILL 18-6

Obtaining a Urine Specimen From an Indwelling Urinary Catheter

Goal: An adequate amount of urine is obtained from the patient without contamination or adverse effect and the patient experiences minimal anxiety during the collection process.

Excellent	Satisfactory	Needs Practice		Comments
___	___	___	1. Identify the patient. Explain procedure to patient. Organize equipment at bedside.	
___	___	___	2. Perform hand hygiene and put on nonsterile gloves.	
___	___	___	3. Close curtains around bed and close door to room if possible.	
___	___	___	4. Clamp the catheter drainage tubing or bend it back on itself distal to the port. If an insufficient amount of urine is present in the tubing, allow tubing to remain clamped up to 30 minutes, to collect sufficient amount of urine, unless contraindicated. Remove lid from specimen container, keeping the inside of the container and lid free from contamination.	
___	___	___	5. **Cleanse aspiration port with alcohol wipe and allow port to air dry.**	
___	___	___	6. Insert the blunt-tipped needle into the port, or attach the syringe to the needleless port. Slowly aspirate enough urine for specimen (usually 10 mL is adequate; check facility requirements). Remove needle or syringe from port. Engage needle guard. **Unclamp drainage tubing.**	
___	___	___	7. If a needle was used on the syringe, remove the needle from the syringe before emptying the urine from the syringe into the specimen cup. Slowly inject urine into specimen container. Replace lid on container. Dispose of needle and syringe appropriately.	
___	___	___	8. Remove gloves. Perform hand hygiene.	
___	___	___	9. Check specimen label with patient identification bracelet. Label should include patient's name and identification number, time specimen was collected, route of collection, identification for person obtaining sample, and any other information required by agency policy. Place label on the container per facility policy. Place container in plastic sealable biohazard bag.	

Obtaining a Urine Specimen From an Indwelling Urinary Catheter *(Continued)*

Excellent	Satisfactory	Needs Practice		Comments
——	——	——	10. Transport specimen to laboratory as soon as possible. If unable to take specimen to laboratory immediately, refrigerate it.	

Skill Checklists to Accompany Taylor's Clinical Nursing Skills:
A Nursing Process Approach, 2nd edition

Name _____ Date _____

Unit _____ Position _____

Instructor/Evaluator: _____ Position _____

SKILL 18-7
Using Venipuncture to Collect a Venous Blood Sample for Routine Testing

Goal: An uncontaminated specimen will be obtained without the patient experiencing undue anxiety and injury.

Excellent	Satisfactory	Needs Practice		Comments
___	___	___	1. Gather the necessary supplies. Check product expiration dates. Identify ordered tests and select the appropriate blood-collection tubes.	
___	___	___	2. Identify the patient. Explain the procedure. Allow the patient time to ask questions and verbalize concerns about the venipuncture procedure.	
___	___	___	3. Close curtains around bed and close door to room if possible.	
___	___	___	4. Provide for good light. Artificial light is recommended. Place a trash receptacle within easy reach.	
___	___	___	5. Assist the patient to a comfortable position, either sitting or lying. If the patient is lying in bed, raise the bed to a comfortable working height. Expose the arm, supporting it in an extended position on a firm surface, such as a table top.	
___	___	___	6. Perform hand hygiene.	
___	___	___	7. Determine the patient's preferred site for the procedure based on his or her previous experience. Apply a tourniquet to the upper arm on the chosen side approximately 3″ to 4″ above the potential puncture site. Apply enough pressure to impede venous circulation but not arterial blood flow.	
___	___	___	8. Assess the veins to determine the best puncture site. Observe the skin for the vein's blue color, or palpate the vein for a firm rebound sensation.	
___	___	___	9. Release the tourniquet. Check that the vein has decompressed.	
___	___	___	10. Attach the needle to the Vacutainer device. Place first blood-collection tube into the Vacutainer, but not engaged in the puncture device in the Vacutainer.	

Using Venipuncture to Collect a Venous Blood Sample for Routine Testing *(Continued)*

Excellent	Satisfactory	Needs Practice		Comments
——	——	——	11. Put on nonsterile gloves. Clean the patient's skin at the selected puncture site with the antimicrobial swab. If using chlorhexidine, use a back-and-forth motion, applying friction for 30 seconds to site, or procedure recommended by the manufacturer. If using alcohol, wipe in a circular motion spiraling outward. Allow the skin to dry before performing the venipuncture.	
——	——	——	12. Reapply the tourniquet approximately 3″ to 4″ above the identified puncture site. Apply enough pressure to impede venous circulation but not arterial blood flow.	
——	——	——	13. Hold the patient's arm in a downward position with your nondominant hand. Align the needle and Vacutainer device with the chosen vein, holding the Vacutainer and needle in your dominant hand. Use the thumb or first finger of nondominant hand to apply pressure and traction to the skin just below the identified puncture site.	
——	——	——	14. Inform the patient that he or she is going to feel a pinch. With the bevel of the needle up, insert the needle into the vein at a 15-degree angle to the skin.	
——	——	——	15. Grasp the Vacutainer securely to stabilize it in the vein with your nondominant hand, and push the first collection tube into the puncture device in the Vacutainer, until the rubber stopper on the collection tube is punctured. You will feel the tube push into place on the puncture device. Blood will flow into the tube automatically.	
——	——	——	16. **Remove the tourniquet as soon as blood flows adequately into the tube.**	
——	——	——	17. Continue to hold Vacutainer in place in the vein and continue to fill the required tubes, removing one and inserting another. Gently rotate each tube as you remove it.	
——	——	——	18. **After you have drawn all required blood samples, remove the last collection tube from the Vacutainer. Place a gauze pad over the puncture site and slowly and gently remove the needle from the vein. Engage needle guard.** Do not apply pressure to site until the needle has been fully removed.	
——	——	——	19. Apply gentle pressure to the puncture site for 2 to 3 minutes or until bleeding stops.	
——	——	——	20. After bleeding stops, apply an adhesive bandage.	

SKILL 18-7

Using Venipuncture to Collect a Venous
Blood Sample for Routine Testing *(Continued)*

Excellent	Satisfactory	Needs Practice		Comments
——	——	——	21. Check specimen labels with patient identification bracelet. Label should include patient's name and identification number, time specimen was collected, route of collection, identification for person obtaining sample, and any other information required by agency policy. Place label on the tubes per facility policy. Place tubes in plastic sealable biohazard bag. Immediately transport to laboratory.	
——	——	——	22. Check the venipuncture site to see if a hematoma has developed.	
——	——	——	23. Discard Vacutainer and needle in sharps container. Remove gloves and perform hand hygiene.	
——	——	——	24. Assist the patient to a comfortable position. If patient's bed was raised, place the bed in the lowest position.	

Skill Checklists to Accompany Taylor's Clinical Nursing Skills:
A Nursing Process Approach, 2nd edition

Name _____   Date _____

Unit _____   Position _____

Instructor/Evaluator: _____   Position _____

Excellent	Satisfactory	Needs Practice	SKILL 18-8 **Obtaining a Venous Blood Specimen** **for Culture and Sensitivity**	
			Goal: An uncontaminated specimen will be obtained without the patient experiencing undue anxiety and injury.	**Comments**
——	——	——	1. Gather the necessary supplies. Check product expiration dates. Identify ordered tests and select the appropriate blood-collection tubes. If tests are ordered in addition to the blood cultures, collect the blood-culture specimens before other specimens.	
——	——	——	2. Identify the patient. Explain the procedure. Allow the patient time to ask questions and verbalize concerns about the venipuncture procedure.	
——	——	——	3. Close curtains around bed and close door to room if possible.	
——	——	——	4. Provide for good light. Artificial light is recommended. Place a trash receptacle within easy reach.	
——	——	——	5. Assist the patient to a comfortable position, either sitting or lying. If the patient is lying in bed, raise the bed to a comfortable working height. Expose the arm, supporting it in an extended position on a firm surface, such as a table top.	
——	——	——	6. Perform hand hygiene.	
——	——	——	7. Determine the patient's preferred site for the procedure based on his or her previous experience. Apply a tourniquet to the upper arm on the chosen side approximately 3″ to 4″ above the potential puncture site. Apply enough pressure to impede venous circulation but not arterial blood flow.	
——	——	——	8. Assess the veins to determine the best puncture site. Observe the skin for the vein's blue color, or palpate the vein for a firm rebound sensation.	
——	——	——	9. Release the tourniquet. Check that the vein has decompressed.	
——	——	——	10. Attach the butterfly-needle extension tubing to the Vacutainer device.	
——	——	——	11. Move collection bottles to a location close to arm, with bottles sitting upright on table top.	

Excellent	Satisfactory	Needs Practice	SKILL 18-8 **Obtaining a Venous Blood Specimen for Culture and Sensitivity** *(Continued)*	Comments
——	——	——	12. Put on nonsterile gloves. Clean the patient's skin at the selected puncture site with the antimicrobial swab. If using chlorhexidine, use a back-and-forth motion, applying friction for 30 seconds to site, or procedure recommended by the manufacturer. Allow the site to dry.	
——	——	——	13. Using a new antimicrobial swab, clean the stoppers of the culture bottles with the appropriate antimicrobial, per facility policy. Cover bottle top with sterile gauze square, based on facility policy.	
——	——	——	14. Reapply the tourniquet approximately 3″ to 4″ above the identified puncture site. Apply enough pressure to impede venous circulation but not arterial blood flow.	
——	——	——	15. Hold the patient's arm in a downward position with your nondominant hand. Align the butterfly needle with the chosen vein, holding the needle in your dominant hand. Use the thumb or first finger of nondominant hand to apply pressure and traction to the skin just below the identified puncture site. Do not touch the insertion site.	
——	——	——	16. Inform the patient that he or she is going to feel a pinch. With the bevel of the needle up, insert the needle into the vein at a 15-degree angle to the skin. You should see a flash of blood in the extension tubing close to the needle when the vein is entered.	
——	——	——	17. Grasp the butterfly securely to stabilize it in the vein with your nondominant hand, and push Vacutainer onto the first collection bottle (aerobic bottle), until the rubber stopper on the collection bottle is punctured. You will feel the bottle push into place on the puncture device. Blood will flow into the bottle automatically.	
			18. **Remove the tourniquet as soon as blood flows adequately into the bottle.**	
——	——	——	19. Continue to hold butterfly needle in place in the vein. Once first bottle is filled, remove the Vacutainer and place on second bottle. After the blood culture specimens are obtained, continue to fill any additional required tubes, removing one and inserting another. Gently rotate each bottle and tube as you remove it.	
——	——	——	20. **After you have drawn all required blood samples, remove last collection tube from the Vacutainer. Place a gauze pad over the puncture site and slowly and gently remove the needle from the vein. Engage needle guard.** Do not apply pressure to site until the needle has been fully removed.	

Excellent	Satisfactory	Needs Practice	SKILL 18-8 **Obtaining a Venous Blood Specimen for Culture and Sensitivity** *(Continued)*	
				Comments
——	——	——	21. Apply gentle pressure to the puncture site with the gauze pad for 2 to 3 minutes or until bleeding stops.	
——	——	——	22. After bleeding stops, apply an adhesive bandage.	
——	——	——	23. Check specimen labels with patient identification bracelet. Label should include patient's name and identification number, time specimen was collected, route of collection, identification for person obtaining sample, and any other information required by agency policy Place label on the culture bottles per facility policy. Place culture bottles and any other collection tubes in plastic sealable biohazard bags, according to facility policy. Immediately transport to laboratory.	
——	——	——	24. Check the venipuncture site to see if a hematoma has developed.	
——	——	——	25. Discard Vacutainer and butterfly needle in sharps container. Remove gloves and perform hand hygiene.	
——	——	——	26. If a second set of blood cultures is ordered, repeat the procedure, collecting from another site or wait the specified time to obtain the specimen.	
——	——	——	27. Assist the patient to a comfortable position. If patient's bed was raised, place the bed in the lowest position.	

Skill Checklists to Accompany Taylor's Clinical Nursing Skills:
A Nursing Process Approach, 2nd edition

Name _____   Date _____

Unit _____   Position _____

Instructor/Evaluator: _____   Position _____

Excellent	Satisfactory	Needs Practice	SKILL 18-9 **Obtaining an Arterial Blood Specimen for Blood Gas Analysis**	
			Goal: The blood sample is obtained from the artery without damage to the artery.	**Comments**
⎯⎯	⎯⎯	⎯⎯	1. Check the patient's identification and confirm the patient's identity. Tell the patient you need to collect an arterial blood sample, and explain the procedure. Tell the patient that the needlestick will cause some discomfort but that he or she must remain still during the procedure. Check the chart to make sure the patient hasn't been suctioned within the past 15 minutes.	
⎯⎯	⎯⎯	⎯⎯	2. Gather equipment and provide privacy.	
⎯⎯	⎯⎯	⎯⎯	3. Perform hand hygiene.	
⎯⎯	⎯⎯	⎯⎯	4. If the patient is on bed rest, ask him or her to lie in a supine position, with the head slightly elevated and the arms at the sides. Ask the ambulatory patient to sit in a chair and support the arm securely on an armrest or a table. Place a waterproof pad under the site and a rolled towel under the wrist.	
⎯⎯	⎯⎯	⎯⎯	5. **Perform Allen's test before obtaining a specimen from the radial artery:**	
⎯⎯	⎯⎯	⎯⎯	a. Have the patient clench the wrist to minimize blood flow into the hand.	
⎯⎯	⎯⎯	⎯⎯	b. Using your index and middle fingers, press on the radial and ulnar arteries. Hold this position for a few seconds.	
⎯⎯	⎯⎯	⎯⎯	c. Without removing your fingers from the arteries, ask the patient to unclench the fist and hold the hand in a relaxed position. The palm will be blanched because pressure from your fingers has impaired the normal blood flow.	
⎯⎯	⎯⎯	⎯⎯	d. Release pressure on the ulnar artery. If the hand becomes flushed, which indicates that blood is filling the vessels, it is safe to proceed with the radial artery puncture. If the hand doesn't flush, perform the test on the other arm.	
⎯⎯	⎯⎯	⎯⎯	6. Perform hand hygiene again and put on gloves.	
⎯⎯	⎯⎯	⎯⎯	7. Locate the radial artery and lightly palpate it for a strong pulse.	

Obtaining an Arterial Blood Specimen for Blood Gas Analysis (Continued)

Excellent	Satisfactory	Needs Practice		Comments
——	——	——	8. Clean the site with the antimicrobial swab. If using chlorhexidine, use a back-and-forth motion, applying friction for 30 seconds to site, or procedure recommended by the manufacturer. Allow the site to dry.	
——	——	——	9. Stabilize the hand with the wrist extended over the rolled towel, palm up. Palpate the artery with the index and middle fingers of your nondominant hand while holding the syringe over the puncture site with your dominant hand. **Do not directly touch the area to be stuck.**	
——	——	——	10. Hold the needle bevel up at a 45-degree angle at the site of maximal pulse impulse, with the shaft parallel to the path of the artery. (When puncturing the brachial artery, hold the needle at a 60-degree angle.)	
——	——	——	11. Puncture the skin and arterial wall in one motion. Watch for blood backflow in the syringe. The pulsating blood will flow into the syringe. Do not pull back on the plunger. Fill the syringe to the 5-mL mark.	
——	——	——	12. After collecting the sample, withdraw the syringe while your nondominant hand is beginning to place pressure proximal to the insertion site with the 2″ × 2″ gauze. Press a gauze pad firmly over the puncture site until the bleeding stops—at least 5 minutes. **If the patient is receiving anticoagulant therapy or has a blood dyscrasia, apply pressure for 10 to 15 minutes; if necessary, ask a coworker to hold the gauze pad in place while you prepare the sample for transport to the laboratory, but do not ask the patient to hold the pad.**	
——	——	——	13. When the bleeding stops and the appropriate time has lapsed, apply a small adhesive bandage or small pressure dressing (fold a 2″ × 2″ gauze into fourths and firmly apply tape, stretching the skin tight).	
——	——	——	14. Once the sample is obtained, check the syringe for air bubbles. If any appear, remove them by holding the syringe upright and slowly ejecting some of the blood onto a 2″ × 2″ gauze pad.	
——	——	——	15. Engage the needle guard and remove the needle. Place the airtight cap on the syringe. Gently rotate the syringe to ensure that heparin is well distributed. Do not shake. Insert the syringe into a cup or bag of ice.	

Excellent	Satisfactory	Needs Practice	SKILL 18-9 **Obtaining an Arterial Blood Specimen** **for Blood Gas Analysis** *(Continued)*	
				Comments
——	——	——	16. Check specimen labels with patient identification bracelet. Label should include patient's name and identification number, time specimen was collected, route of collection, identification for person obtaining sample, amount of oxygen patient is receiving, and any other information required by agency policy. Place label on the syringe per facility policy. Place iced syringe in plastic sealable biohazard bag. Immediately transport to laboratory.	
——	——	——	17. Discard needle in sharps container. Remove gloves and perform hand hygiene.	
——	——	——	18. Continue to monitor the patient's vital signs, and monitor the extremity for signs and symptoms of circulatory impairment such as swelling, discoloration, pain, numbness, or tingling. Watch for bleeding at the puncture site. Advise the patient not to use the affected extremity for vigorous activity for at least 24 hours.